Complementary/ Alternative Therapies in Nursing

3rd Edition

Mariah Snyder, PhD, RN, FAAN
Ruth Lindquist, PhD, RN

Springer Publishing Company

Springer Publishing Company, Inc.
536 Broadway
New York, NY   10012-3955

Cover design by Margaret Dunin
Acquisitions Editor: Ruth Chasek
Production Editor: T. Orrantia

98 99 00 01 02 / 5 4 3 2 1

Library of Congress Cataloging-in-Publication Data

Complementary/alternative therapies in nursing 3rd edition / edited by Mariah
    Snyder and Ruth Lindquist.
      p.   cm.
      Rev. ed. of: Independent nursing interventions / edited by Mariah
    Snyder. 2nd ed. Albany, NY: Delmar Publishers, c1992.
      Includes bibliographical references and index.
      ISBN 0-8261-1169-6
      1. Holistic nursing. 2. Nurse and patient. 3. Alternative
    medicine. I. Snyder, Mariah. II. Lindquist, Ruth.
    III. Independent nursing interventions.
      [DNLM: 1. Alternative Medicine—nurses' instruction. 2. Nursing Care.
    3. Holistic Health. WB 890 C7377 1998]
    RT41.I53   1998
    610.73—dc21
    DNLM/DLC
    for Library of Congress   97-37261
                                                                    CIP

Contents

Contributors

Donna Brauer, PhD, RN
School of Nursing
University of Minnesota
Minneapolis, MN

Linda Chlan, PhD, RN
School of Nursing
University of Iowa
Iowa City, IO

WenYun Cheng, MS, RN
School of Nursing
University of Minnesota
Minneapolis, MN

Jacqueline Corso, MS, RN
School of Nursing
University of Minnesota
Minneapolis, MN

Jessie S. Daniels, MA, RN
School of Nursing
University of Minnesota
Minneapolis, MN

Paula Dicke, MS, RN
Fairview University Medical
Center
Minneapolis, MN

Ellen Egan, PhD, RN, FAAN
School of Nursing
University of Minnesota
Minneapolis, MN

Marion Good, PhD, RN
Francis Payne Bolton School of
Nursing
Case Western Reserve University
Cleveland, OH

Marilyne Gustafson, PhD, RN
School of Nursing
University of Minnesota
Minneapolis, MN

Kirsten James, BA, RN
Victoria University
Melbourne, Australia

Merrie Kaas, DNSc, RN, CS
School of Nursing
University of Minnesota
Minneapolis, MN

Mary Jo Kreitzer, PhD, RN
School of Nursing
University of Minnesota
Minneapolis, MN

Ruth Lindquist, PhD, RN
School of Nursing
University of Minnesota
Minneapolis, MN

Daniel L. Mark, BS
School of Nursing
University of Minnesota
Minneapolis, MN

Michaelene Mirr, PhD, RN
School of Nursing
University of Wisconsin
Eau Claire, WI

Susan Moch, PhD, RN
School of Nursing
University of Wisconsin
Eau Claire, WI

Margo Nelson, PhD, RN
Department of Nursing
Augustana College
Sioux Falls, SD

Yoshiko Nojima, BA, RN
Department of Nursing
Hiroshima University
Hiroshima, Japan

Janice Post-White, PhD, RN
School of Nursing
University of Minnesota
Minneapolis, MN

Mary Fern Richie, DSN, RN, CS
School of Nursing
Vanderbilt University
Nashville, TN

Sharon Ridgeway, PhD, RN
School of Nursing
University of Minnesota
Minneapolis, MN

Jo Ann B. Ruiz-Bueno, PhD, RN
School of Nursing
University of Cincinnati
Cincinnati, OH

Muriel B. Ryden, PhD, RN, FAAN
School of Nursing
University of Minnesota
Minneapolis, MN

Carol Schaefer, MSN, RN
Division of Supportive Living
Wisconsin Bureau of Quality
  Assurance
Madison, WI

Kevin Shaller, Captain
US Department of Army
Columbia, SC

Kevin Smith, MS, RN,
School of Nursing
University of Minnesota
Minneapolis, MN

Mariah Snyder, PhD, RN, FAAN
School of Nursing
University of Minnesota
Minneapolis, MN

Mary Steffes, MS, RN
School of Nursing
University of Minnesota
Minneapolis, MN

Lois Taft, PhD, RN
Institute for Women's Health
Evanston Northwestern Healthcare
Evanston, IL

Mary Fran Tracy, MS, RN
Fairview University Medical Center
Minneapolis, MN

Diane Treat-Jacobson, RN, MS
Minnesota Vascular Disease Center
University of Minnesota
Minneapolis, MN

JingJy Wang, MS, RN
School of Nursing
University of Minnesota
Minneapolis, MN

Introduction

This is the third edition of a book that was titled *Independent Nursing Interventions* when it was first published in 1985. At the time it seemed an apt title for a compendium of approaches to wellness and healing that nurses could use which did not involve medication, surgery, or physicians. Many were therapies that were traditionally part of nursing's armamentarium, such as massage and application of heat and cold, but most fell within an evolving category now identified as "alternative" or "complementary."

Thus, this third edition has a new title. Times have changed, and there is a greater demand by individuals and health professionals for this kind of information than ever. It is the premise of this book that nurses are natural providers of these kinds of holistic services, and this book provides accessible, practical, research-based descriptions of the techniques that they needed in twenty-eight alternative/complementary interventions described in the book.

With an increasing number of persons seeking complementary/ alternative therapies, a revolution is occurring in health care. Although use of alternative/complementary therapies may appear to challenge the allopathic system of care that has predominated in Western health care, these therapies are frequently used in conjunction with allopathic therapies. A weakness of the allopathic system has been its lack of attention to the psychosocial and spiritual aspects of care. One of the major reasons persons use complementary/alternative therapies is for healing of mind, body, and spirit. Now is the opportune time for nurses to deliver to society the type of health care society desires. Interventions described in this book will assist nurses in achieving this goal.

Nursing is concerned with preventing and alleviating health problems, managing symptoms, and healing the entire person. Healing focuses on achieving increased harmony within a person. Nursing is also concerned with empowering persons to assume more responsibility for their own health and well-being. The majority of the therapies included in this book require active participation by the client, with individuals eventually assuming responsibility for incorporation of the therapies into their lives.

Nursing is both an art and a science. Therefore, the research base for the interventions, to the extent that it is available, is described. To prompt students, clinicians, and researchers to conduct more research, the authors have identified several of the many areas in which additional research is needed.

A similar format is used for all of the chapters. Authors first supply a definition and scientific basis for the treatment, followed by a description of the intervention, its uses and precautions, research questions, and references. Readers have found this feature of the previous editions to be useful in comparing and contrasting the various interventions for use with specific populations.

As we approach the 21st century, it is our hope that this book will continue to assist nurses in the provision of quality nursing care that encompasses the art and science of nursing. Both nursing students (undergraduate and graduate) and practicing nurses can glean knowledge about interventions appropriate for clients in a wide variety of settings (e.g., hospitals, nursing homes, homes, schools, prisons, industry).

We wish to thank our many students, nursing colleagues, and clients who have shared their experiences with us. Their input has both validated the intense interest in the interventions we describe and the contributions that these methods have made to the health and well-being of our clients. We are confident that nurses' use of complementary/alternative therapies will continue to increase and thus position the nurse as a sought-after provider of these therapies.

Mariah Snyder, PhD, RN, FAAN
Ruth Lindquist, PhD, RN

1

Progressive Muscle Relaxation

Mariah Snyder

Progressive muscle relaxation (PMR), a technique developed by Edmund Jacobson (1938), is one of the most widely used interventions for reducing high levels of stress and preventing the occurrence of high stress levels. It is often a component of many other stress management interventions. Progressive muscle relaxation provides persons with a means to control tension and anxiety. Thus, it is congruent with nursing's tenets of self-care and health promotion.

DEFINITION

Progressive muscle relaxation (PMR) is defined as the progressive tensing and relaxing of successive muscle groups. A person's attention is drawn to discriminating between the feelings experienced when the muscle group is relaxed and when it is tensed. With continued use of PMR, an individual can sense muscle tension without having to progress through the tensing and relaxing of specific muscle groups.

SCIENTIFIC BASIS

When a person perceives a situation to be a stressor, a sympathetic nervous system response occurs that is often referred to as the *fight-flight response*. The sympathetic nervous system response includes dilation of pupils, shallowness of respirations, increased heart rate, and tensing of muscles. This response assists humans to react to short-term stressful situations. However, if the perceived stressor persists over time, the repeated psychophysiological stress response can have deleterious effects on the body. Stress is a part of every person's life. The desired outcome of relaxation strategies is the mitigation of persisting high levels of stress, or the avoidance of high stress levels.

Brown (1977) noted that the stress response is part of a closed feedback loop between the muscles and the mind. Appraisal of stressors results in tensing of muscles; the tensed muscles in turn send stimuli to the brain. Thus, a feedback loop is established. Relaxing muscles interrupts this feedback loop.

Jacobson (1938) reported that PMR decreases the body's oxygen consumption, metabolic rate, respiratory rate, muscle tension, premature ventricular contractions, systolic and diastolic blood pressure, and increases alpha brain waves. Subsequent studies (Gift, Moore, & Soeken, 1992; Hahn et al., 1993) have validated Jacobson's findings.

INTERVENTION

Numerous techniques for PMR have evolved since Jacobson first publicized his technique. Active muscle relaxation (Bernstein & Borkovec, 1973; Jacobson, 1938), passive muscle relaxation (Haynes, Moseley, & McGowan, 1975), self-control relaxation (Lichstein, 1988), and rapid relaxation (Deffenbacher & Snyder, 1976) are some of the techniques that have been used. The technique developed by Bernstein and Borkovec (1973) is one of the most widely used PMR techniques and its efficacy has been explored in multiple studies. Differences among techniques include the method for relaxing muscle groups, groups of muscles to which attention is given, type of instruction (live vs. tape), number of teaching sessions used, and the environment in which the teaching is done. Although the majority of findings from studies exploring the efficacy of PMR techniques have substantiated the effectiveness of PMR in producing positive outcomes, findings from some studies have not shown PMR to be efficacious. One or a combination of the variables noted above may have had an impact on the outcomes achieved.

Another factor that may impact results is the personal characteristics of the patients. Smith (1989) advocated fitting the stress management intervention with the personal characteristics of a person. Because few studies have explored the characteristics of persons for whom PMR would be most useful, it is not known whether this factor may also have an impact on outcomes achieved.

Technique

Instructions that apply for all PMR techniques will be described before detailing Bernstein and Borkovec's technique.

Lichstein (1988), based on a review of the literature, found the following to be factors for persons not continuing to use a relaxation technique:

- not enough time
- forgetting to use it
- uncertainty about relaxation procedure
- failure to achieve relaxation
- lack of a quiet place for practice
- changing interest in relaxation

These factors guide the instructor in teaching PMR to patients. Not only is it essential for persons to master the technique to achieve relaxation, but persons also need assistance to integrate PMR into their daily lives.

A quiet atmosphere facilitates persons' concentrating on the instructions for PMR. The instructor assists the patient in identifying a space at home that would be most conducive for practice of PMR. Strategies to eliminate interruptions are needed: Telephones, persons entering the room, and loud noises need to be removed. If PMR is being taught in a hospital room, a sign on the door will help reduce interruptions. When it is impossible to eliminate noises and conversations, quiet music may help to dampen the effect of these noises.

Another environmental factor to consider is lighting. Reduced lighting promotes relaxation; however, during instruction adequate lighting is needed so that the teacher can determine the degree of relaxation a patient is obtaining.

A reclining chair is ideal for PMR as it is comfortable and also supports the body. Pender (1985) used lawn recliners when teaching PMR to groups. A bed or couch may be used, but the tendency to sleep increases when the patient is in the supine position. Adaptations in the technique are needed for patients who are bedfast.

Comfortable, unrestrictive clothing allows the patient to tense and

TABLE 1.1   Guidelines for Fourteen Muscle Group Progressive Muscle Relaxation

General Information
Persons are instructed to tense the specific muscle group when they hear "Tense," and to release the tension when they hear "Relax." Tension is held for 7 seconds. Patter is used to draw attention to the feelings of tension and relaxation. When muscles are relaxed, attention is drawn to the differences noted between the relaxed state and the tensed state.

Tension of Specific Muscle Groups
Dominant hand and forearm: Make a tight fist and hold it.
Dominant upper arm: Push elbow down against the arm of the chair.
Instructions are repeated for nondominant arm.
Forehead muscles: Lift eyebrows as high as possible.
Muscles of central face (cheek, nose, eyes): Squint eyes and wrinkle nose.
Lower face and jaw: Clench teeth and widen mouth.
Neck: Pull chin down toward chest, but do not touch chest.
Chest, shoulders, and upper back: Take deep breath, hold it, pull shoulder blades toward back.
Abdomen: Pull stomach in and try to protect it.
Dominant side thigh: Lift leg and hold it out straight.
Dominant side calf: Point toes toward ceiling.
Instructions repeated for thigh and calf of nondominant side.

Adapted from Bernstein & Borkovec (1973).

relax muscles without feeling the tug or pull of clothing. Shoes are removed prior to the PMR session. Likewise, glasses and contact lenses are removed. Since sessions, particularly the initial sessions, last 45–60 minutes, the patient may wish to use the bathroom before beginning a PMR session.

At the first session, the rationale for the PMR is provided. This includes information about stressors, the impact stress has on the body, and signs and symptoms of high levels of stress. The instructor describes and then demonstrates how each muscle group is tensed. Patients practice tensing each of the muscle groups. If difficulty is encountered in achieving tension, an alternate method for achieving tension of that muscle group can be tried.

Bernstein and Borkovec Technique.   In the technique developed by Bernstein and Borkovec (1973), 16 muscle groups are initially tensed and relaxed. Fourteen of these groups are detailed in Table 1.1, which is adapted from Bernstein and Borkovec (1973). Although Bernstein and Borkovec also included tensing muscles of the feet, these are not included in the table because tensing foot muscles produces muscle spasms in many persons. The 14 muscle groups are combined into 7 and then 4 groups at subsequent sessions. The ultimate goal is for the person to achieve muscle relaxation without having to tense the specific muscle groups.

After progressing through all of the muscle groups, the instructor asks the patient to identify tension remaining in any of the muscle groups. The instructor observes the patient to assess if general relaxation has occurred. Indicators of relaxation are:

- slowed, shallower breathing
- arms relaxed and shoulders forward
- feet apart with toes pointing out

Two or three minutes are provided at the conclusion of the session for the patient to enjoy the feelings associated with relaxation.

Termination of relaxation is done gradually. The instructor counts backward from four to one. On the count of four, patients are instructed to move their hands and feet; on three, arms and legs; on two, head and neck; and on the count of one, open eyes. Opportunity

TABLE 1.2 Content for Ten Teaching Sessions

Session	Content
1	Rationale for technique
	Demonstrate tensing/relaxing 16 muscle groups
	Practice tensing and relaxing muscle groups
	Determine time for home practice
2-3	Practice tensing/relaxing 16 muscle groups
	Discuss problems encountered
4	Introduce and practice 7 muscle group relaxation
	Discuss adaptations and concerns
5	Practice tensing/relaxing 7 muscle groups
6	Introduce and practice 4 muscle group relaxation
	Discuss adaptations and concerns
7	Practice tensing/relaxing 4 muscle groups
8	Practice tensing/relaxing 4 muscle groups
	Discuss problems encountered
	Introduce recall technique and life application
9	Practice tensing/relaxing 4 muscle groups
	Use recall technique
10	Practice recall technique
	Discuss problems and arrange follow-up sessions as needed

Adapted from Bernstein & Borkovec (1973).

is provided for the patient to ask questions or discuss feelings experienced.

Ten teaching sessions are proposed by Bernstein and Borkovec (1973). Content for sessions is presented in Table 1.2, which is adapted from Bernstein and Barkovec (1973). The number of sessions is often fewer than the 10 proposed by Bernstein and Borkovec. In studies by Gift, Moore, & Soeken, 1992; Renfroe, 1988; and Sloman, Brown, Aldana, & Chee, 1994, positive outcomes were achieved when three to six sessions were used. In a review of studies in which PMR was used, Borkovec and Sides (1979) found that better results occurred when four or more teaching sessions were used. A critical factor in determining the number of teaching sessions needed is ensuring that persons have mastered relaxing muscle groups and have integrated PMR into their lifestyles.

Critical to the effectiveness of PMR is daily practice sessions. At least one 15–minute practice session a day is necessary to master the technique and to achieve relaxation. Two sessions a day would be ideal. Helping patients find a time of day to practice relaxation is an important element of the instruction sessions. The time of day PMR is practiced is not important, but it must become a part of the person's daily routine.

Measurement of Effectiveness

A variety of outcomes has been used to measure the efficacy of PMR. Because the technique has been used with persons having diverse problems, the measurements appropriate for each vary.

Common physiological measurements used include systolic and diastolic blood pressure (Pender, 1984), heart rate, body posturing (Luiselli, Steinman, Marholin, & Steinman, 1983), respiratory rate, dyspnea (Renfroe, 1988), and muscle tension (Jones & Evans, 1981). Frequently, electromyogram readings of the frontalis and forearm muscles are taken to determine the degree of tension present in the entire body. According to Jones and Evans (1981), however, this measurement is not indicative of reduced tension in muscles throughout the body.

Changes in vital signs are frequently used to measure the impact of PMR (Snyder, 1993). Because the autonomic nervous system is intimately involved in the stress response, reduction of stress would be manifested in reduced blood pressure, heart rate, and respirations. However, practitioners need to be alert to underlying pathology or medications that may interfere with reductions in these and other physiological parameters.

Anxiety is the variable most frequently measured to determine the efficacy of PMR (Snyder, 1993). The State-Trait Anxiety Self-Questionnaire (Spielberger, Gorusch, Luschene, Vagg, & Jacobs, 1983), two 20–item inventories that measure state and trait anxiety has been widely used. State anxiety is a measurement of a person's feelings at a particular point in time while trait anxiety is a measurement of a person's overall view. Four items of the state anxiety inventory have been found to have a good correlation with the 20–item inventory (O'Neil, Spielberger, & Hansen, 1969). These four items could be readily used in clinical settings to determine the efficacy of PMR (Stewart, 1989).

Other instruments used to measure subjective response to PMR have included the Profile of Mood States (POMS) (McNair, Lorr, & Droppleman, 1971), Adjective Affective Checklist (AACL), (Zuckerman, 1960), depression, and various cognitive status exams (Yesavage, 1984). Patient self-report of feelings of relaxation have also been used in some studies. Patient feelings of relaxation may be a strong indicator on whether a person will continue to use PMR.

In the majority of studies the effect of PMR has been evaluated immediately following administration of the intervention. Longitudinal measurements are needed to determine if PMR produces ongoing positive results. Such measurements are particularly needed when PMR is taught to persons with hypertension, dyspnea, and other chronic health conditions.

USES

Progressive muscle relaxation has been used to achieve many outcomes in diverse populations. Table 1.3 lists conditions/populations for which PMR has been tested. Attention will focus on the use of PMR for health promotion, relief of pain, and reduction of stress for specific conditions.

Health Promotion

As a profession, nursing has taken a foremost position in intervening to promote health. Teaching patients interventions to maintain or improve their health is a key role for nurses in all settings:

TABLE 1.3   Conditions in Which PMR has been Used

Stress Reduction
  Insomnia (Borkovec, Kaloupek, & Slama, 1975)
  Asthma (Freedberg, Hoffman, Light, & Kreps, 1987)
  Reduction of seizures (Snyder, 1983; Whitman et al., 1990)
  Hypertension (Hahn et al., 1993; Pender, 1985)
  Chronic obstructive pulmonary disease (Gift et al., 1992; Renfroe, 1988)
  Functional outcomes following head injury (Lysaght & Bodenhamer, 1990)

Pain Reduction
  Cancer (Sloman et al., 1994)
  Postoperative (Wells, 1982)
  Headache (Blanchard et al., 1991)

Health Promotion
  Relief of nausea and vomiting (Cotanch, 1983)
  Diagnostic procedures (Rice, Caldwell, Butler, & Robinson, 1986)
  Nurses (Tsai & Crockett, 1993)

hospitals, clinics, homes, schools, prisons, and work. Studies on PMR in healthy persons has shown that the intervention has little or no effect in lowering blood pressure or reducing heart rate (Glaister, 1982; Shapiro & Lehrer, 1980). However, these findings do not negate teaching PMR to healthy persons, as it can used to maintain their health condition.

Pain

Progressive muscle relaxation has been used extensively in the management of multiple causes of pain: headache, postoperative pain, labor pain, and chronic pain such as low back pain. Muscle tension increases the perception of pain; thus, the lessening of anxiety and tension reduces the pain experienced. Use of PMR may provide persons with a sense of control over their pain.

PMR is frequently used as an adjunct or complementary therapy in the management of pain. This is particularly true with patients who have cancer. Sloman and colleagues (1994) found that patients who were taught PMR reported subjectively less pain than patients in the control group. Likewise, patients receiving PMR used less non-opiate analgesics. Nurses may find PMR to be a helpful intervention for persons with cancer who are undergoing radiation or chemotherapy.

Tension headaches are a commonly found problem in today's society. Progressive muscle relaxation has been shown to be efficacious in decreasing the pain of tension headaches. Blanchard and colleagues (1991) reported that subjects with tension headaches who had received 8 weeks of PMR training had improvements that were significantly different from those of subjects in the control group. Persons prone to tension headaches can be taught to use PMR on a regular basis so as to avoid their occurrence.

Several earlier studies in nursing used a modified relaxation technique, the jaw drop (Flaherty & Fitzpatrick, 1978; Horowitz, Fitzpatrick, & Flaherty, 1984). Patients using this technique reported decreased pain following surgery. The jaw relaxation procedure instructs patients to smile as widely as possible and to hold this tension for a few seconds before releasing the tension. Next, they press their lips into an "O" shape and concentrate on the tension before relaxing the muscles. Lastly, tension in the throat muscles is achieved by clenching the jaw, biting down hard, and pressing the tongue against the roof of the mouth; these muscles are then relaxed.

Reduction of Stress

As noted in Table 1.3, PMR has been used to reduce stress associated with a number of conditions. It has been used for years as an adjunct therapy in the treatment of hypertension. Although fewer studies have been done on the use of PMR as an antiseizure adjunct therapy, several studies have documented its efficacy (Snyder, 1983; Whitman, Dell, Legion, Eibhlyn, & Staatsinger, 1990). Many persons who have experienced seizures have high stress levels due to their concerns about another seizure occurring or others finding out that they have epilepsy. Thus, reduction of high stress is an important outcome for this population. Whitman and colleagues reported a 54% decrease in persons who used PMR as an adjunct to their anticonvulsant.

Precautions

Although PMR has been used with multiple populations and has been proven to be an efficacious nursing intervention, nurses need to have an awareness of precautions for its use.

It is important for practitioners to know if patients practice PMR on a regular basis, as this use may affect the pharmacokinetics of medications. Trophotropic reactions may occur (Lichstein, 1988). This reaction potentiates the effects of some medications and may result in a toxic level of the medication. Because of a relaxed state, a lower dose of a medication may be indicated. This is particularly true for insulin, since an overdose results in a hypoglycemic state.

Complete relaxation may produce a hypotensive state. Persons need to be taught to remain seated for a few minutes after practicing PMR. Movement in place and gradual resumption of activities helps overcome the hypotensive state. Taking persons' blood pressures at the conclusion of teaching sessions may help to identify persons prone to hypotensive states.

Herman (1987, 1989) studied the effect of PMR on inducing the Valsalva response in healthy adults. She reported that the Valsalva response occurred in 43% of the subjects studied in the first study and 18% in the second study. Implications are that nurses need to assess patients during the teaching sessions to identify those who are holding their breath during the tensing of muscles and to provide instructions about avoiding the Valsalva response.

Some persons with chronic pain have reported heightened awareness of pain following use of PMR. Concentration on the tension and relaxation of muscles tends to draw the person's attention to the pain present rather than to the muscle sensation being experienced. Thus, good assessment of individuals is needed.

Persons with cardiac conditions should not practice the seven and four muscle group tensing and relaxing that is part of the Bernstein and Borkovec technique (1973). Tensing and then relaxing the large muscle groups results in large volumes of blood being placed in circulation at one time. This volume places an unduly heavy load on the damaged heart muscles.

RESEARCH QUESTIONS

Progressive muscle relaxation has been used as a single nursing intervention and in conjunction with other interventions. A body of literature is emerging in nursing and in other disciplines to guide use of PMR. However, there is considerably more work to do. A few of the areas in which research is needed include the following areas:

1. Few studies have examined the characteristics of persons who "like" PMR. Obtaining data on psychological variables of subjects would be helpful. McGrady and Roberts (1992) reported different findings from use of PMR for racially different groups.

Lerman et al. (1990) reported different responses to PMR between persons who were "blunters" or "monitors."

2. What are the long-term effects of the use of PMR? How many persons continue to use it after three months? Six months? One year?

3. Do persons who learn PMR for one purpose, such as pain control, apply it to other areas of their life, such as insomnia? This information would be helpful in promoting overall health of individuals.

4. Additional studies are needed to determine the efficacy of PMR in comparison to other stress management interventions. Also, explorations of the efficacy of PMR in combination with other stress management techniques are needed. A number of studies have examined PMR used in conjunction with biofeedback.

REFERENCES

Bernstein, D., & Borkovec, T. (1973). *Progressive relaxation training.* Champaign, IL: Research Press.

Blanchard, E. B., Nicholson, N. L., Taylor, A. E., Steffek, B. D., Radnitz, C., & Appelbaum, K. A. (1991). The role of regular home practice of relaxation treatment for tension headache. *Journal of Consulting and Clinical Psychology, 59,* 467–470.

Borkovec, T., & Sides, J. (1979). Critical procedural variables related to the physiological effects of progressive muscle relaxation: A review. *Behavior Research and Therapy, 17,* 119–125.

Borkovec, T., Kaloupek, D., & Slama, K. (1975). The facilitative effect of muscle tension-release in the relaxation treatment of sleep disorders. *Behavior Therapy, 6,* 301–309.

Brown, B. (1977). *Stress and the art of biofeedback.* New York: Bantam.

Cotanch, P. (1983). Relaxation training for control of nausea and vomiting in patients receiving chemotherapy. *Cancer Nursing, 6,* 272–282.

Deffenbacher, J., & Snyder, A. (1976). Relaxation and self-control in the treatment of test and other anxieties. *Psychological Reports, 39,* 379–385.

Flaherty, G., & Fitzpatrick, J. (1978). Relaxation technique to increase comfort level of postoperative patients: A preliminary study. *Nursing Research, 27,* 352–355.

Freedberg, P. D., Hoffman, L. A., Light, W. C., & Kreps, M. K. (1987). Effect of progressive muscle relaxation on the objective symptoms and subjective responses associated with asthma. *Heart & Lung, 16,* 24–30.

Gift, A. G., Moore, T., & Soeken, K. (1992). Relaxation to reduce dyspnea and anxiety in COPD patients. *Nursing Research, 41,* 242–246.

Glaister, B. (1982). Muscle relaxation training for fear reduction of patients with psychological problems: A review of controlled studies. *Behavior Research Therapy, 20,* 493–504.

Hahn, Y. B., Ro, Y. J., Song, H. H., Kim, N. C., Sim, H. S., & Yang, S. Y. (1993). The effect of thermal biofeedback and progressive muscle relaxation training in reducing blood pressure of patients with essential hypertension. *Image: Journal of Nursing Scholarship, 25,* 204–207.

Haynes, S., Moseley, D., & McGowan, W. (1975). Relaxation training and biofeedback in the reduction of frontalis muscle tension. *Psychophysiology, 12,* 547–552.

Herman, J. (1987). The effect of progressive relaxation on Valsalva response in health adults. *Research in Nursing and Health, 10,* 171–176.

Herman, J. (1989). Valsalva response during progressive relaxation. *Scholarly Inquiry for Nursing Practice, 3,* 217–232.

Horowitz, B. F., Fitzpatrick, J. J., & Flaherty, G. G. (1984). Relaxation techniques for relief of pain after open heart surgery. *Dimensions of Critical Care Nursing, 3,* 364–371.

Jacobson, E. (1938). *Progressive relaxation.* Chicago: University of Chicago Press.

Jones, G., & Evans, P. (1981). Effectiveness of frontalis feedback training in producing general body relaxation. *Biological Psychology, 12,* 313–320.

Lerman, C., Rimer, B., Blumberg, B., Cristinzio, S., Engstrom, P. F., MacElwee, N., O'Connor, K., & Seay, J. (1990). Effects of coping style and relaxation on cancer chemotherapy side effects and emotional responses. *Cancer Nursing, 13,* 308–315.

Lichstein, K. L. (1988). *Clinical relaxation strategies.* New York: Wiley.

Luiselli, J. K., Steinman, D. L, Marholin, D., & Steinman, W. M. (1981). Evaluation of progressive muscle relaxation with conduct-problem learning disabled children. *Child Behavior Therapy, 3,* 41–55.

Lysaght, R., & Bodenhamer, E. (1990). The use of relaxation training to enhance functional outcomes in adults with traumatic head injuries. *American Journal of Occupational Therapy, 44,* 797–802.

McGrady, A., & Roberts, G. (1992). Racial differences in the relaxation response of hypertensives. *Psychosomatic Medicine, 54,* 71–78.

McNair, D. M., Lorr, M., & Dropplemann, L. F. (1971). *Profile of mood states.* San Diego: Educational and Industrial Testing Service.

O'Neil, H. F., Spielberger, C. D., & Hansen, D. N. (1969). The effects of state anxiety and task difficulty on computer-assisted learning. *Journal of Educational Psychology, 60,* 343–350.

Pender, N. (1985). Effects of progressive muscle relaxation training on anxiety and locus of control among hypertensive adults. *Research in Nursing and Health, 8,* 67–82.

Renfroe, K. (1988). Effect of progressive muscle relaxation on dyspnea and state anxiety in patients with chronic obstructive pulmonary disease. *Heart & Lung, 17,* 408–413.

Rice, V. H., Caldwell, M., Butler, S., & Robinson, J. (1986). Relaxation training and response in cardiac catheterization. *Nursing Research, 35,* 39–43.

Shapiro, S., & Lehrer, P. (1980). Psychophysiological effects of autogenic training and progressive relaxation. *Biofeedback and Self-Relaxation, 5,* 249–255.

Sloman, R. (1995). Relaxation and the relief of cancer pain. *Nursing Clinics of North America, 30,* 697–709.

Sloman, R., Brown, P., Aldana, E., & Chee, E. (1994). The use of relaxation for the promotion of comfort and pain relief in persons with advanced cancer. *Contemporary Nurse, 3*(1), 6–12.

Smith, J. C. (1989). *Relaxation dynamics.* Charles, IL: Research Press.

Snyder, M. (1983). Effect of relaxation on psychosocial functioning in persons with epilepsy. *Journal of Neurosurgical Nursing, 15,* 250–254.

Snyder, M. (1993). The influence of interventions on the stress-coping linkage. In J. Barnfather and B. Lyon (Eds.), *Stress and coping: State of the science and implications for nursing theory, research, and practice* (pp. 159–170). Indianapolis, IN: Sigma Theta Tau International.

Spielberger, C., Gorusch, R., Luschene, R., Vagg, P., & Jacobs, G. (1983). *Manual for STAI.* Palo Alto, CA: Consulting Psychological Press.

Stewart, C. (1989). *Effectiveness of sensory information and relaxation information as interventions in the reduction of cardiac catheterization stress.* Unpublished master's thesis, University of Minnesota, Minneapolis, MN.

Tsai, S., & Crockett, M. S. (1993). Effects of relaxation training, combining imagery and meditation, on the stress level of Chinese nurses working in modern hospitals in Taiwan. *Issues in Mental health Nursing, 14,* 51–66.

Wells, N. (1982). The effect of relaxation on postoperative muscle tension and pain. *Nursing Research, 31,* 236–238.

Whitman, S., Dell, J., Legion, V., Eibhlyn, A., & Staatsinger, J. (1990). Progressive relaxation for seizure reduction. *Journal of Epilepsy, 3,* 17–22.

Yesavage, J. A. (1984). Relaxation training and memory training in 39 elderly patients. *American Journal of Psychiatry, 141,* 778–781.

Zuckerman, M. (1960). The development of an adjective checklist for the measurement of anxiety. *Journal of Consulting Psychology, 24,* 457–462.

2

BREATHING

JingJy Wang and Mariah Snyder

Breathing techniques have been used as forms of therapy since ancient times (Jencks, 1984). Reports on the use of breathing therapy by the Chinese date to the sixth century B.C. Records from the second century B.C. in India reveal that *hatha yoga* incorporated breathing techniques to achieve hypnosis. Early Christian monks used a rhythmic form of breathing during prayers. Breathing was not an important component of Western medicine until the 1900s, when psychotherapy began to incorporate breathing techniques. Bonnet (cited in Jencks, 1984) instructed his patients to repeat hypnotic formulas in rhythm with their breathing patterns. Schultz (1957), the father of the autogenic technique, observed that irregular breathing was present during stress. He incorporated the phrase, or mantra, "It breathes me," for persons to use during the autogenic technique to provide a passive focus on breathing.

For many years nursing has used breathing techniques to achieve many different outcomes. Fundamentals of nursing texts provide instructions on using deep breathing to reduce preoperative anxiety and to decrease postoperative pain and complications. Nursing also has made considerable use of breathing patterns as part of relaxation techniques, such as the LeMaze techniques used during birthing. Increasingly, more and more nurses are using breathing techniques with many patient populations, helping pediatric patients master the stress of painful procedures and producing positive lung function in cystic fibrosis patients, for two examples. Although nursing has used techniques for breathing for various purposes, nursing has given little attention to breathing as a specific intervention.

DEFINITION

Breathing is defined as drawing air into and expelling it from the lungs. Inhalation and exhalation comprise breathing. The term is sometimes preceded by an adjective that identifies the muscles being used in respiration: diaphragmatic, intercostal, or accessory muscles breathing. Diaphragmatic breathing is the most efficient and relaxed type of breathing. Damage to the spinal cord in the high cervical region damages the phrenic nerve and often necessitates continuous ventilator assistance. Intercostal muscles are involved in the expansion of the chest cavity. However, reliance on the intercostal muscles for breathing is very taxing. Accessory muscles are used primarily when there is interference with diaphragmatic breathing.

Emotional states associated with particular patterns of breathing have also been used to classify breathing. Smith (1989) noted that a person breathes quickly and choppily when angry, holds one's breath when fearful, and gasps when shocked. Thus, breathing reveals much about a person's emotional state. When persons are fearful or anxious, the respiration rate increases. Stamford (1992) introduced some breathing patterns to accommodate the increased demands of exercise: deep versus fast breathing; chest versus belly breathing; and nose versus mouth breathing.

SCIENTIFIC BASIS

The character of one's breathing has a profound influence on a person's quality of life (Speads, 1986). Proper breathing improves circulation, normalizes muscle tone, and enhances clear thinking. These effects often result in a more positive mood. According to Speads, the effect of breathing on physiological and psychological functioning supports the total harmony within an individual. Research findings suggest that respiratory muscle feedback and breathing retraining improve lung function in patients with cystic fibrosis (Delk, Gevirtz, Hicks, Carden, & Rucker, 1994).

Breathing is an automatic, self-regulatory function. However, many variables influence breathing patterns. Attention to these variables will assist the person in being able to change his or her breathing patterns so as to promote more effective and healthy breathing.

INTERVENTION

Breathing techniques vary depending on the purpose for which they are used. Most fundamentals of nursing texts include descriptions of deep breathing techniques to use for postoperative and immobilized patients. Breathing techniques are also widely used in birthing to facilitate the labor process and help women to relax during contractions. Also, breathing techniques are used as interventions to reduce dyspnea. One breathing strategy for patients with obstructive lung disease is pursed-lip breathing. Pursing the lips during exhalation slows the rate of breathing.

Numerous breathing techniques have been incorporated into relaxation interventions: A breathing technique is one of the key elements of yoga (Fields, 1995). Yoga is a way of working with the mind and body, with breathing serving as the link to help people to become calm and relaxed, to release tension, and to increase the healthy flow of energy throughout the body. Some techniques are very simple, such as having a patient focus on inhalation and exhalation. An accompanying message is "Let tension escape with the exhalation." Other breathing techniques, such as the integrative breathing technique of Smith (1989), are more complex. This latter technique will be described.

Techniques

Table 2.1 provides the guidelines for the integrative breathing technique (Smith, 1985). According to Smith (1989), integrative breathing helps in distinguishing relaxed and tense breathing, encourages use of the diaphragm, and facilitates an appropriate breathing pattern. This exercise can be practiced in either a standing or sitting position depending on which works best for the person.

Although the integrative breathing technique of Smith (1989) comprises 12 segments, any one or a combination of the segments may be used for producing relaxation. Modifications may need to be made for patients depending upon their health status and limitations. For patients on bed rest or with functional deficits, the stretching exercises would not be feasible. Working with the breath is more difficult for smokers and for patients with respiratory illnesses. However, the focused breathing segment and the verbal thought segment could easily be used by these patients.

TABLE 2.1   Guidelines for Integrative Breathing Technique

1. Sit in chair with feet flat on floor. Close eyes and let body become comfortable. Take a deep breath and slowly exhale; this is done several times.
2. Circle arms behind the body while inhaling and circle arms to the front of the body while exhaling. These actions are repeated several times. Conclude with arms limp by one's side.
3. Stretch back and let the head tilt back while inhaling. Arms remain hanging at sides. Relax and bring body back into a comfortable upright position with each exhalation. The head may bend slightly forward. These actions are repeated several times.
4. Arch back as in the previous segment, but during the exhaling portion bend forward with the head and chest moving toward the knees. Arms hang limply at sides. Take several shorter breaths. Take a deep breath while sitting upright. Take several deep breaths in the sitting position with the exhalations being very slow and deliberate.
5. Arch back and gently circle both arms toward the sky, like the wings of a bird. When ready to exhale, let the arms slowly circle down so that they are hanging heavily at the sides. Bow forward and remain in that position for a short period of time; breathe in whatever manner seems comfortable. Place the arms in the lap and breathe in a natural manner. Repeat this sequence twice.
6. Spread palms of hands across the abdomen with the thumbs touching the bottom of the chest. Taking a deep breath, press hands firmly against the abdomen to assist in expelling air from the lungs. Fingers are relaxed during inhalation. This sequence is repeated several times.
7. Using diaphragmatic breathing, the hands remain gently on the stomach during both inhalation and exhalation. After the exhalation, pull stomach in as if to push out any remaining air. These actions are repeated several times.
8. While inhaling, imagine sniffing a delicate flower. The inhalation should be smooth and gentle. Exhalation is done naturally.
9. Attention is drawn to air moving through the nostrils and into the body. Exhale through the lips as if blowing out a candle flame. The inhalations and exhalations are repeated several times.
10. Focus attention on the air entering and leaving the body; let breathing be effortless. Relax and just think of the word *one* for a minute.
11. Finally, use a word of your choosing to repeat during exhalation. Let the word repeat effortlessly as your inhale and exhale. Then, just let it float away like a cloud.

Note. From *Relaxation dynamics* by J. C. Smith, 1989. Champaign, IL: Research Press. Copyright 1989 by Research Press. Adapted by permission.

Measurement of Effectiveness

Parameters that can be used to measure the effectiveness of breathing include subjective and objective reports such as observed and self-reported emotions, overall well-being, behavioral indexes of relaxation, and biochemical indexes results, such as lung function or arterial blood gas value. Subjective reports of well-being may be the most useful indicator.

USES

Few nursing studies on the use of breathing were found. Often, when breathing techniques were used, they were incorporated into another intervention, making it difficult to determine the specific effects resulting from the breathing techniques. However, breathing techniques have been used with a wide variety of patient populations.

One of the most frequent uses has been to decrease anxiety and the symptoms associated with increased anxiety. Jencks (1984) reported that providing directions on breathing and relaxation to adults during blood drawing helped to reduce anxiety. A simple breathing and relaxation method was found to be effective in reducing the stress experienced by hospitalized children who had pain and high anxiety (McDonnnell & Bowden, 1989). Biofeedback-assisted breathing retraining produced a significant improvement in lung function in patients with cystic fibrosis (Delk et al., 1994). Attention to breathing may have served to decrease anxiety and improve overall respiration. Another population for whom breathing techniques have been used is persons with chronic obstruction pulmonary disease; breathing techniques helped to reduce dyspnea. Temporary improvement of arterial blood gas values also occurred (Miller & Petty, 1990).

Breathing has been used to reduce pain. Miller and Perry (1990) described use of a simple, slow, rhythmic, deep-breathing technique to decrease pain in subjects who had undergone coronary artery bypass graft surgery. Statistically significant, but not clinically significant, decreases in systolic and diastolic blood pressure occurred in the experimental group. Most important, the majority of persons using the breathing relaxation technique reported that it was beneficial in lessening postoperative pain.

Precautions

Breathing patterns and techniques need to be personalized for each patient. Helping persons gain awareness of their breathing will assist them in developing the technique with which they are most comfortable. During the initial sessions, the nurse needs to be attentive to how a patient is breathing so as to prevent shallow breathing and hyperventilation.

RESEARCH QUESTIONS

As was indicated earlier, few nurse researchers have explored breathing as a specific intervention. Therefore, the following projects are suggested:

1. Compare the effectiveness of breathing with other relaxation techniques and determine with which populations it is the intervention of choice.
2. Determine the problems encountered in the use of the intervention so that complications can be avoided.
3. Compare and contrast the effectiveness of various breathing techniques.
4. Design and validate specific breathing techniques for patient with respiratory disorders.

REFERENCES

Delk, K. K., Gevirtz, R., Hicks, D. A., Carden, F., & Rucker, R. (1994). The effects of biofeedback-assisted breathing retraining on lung functions in patients with cystic fibrosis. *Chest, 105*(1), 23–28.

Fields, N. (1995). Teaching the gentle way to labour. *Nursing Times, 91*(6), 44–45.

Jencks, B. (1984). Using the patient's breathing rhythm. In W. C. Wester & A. Smith (Eds.), *Clinical hypnosis: A multidisciplinary approach* (pp. 29–41). Philadelphia: Lippincott.

McDonnell, L., & Bowden, M. L. (1989). Breathing management: A simple stress and pain reduction strategy for use on a pediatric service. *Issues in Comprehensive Pediatric Nursing, 12*, 339–344.

Miller, K. M., & Perry, P. A. (1990). Relaxation technique and postoperative pain in patients undergoing cardiac surgery. *Heart & Lung, 19,* 136–146.

Schultz, J. H. (1957). Autogenous training. In J. H. Masserman & J. L. Moreno (Eds.), *Progress in psychotherapy* (Vol. 2, pp. 173–176). New York: Grune & Stratton.

Smith, J. C. (1989). *Relaxation dynamics.* Champaign, IL: Research Press.

Speads, C. (1986). *Ways to better breathing.* Great Neck, NY: Morrow.

Stamford, B. (1992). Tips for better breathing. *The Physician and Sports-medicine, 20*(9), 201–202.

3

EXERCISE

Diane Treat-Jacobson and Daniel L. Mark

Exercise is rapidly becoming recognized as a lifelong endeavor essential for energetic, active, and healthy living. The research supporting the benefits of exercise is substantial. The effects of exercise and its benefits have been linked to many physiological and psychological responses, from reduction in the stress response to an increased sense of well-being (Pender, 1996; Crews & Landers, 1987).

Despite the tremendous benefits of exercise, it is, surprisingly, an activity largely ignored by the general population. Indeed, the Surgeon General (U.S. Surgeon General, 1996) has issued a report identifying millions of inactive Americans as being at risk for a wide range of chronic diseases and ailments including coronary heart disease (CHD), adult onset diabetes, colon cancer, hip fractures, hypertension, and obesity.

Nurses need to recognize the importance of exercise as being essential to the health of the population as a whole. They need to take responsibility for using current and emerging knowledge to assist clients to develop lifelong exercise habits appropriate to their age and physical condition. Exercise must be an integral part of personal lifestyle if it is to have optimum effects on health. Maintaining physical fitness can be enjoyable and rewarding for persons of all ages and can contribute significantly to extending longevity and improving quality of life. Knowledge of exercise and its application in multiple populations will assist in the delivery of expert nursing care. This chapter discusses the definition, physiological basis, and application of exercise as a nursing intervention.

DEFINITION

Physical activity is defined as "any bodily movement produced by skeletal muscles that results in caloric expenditure" (Pender, 1996, p. 185; Caspersen, Powell, & Christenson, 1986). Definitions of exercise are complex and vary according to discipline, however they all incorporate physical activity into their descriptions.

Commonly, exercise is classified according to whether oxygen is consumed during the activity. Exercise is considered to be *aerobic* when the energy needed is supplied by the oxygen (O_2) inspired (Kisner, 1996). In general, aerobic exercise increases demand on the respiratory, cardiovascular and musculoskeletal systems. Sustained periods of work require aerobic metabolism of energy at a level compatible with the body's oxygen supply capabilities. *Anaerobic* exercise is exercise during which the energy needed is provided without utilization of inspired oxygen (Kisner & Colby, 1996). This occurs during short, vigorous bouts of exercise or when the body's oxygen supply capabilities cannot meet the metabolic demands of the exercise.

SCIENTIFIC BASIS

Better understanding of exercise physiology and the body's response to various stages of physical activity will assist in the development of exercise programs appropriate for the individual and the goal of the exercise. The response of the body to exercise occurs in stages. Eight to ten seconds after the initiation of exercise, a large sympathetic outburst occurs and the heart overshoots the rate needed, but then returns to the rate required for increased activity. Impulses from muscles being exercised are sent to the brain; an increase in the heart rate is initiated (Fletcher, 1982). During this phase, there is a sluggish adjustment of respiration and circulation, resulting in an O_2 deficit; exercise is fueled by the anaerobic metabolism of creatine phosphate and glucose (Kisner & Colby, 1996).

As exercise continues, oxygen consumption (VO_2) increases. Cardiac output (CO) is increased to meet the increased O_2 demands of the working muscle. The increase in CO is due to increased stroke volume (SV) and heart rate (HR), increased myocardial contractibility (from positive inotropic sympathetic impulses to the heart), increased venous return, and a decreased peripheral resistance offered by the exercising muscles (Fletcher, 1982). In normal individuals, CO can increase 4–5 times normal, allowing for increased delivery of O_2 to exercising muscle beds and facilitating removal of lactate, carbon dioxide (CO_2) and heat. Respiration increases to deliver O_2 and to allow for elimination of CO_2 (Shepard, 1992; Holloszy, 1976). Blood pressure increases as a result of increased cardiac output and the sympathetic vasoconstriction of vessels in the non-exercising muscles, viscera, and skin. During this "steady state" exercise phase, O_2 uptake equals O_2 tissue requirement, aerobic metabolism of glucose and fatty acids occurs, and there is no accumulation of lactic acid.

As exercise becomes more strenuous, there is a shift toward anaerobic metabolism of glucose, resulting in increased production of lactic acid (Balady & Weiner, 1992). The anaerobic threshold is a point during exercise at which ventilation abruptly increases despite linear increases in work rate. At a given work rate, the O_2 supply does not meet the oxygen requirement. This increases anaerobic glycolysis for energy generation and increases lactate production. Accumulation of lactic acid can lead to symptoms of dyspnea and fatigue. Shortly beyond the anaerobic threshold, fatigue ensues and work ceases. Exercise at a level which allows for aerobic metabolism and reduces the need for anaerobic metabolism reduces the production of lactic acid and may delay onset of these symptoms.

INTERVENTION

According to the National Institutes of Health consensus statement (NIH, 1995), exercise is considered to be beneficial to health. The benefits of exercise are well documented. The U.S. Surgeon General (1996) has recently released a report detailing the impact of physical activity and inactivity in our society. In this report the list of benefits of physical activity to the general health and well-being of Americans include:

1. decreased the risk of premature death
2. decreased risk of premature death from heart disease
3. decreased the risk of acquiring Type II diabetes
4. decreased risk of incurring high blood pressure
5. decreased high blood pressure in hypertensive individuals
6. decreased risk of acquiring colon cancer
7. decreased feelings of uneasiness and despair
8. improved weight control

9. strengthening and maintenance of muscles, joints and bones
10. improved balance and mobility in older adults
11. feelings of psychological well-being.

Given that the benefits of exercise apply to all age groups across a broad spectrum of health and disease, it is important for nurses to recognize opportunities to promote exercise as a nursing intervention. There are countless activities included under the "umbrella" of exercise. Finding the activity that fits an individual's capabilities and meets the purposes for which exercise is prescribed is key to the success of the intervention (Gavin, 1988). When prescribing an intervention, it is important to take into account the recommended exercise intensity for the patient population being served. This can range from children to adults to elderly or those with chronic disease.

Evidence suggests that exercise is more likely to be initiated if the individual (a) recognizes the need to exercise, (b) perceives the exercise to be beneficial and enjoyable, (c) perceives that the exercise has minimal negative aspects such as expense, time burden, negative peer pressure, (d) feels capable and safe engaging in the exercise, and (e) has ready access to the activity and can easily fit it in to the daily schedule (NIH Consensus Statement, 1995).

Technique

An exercise session should involve three phases, including warming up, aerobic exercise, and cooling down. The phases of exercise are designed to allow the body opportunity to sustain internal equilibrium by gradually adjusting its physiological processes to the stress of exercise and thus maintaining homeostasis.

Phases of an Exercise Session.

Warm up phase. The goal of the warm-up is to allow the body time to adapt to the rigors of aerobic exercise. Warming up results in an increase in muscle temperature, a higher need for oxygen in order to meet the increased demands of the exercising muscles, dilatation of capillaries resulting in increased circulation, adjustments within the neural respiratory center to the demands of exercise, and a shifting of blood flow centrally from the periphery resulting in increased venous return (Kisner, 1996). In addition, a good warm-up increases flexibility, and decreases or prevents arrhythmias and ischemic ECG changes

(Kisner, 1996). Warm-up exercises should be done for 10 minutes, involve all major body parts, and achieve a heart rate within 20 beats per minute of the target heart rate for the following aerobic exercise (Kisner, 1996). In addition a good warm-up should incorporate stretching exercises. Stretching exercises are done at a slow, steady pace and help maintain a full range of motion in body joints, and strengthen tendons, ligaments and muscles.

Aerobic exercise phase. The aerobic phase of exercise has four components: intensity, frequency, duration, and mode of exercise. The combination of these components determines the effectiveness of the exercise. A balance needs to be achieved to obtain maximal benefit at least risk and discomfort. Adjustment of intensity is important not only for safety reasons, but also for comfort and enjoyment of the activity (Foster & Tamboli, 1992). If exercise can be kept at a level that is comfortable, the individual is more likely to continue to perform the activity. As exercise tolerance develops, any or all of the exercise components can be increased to meet the individual's aerobic capacity. For example if an individual is comfortable with the intensity of the exercise, the duration and frequency can be increased to further improve training effect.

Cool down. Immediately following the endurance exercises, the person should engage in a cooling down period. This allows the body to adjust to normal conditions and to eliminate the lactic acid that may have accumulated in the muscle tissue during exercise. Five to ten minutes are needed for the body to adjust to a slower pace. Cooling down exercises may include walking slowly, deep breathing, and stretching exercises.

Maintenance. Maintaining the exercise program is the key to the effectiveness of the intervention. Setting both short- and long-term goals helps improve adherence. The individual can experience a sense of accomplishment upon meeting short-term goals while still striving for overall goals. Keeping a record or graph provides a visual demonstration of progress and may provide insight into possible adjustments to the exercise program which may assist in achievement of goals.

Specific technique: Walking. Walking is one exercise in which persons in all age groups and with varying levels of disability can engage to improve endurance. A major advantage is that walking requires no special equipment, facilities, or new skills. It is also safer and easier to maintain than many other forms of exercise. Intensity, duration, and frequency are easily regulated and adjusted to accommodate a wide range of physical capabilities and limitations. The initial intensity should be outlined at the start of the program and is dependent on baseline level of conditioning, physical or disease-related limitations or precautions, and outcome goals.

A walking program can be approached in two ways. The exercise can be completed in one or multiple daily sessions. For example, a previously sedentary individual may wish to begin an exercise program consisting of 2-minute brisk walks throughout the day. This could be increased to 5-minute walks, and then 10-minute walks as stamina increases. The more traditional alternative would be to engage in one longer session at least 3 times per week. These sessions would include a warm-up session for 5–10 minutes, an aerobic period of 10–15 minutes initially, gradually increasing to 30–60 minutes in length, and a cool down period of 5–10 minutes (American Heart Association [AHA], 1995).

The exercising individual should monitor the body's response to the activity to ensure that the intensity is appropriate for the individual. Several methods have been used.

Monitor target heart rate. The target heart rate should be between 50% and 75% of the maximal heart rate, which is calculated by subtracting one's age from 220 (AHA, 1995). The heart rate should be assessed one third to one half of the way through the exercise session and immediately after stopping exercise. Exercise intensity can be increased or decreased based on this measurement.

The Talk Test. The talk test can replace target heart rate monitoring when an individual is exercising at a moderate intensity. If the exercise prevents the individual from talking comfortably, the intensity should be decreased.

Rating of Perceived Exertion. This is a scale which describes the sense of effort during the exercise. This scale can be ranked from one to ten with one being no effort and ten being maximal effort (AHA, 1995).

Conditions/Populations in Which the Intervention Has Been Used

The Surgeon General (1996) and the NIH (1995) have both recently released documents discussing the statistics related to exercise behav-

TABLE 3.1 Nine Tips for Fitness Walking

Warm up by performing a few stretches.

Think tall as you walk. Stand straight with your head level and your shoulders relaxed.

Your heel will hit the surface first. Use smooth movements rolling from heel to toe.

Keep your hands free and let your arms swing naturally in oppostion to your legs.

When you're ready to pick up the pace, quicken your step and lengthen your stride. But don't compromise your upright posture or smooth, comfortable movements.

To increase your intensity, burn more calories, and tone your upper body, bend your arms at the elbows and pump your arms. Keep your elbows close to your body.

Breathe in and out naturally, rhythmically, and deeply.

Use the "Talk Test" to check your intensity, or take your pulse to see if you are within your target heart rate.

Cool down during the last three to five minutes by gradually slowing your pace to a stroll.

American Heart Association (1995).

ior, the benefits of exercise, and the dangers of a sedentary lifestyle for individuals of all ages. Initiating exercise programs with children and young people will have a major impact on the health of the nation. It is important to maintain exercise habits throughout adulthood. Exercise programs have been used in numerous chronic disease populations including individuals with diabetes and in those with mobility deficits.

Two populations in which exercise is particularly beneficial include the elderly and individuals with heart disease. The application and demonstrated effects of exercise intervention in each of these populations will be discussed below.

Elderly. The elderly are especially prone to the "hazards of immobility" which affect many of the body's systems. Exercise results in increased bone strength (Smith & Reddan, 1976), and increased total body calcium (Dalsky et al., 1988), as well as improved coordination which may result in a reduction in falls (Bassett, McClamrock, & Schmelzer, 1982). Such improvements would facilitate movement and activities and promote self-care by the elderly.

Exercise has also been shown to improve body functioning and overall well-being. Blumenthal, Schocken, Needles, & Hindl (1982) reported that 40% of the elderly in their study who exercised felt healthier, were more satisfied with life, had more self-confidence, and were in a better mood than before the program began.

While it is important to tailor exercise programs for all persons, this is particularly true for the elderly, who may have specific limitations. Exercise needs to be initiated at lower levels and increased gradually. Participants need to be taught to notice and listen to the body's response to the activity and to adjust accordingly. Previously sedentary elderly individuals may be more comfortable initiating an exercise program with some supervision which allows them to become accustomed this new level of activity in a safe environment. Group exercise may be especially appealing to the older person.

Heart Disease. Exercise rehabilitation is a common intervention for those with (CHD) with or without coronary artery bypass graft surgery (CABG). Cardiac rehabilitation (CR) provides a safe environment for the initiation of an exercise program. Programs usually have several phases and are tailored to the specific needs, limitations, and characteristics of individual patients. The exercise prescription changes as fitness levels improve. The goal of CR is to help patients resume active and productive lives (Foster & Tamboli, 1992; Hamm & Leon, 1992).

Exercise training has been shown to improve symptom-limited exercise capacity in CHD and CABG patients as a result of cardiovascular changes, which include: improved left ventricular function and CO, reduced serum catecholamines (leading to reduced blood pressure), decreased resting and submaximal HR, higher arterial O_2 content, increased O_2 extraction from exercising muscle (thus increased A-VO_2 difference), decreased cardiac work, increased ischemic threshold, VO_{2max} and exercise tolerance (Detry et al., 1971; Ferguson et al., 1982; Juneau, Beneau, Marchand, & Brosseau, 1991; Wenger, 1993). Improvements in SV and CO are changed with more intense training levels and show less change in older and more frail individuals (Detry et al., 1971). Patients with CHD have a low skeletal muscle oxidative capacity which is significantly improved with training, despite relatively low workloads and exercise intensities, consistent with other non–heart disease populations (Ferguson et al., 1982). Trained cardiac patients function further from the ischemic threshold in performing activities of daily living (ADLs) and require a lower percentage of maximal effort to perform activities (since maximal effort is increased). Thus, training increases stamina and endurance and helps to maintain independence (Wenger, 1993). Even patients with congestive heart failure (CHF), who typically have very poor cardiac function, have found rehabilitation to be beneficial, improving exercise tolerance through improvement in peripheral mechanisms that enable them to aerobically metabolize substrates more efficiently (Koch, Douard, & Broustet, 1992; Sullivan, 1994).

Submaximal endurance has been reported to improve to a much greater degree than maximal performance (Ades, Waldmann, Poehlman, Gray, Horton, & LeWinter, 1993). Prior to training, older coronary patients are often unable to perform ADLs without dyspnea, angina or fatigue. Results of one study of patients with CHD showed that activities which were exhaustive prior to training, were able to be performed for long periods of time after training (Ades et al., 1993).

Measurement of Effectiveness

The appropriate measure of the effectiveness of an exercise intervention depends on the specific exercise prescribed and the goals of the intervention. If cardiovascular fitness is the targeted outcome, an aerobic exercise program would be prescribed and changes in the cardiovascular system would be used to determine the effectiveness of the intervention. With aerobic exercise, the intensity of the aerobic phase of exercise must be great enough to generate a stress on the system sufficient to provide a training effect (i.e., increased stroke volume and cardiac output, increased anaerobic threshold, and improved local circulation [Halfman & Hojnacki, 1981]). Exercise prescribed to improve function may use parameters such as improved joint mobility, prevention or reduction of osteoporosis, and improved strength in determining exercise effectiveness (Benison & Hogskel, 1986; Compton, Eisenman, & Henderson, 1989). These would be appropriate especially in elderly individuals.

Studies have shown that for older and very sedentary individuals exercise at lower intensities can be beneficial. Exercising at lower levels of intensity has resulted in improvements in fitness in older sedentary men and women (Belman & Gaesser, 1991; Foster, Hume, Burns, Dickenson, & Chatfield, 1989; Stevenson & Topp, 1990).

It has been argued that low-intensity training regimens may produce more gradual change and show only small changes in fitness, but these programs may have greater patient compliance with activity and may be safer for a relatively frail population. In addition, there can be large changes in function with relatively small changes in fitness, especially in populations of older, sedentary individuals (Buchner, Beresford, Larson,

LaCroix, & Wagner, 1992). Buchner and colleagues (1992) elaborate on the concept of a functional "threshold," below which an individual is not able to completely carry out all ADLs. Even small improvements in fitness can keep an individual above that threshold or provide a greater "margin of safety," and may mean the difference between being able to independently carry out daily requirements and becoming dependent on a caregiver (Foster et al., 1989).

In addition to fitness changes, programs should assess changes in physical functioning and disability, ability to perform ADLs and changes in symptoms and activity tolerance. All are variables that are meaningful to the patient in terms of functioning in daily life. Lower intensity programs, which may not demonstrate great changes in maximal exercise capacity, might produce sufficient changes in these outcome variables to make a difference in the individual's quality of life. Development and implementation of programs designed to meet the specific needs of patients can help maximize functional and quality-of-life outcomes.

PRECAUTIONS

It is important that prior to beginning a program both the nurse and the patient to be aware of the signs of overexercising. Usually symptoms result from excessive intensity, duration, or frequency of exercise before the body is ready. It is important to begin an exercise program slowly, to follow safety guidelines, and to exercise consistently, several times per week. The American Heart Association (1995) has listed general guidelines to follow to help ensure exercise safety. These include:

1. Stretch the muscles and tendons prior to beginning exercise, especially those that are the focus of the exercise.
2. Ensure that footwear appropriate for the exercise is worn.
3. Exercise on a surface with some "give" to it to help prevent injury to joints. This is especially important for high-impact activities.
4. Learn to do the exercise properly and continue good form even when increasing speed or intensity of the exercise.

Previously sedentary elderly individuals and those with chronic disease, especially heart disease, should consult a physician prior to initiating an exercise program. It may be necessary to initiate the exercise in a monitored setting or to have an exercise stress test to ensure safety and confirm that the appropriate level of exercise has been prescribed. Information on the warning signs of heart disease is an essential educational component prior to initiation of an exercise program, especially for those in high-risk categories.

There are other noncardiac risks and potential exercise-related injuries. These include muscle and joint pain, cramps, blisters, shin splints, low back pain, tendinitis, and other sprains or muscle strains. Many of these problems can be avoided by starting an exercise program slowly and by following safety precautions. Should any of these problems arise, they can usually be treated with one or a combination of therapies, including rest, ice, compression, and elevation (AHA, 1995).

FUTURE RESEARCH

There are many gaps in our knowledge related to exercise, its measurement, the benefits, and methods to improve exercise adherence. Specific research areas needed include:

1. Development of measures of exercise behavior which are valid and reliable in different populations and with various levels of activity.
2. Development and testing of specific interventions to increase exercise adherence in multiple populations
3. Assessment of the impact of exercise interventions in multiple populations through controlled longitudinal studies.
4. Investigation of the influence of numerous factors such as environment, social factors, and heredity on adoption of and adherence to exercise.
5. Development of accurate methods of cost/benefit analysis to evaluate the long-term benefits of exercise.
6. Determination of minimum requirements for exercise intensity, duration etc. in order to achieve benefit. Make these requirements population, age, and condition specific.

REFERENCES

Ades, P., Waldmann, M., Poehlman, E., Gray, P., Horton, E., Horton, E., & LeWinter, M., (1993). Exercise conditioning in older coronary patients. Submaximal lactate response to endurance capacity. *Circulation, 88*(2), 72–577.

American Heart Association (1995). *Your Heart, an Owner's Manual.* Englewood Cliffs, NJ: Prentice Hall.

Balady, G., & Weiner, D. (1992). Physiology of exercise in normal individuals and patients with coronary heart disease. In N. Wenger and H. Hellerstein (Eds.) *Rehabilitation of the Coronary Patient.* (pp. 103–122). New York: Churchill Livingstone.

Bassett, C., McClamrock, E., & Schmelzer, M. (1982). A 10–week exercise program for senior citizens. *Geriatric Nursing, 3,* 103–105.

Belman, M., & Gaesser, G. (1991). Exercise training below and above the lactate threshold in the elderly. *Medicine and Science in Sports and Exercise, 23,* 562–568.

Benison, B., & Hogstel, M. (1986). Aging and movement therapy: Essential interventions for the immobile elderly. *Journal of Gerontological Nursing 12(12),* 8–16.

Blumenthal, J., Schocken, D., Needles, T., & Hindle, P. (1982). Psychological and physiological effects of physical conditioning on the elderly. *Journal of Psychosomatic Medicine 26,* 505–510.

Buchner, D., Beresford, S., Larson, E., LaCroix, A., & Wagner, E. (1992). Effects of physical activity on health status in older adults. II: Intervention studies. *Annual Review of Public Health, 13,* 469–488.

Caspersen C., Powell K., & Christenson G. (1986). Physical activity, exercise and physical fitness: Definitions and distinctions for health-related research. *Public Health Reports,101,* 126–131.

Compton, D., Eisenman, P., & Henderson, H., (1989). Exercise and fitness for persons with disabilities. *Sports Medicine, 7,* 150–162.

Crews, D., & Landers, D. (1987). A meta-analytic review of aerobic fitness and reactivity to psychosocial stressors. *Medicine and Science in Sports and Exercise 19(suppl),* S114–S120.

Dalsky, O., Stocke, K., Ehsani, A., Slatopolsky, E., Lee, W., & Birge, S. (1988). Weight-bearing exercise training and lumbar bone mineral content in postmenopausal women. *Annals of Internal Medicine, 108,* 824–829.

Detry, J., Rosseau, M., Vandenbroucke, G., Kusumi, F., Brasseur, L., & Bruce, R. (1971). Increased arteriovenous oxygen difference after physical training in coronary heart disease. *Circulation, 64,* 109–118.

Fletcher, G., (1982). *Exercise in the practice of medicine.* Mount Kisco, NY: Futura.

Ferguson, R., Taylor, A., Cote, P., Charlebois, J., Dinelle, Y., Perionnet, F., Dechamplain, J., & Bourassa, M. (1982). Skeletal muscle and cardiac changes with training in patients with angina pectoris. *American Journal of Physiology, 243,* H830–H836.

Foster, V., Hume, G., Byrnes, W., Dickenson, A., & Chatfield, S. (1989). Endurance training for elderly women: Moderate vs. low intensity. *Journal of Gerontology, 44*(6), M184–178.

Foster, C., & Tamboli, H. (1992). Exercise prescription in the rehabilitation of patients following coronary artery bypass graft surgery and coronary angioplasty. In R. Shepard and H. Miller (Eds.), *Exercise and the heart in health and disease* (pp. 283–298). New York: Dekker.

Gavin, J. (1988). Psychological issues in exercise prescription. *Sports Medicine, 6*, 1–10.

Halfman, M., & Hojnacki, L. (1981). Exercise and the maintenance of health. *Topics in Clinical Nursing, 3*(2), 1–10.

Hamm, L., & Leon, A. (1992). Exercise training for the coronary patient. In N. Wenger and H. Hellerstein (Eds.), *Rehabilitation of the coronary patient* (pp. 367–402). New York.

Holloszy, J. (1976). Adaptations of muscular tissue to training. *Progress in Cardiovascular Disease, 18*, 445–458.

Juneau, M., Geneau, S., Marchand, C., & Brosseau, R. (1991). Cardiac rehabilitation after coronary artery bypass surgery. *Cardiovascular Clinics, 12*(2), 25–42.

Kisner, C., & Colby, L. (1996). *Therapeutic exercise: Foundations and techniques,* (3rd ed.). Philadelphia: Davis.

Koch, M., Douard, H., & Broustet, J-P. (1992). The benefit of graded physical exercise in chronic heart failure. *Chest, 101*(5 suppl.), 231S–235S.

National Institutes of Health Consensus Statement. (1995). *Physical activity and cardiovascular health, Dec. 18–20, 13*(3), 1–17.

Pender, N. (1996). *Health promotion in nursing practice* (3rd ed.). Stamford, CT: Appleton & Lange.

Shepard, R. (1992). Physiological, biochemical, and psychological responses to exercise. In R. Shepard and H. Miller (Eds.), *Exercise and the heart in health and disease.* New York: Dekker.

Smith, E., & Reddan, W. (1976). Physical activity—a modality for bone accretion in the aged. *American Journal of Roentgenology, 126*, 1297.

Stevenson, J., & Topp, R. (1990). Effects of moderate and low intensity long-term exercise by older adults. *Research in Nursing and Health, 13*, 209–218.

Sullivan, M. (1994). New trends in cardiac rehabilitation in patients with chronic heart failure. *Progress in Cardiovascular Nursing, 9*(1), 13–21.

U.S. Surgeon General. (1996). *Report on physical activity and health* [Online] Available: http://www.cde.800/nccdphd/sgr/mm.htm

Wenger, N. (1993). Modern coronary rehabilitation. New concepts in care. *Postgraduate Medicine, 94*(2), 131–141.

4

TAI CHI/MOVEMENT THERAPY*

Kevin Shaller

An ancient Chinese proverb says: "A door-pivot will never be worm-eaten and flowing water will never become putrid" (Man-Ch'ing, 1981, p. 20). The Chinese culture, with its rich traditions in the martial arts and holistic healing, has long advocated the importance of movement for health and longevity. Tai chi is a centuries-old system of movements, or "forms," that is designed to mobilize and direct the flow of chi (internal energy) throughout the body while improving balance, strength, coordination, and flexibility. It has been said that practitioners of tai chi "will gain the pliability of a child, the health of a lumberjack, and the peace of mind of a sage" (Man-Ch'ing & Smith, 1983, p. 1).

Tai chi and other movement therapies such as dance and yoga are rapidly becoming more popular in the United States as more Americans strive to keep both the body and mind fit. The purpose of this chapter is to introduce and describe tai chi as a movement therapy.

Movement therapy emphasizes the holism of human beings. In particular, tai chi and yoga focus on the relaxation of the entire body with progressive and systematic movement in coordination with deep steady breathing. This combination of movement and breathing engages both body and mind (Berg, 1995). This holistic mind-body connection is a key component in many nursing theories and models.

---

*Disclaimer: The views expressed in this article are those of the author and do not reflect the official policy or position of the Department of Army, Department of Defense, or the U.S. Government.

Goldberg and Fitzpatrick (1980) contended that nursing, more than any other profession, is oriented to the wholeness of persons. Thus, interventions that promote the integration of the total person should be emphasized in nursing. Nurses working in institutions, communities, and homes have a great opportunity to influence clients towards movement therapy.

DEFINITION

Tai chi, translated as "the ultimate" or "supreme ultimate" means improving and progressing toward the unlimited (Liao, 1990). Tai chi began over 1,700 years ago as a philosophy or way of life influenced by the theory of opposites: the yin and the yang (Liao, 1990). It was not until the 13th century, however, that the philosophy was integrated with physical movement and meditation. Chang San-feng, a Taoist monk, developed a series of forms or postures based on the movements of fighting animals. These postures were linked to form a series of movements that were intended to exercise internal organs in an effort to develop internal energy or chi (Man-Ch'ing, 1981).

According to Liao (1990), the original yin-yang principles of tai chi were easily applied to the martial arts. Many periods of conflict and unrest throughout Chinese history produced the external, or self-defense, tai chi. The pure, or internal, tai chi was maintained by a small number of masters who taught only select families. Continued turmoil in China up through the early 20th century relegated tai chi to an almost completely external exercise devoid of its original intentions (Liao, 1990).

The Yang style short form, consisting of 37 movements, is the most popular form practiced today. It was developed by Master Cheng Man-ch'ing and brought to the United States in the early 1940s (Man-ch'ing & Smith, 1983). Tai Chi Chih, a modified form of the Yang style, was developed by tai chi master Justin Stone. Tai Chi Chih (TCC) consists of 20 simple, repetitive, nonstrenuous movements that involve no physical contact and emphasize a soft continuity of motion (Stone, 1994). Stone (1994) developed TCC after finding that many students could not master the complex Yang style movements. While the Yang style remains popular, simpler, less strenuous variations such as TCC may be more adaptable to those students with some degree of physical or functional limitation.

SCIENTIFIC BASIS

Most of the evidence related to the benefits of tai chi has been anecdotal. Reports of miraculous recoveries from conditions like arthritis and chronic back pain are common. Advertisements for tai chi classes claim benefits of relaxation, improved breathing, circulation, balance, flexibility, fitness, and blood pressure. Several recent studies, to be discussed in a later section, have provided support for some of the above claims.

The FICSIT (Frailty and Injuries: Cooperative Studies of Intervention Techniques) trial site in Atlanta used tai chi movements because they were thought to "dynamically tax balance mechanisms while facilitating concentration of body position within the immediate environment" (Wolf, Barnhart, Kutner, McNeeley, Coogler, & Tingsen, 1996, p. 490). Tse and Bailey (1992) reported that regular tai chi practice significantly improved balance control in three of five tests and advocated the following factors as an explanation for the improvements.

1. All t'ai chi movements are circular, slow, continuous, even, and smooth. Patterns of movement flow from one to the next. The even, slow tempo facilitates a sensory awareness of the speed, force, trajectory, and execution of movement throughout the exercise.
2. Because movements are well controlled, all unnecessary exertion is avoided, and only sufficient effort is used to overcome gravity. Muscle coordination instead of rigid contraction can therefore be promoted.
3. Throughout the exercises, the body is constantly shifted from one foot to the other. This is likely to facilitate improvement of dynamic standing balance.
4. Throughout the exercises, different parts of the body take turns in playing the role of stabilizer and mover, allowing smooth movements to be executed without compromising the balance and stability of the body. (p. 297)

The practice of continuously interchanging the roles between weight bearing and non–weight bearing legs may enhance balance by affecting motor control mechanisms in the brain (Tse & Bailey, 1992).

Exercise intensity, classified as low, moderate, and high, is often used to gauge the cardiorespiratory benefit of an activity. Several studies have determined that tai chi can be classified as a moderately intensity activity similar to brisk walking (Brown, Mucci, Hetzler, &

Knowlton, 1989; Lai, Lan, Wong, & Teng, 1995; Schneider & Leung, 1991).

INTERVENTION

Many variations of the original tai chi are taught and practiced. Recent popularity of tai chi as a primary or adjunctive exercise has spawned numerous books, videos, clubs, and television programs. Tai chi classes have become standard at many health clubs, senior centers, YMCAs, and college campuses (Meditation in motion, 1994). Although the important movements and postures have been maintained in most tai chi variations, it critical for nurses to provide guidelines to clients for choosing a particular tai chi class or style. These guidelines will be presented in the "Precautions" section.

Technique

Learning and practicing TCC in accordance with the principles of yin-yang is essential for maximizing benefits. The yin (negative, receptive, cold, insubstantial) and the yang (positive, creative, hot, substantial) forces circulate and balance the chi or internal energy during TCC movements (Stone, 1994). Cultivation of chi is the ultimate means of maintaining health and wellness.

Chi circulates along a complex system of meridians or channels throughout the body. Other traditional Chinese therapies, such as acupuncture, access these meridians and attempt to improve the flow of chi. According to Stone (1994), the yin and yang are divided with the beginning motions of TCC, balanced during practice, and reunited at the finish. The emphasis on softness, continuity, and relaxation allows the chi to move freely along meridians. Postures and movements should be performed with the feeling of "swimming through very heavy air" (Stone, 1994 p. 31). The essential principles of movement for TCC are listed below (Stone, 1994):

1. Begin and maintain complete relaxation with natural breathing.
2. Stand with the tailbone pressed slightly forward and with the head and torso erect as if suspended from above by wire.
3. Shoulders are relaxed with slight drooping; fingers are spread apart and slightly cupped.

TABLE 4.1 Description of "around the platter," a Tai Chi form.

1. Hands are held at the chest, wrists slightly bent and elbows close to sides. Fingers are spread apart. Legs are slightly apart and bent with the right in front of the left. Weight is equally distributed between legs.
2. Begin to rock forward shifting weight to right leg with hands moving to the right. (Imagine a round platter at the chest, and the hands circling around the platter from right to left).
3. As most of the weight shifts to the right leg and the hands are directly in front of the body, the left heel comes off the ground. As the hands move left of midline the weight begins to shift back toward the left leg. When the hands have completed a full circle (held at the chest), most of the weight is on the left leg and the right toe is off the ground.
4. This movement can be repeated 6–9 times and then repeated again going from left to right.

Note. From *T'ai Chi Chih: Joy Through Movement,* by J. F. Stone, 1994, Fort Yates, Good Karma Publishing, Inc.

4. Concentration is on the soles of the feet or the t'an t'ien (area slightly below the umbilicus).
5. Knees are slightly bent with the weight being shifted from right to left and forward and back.

A description of how to perform the movement called "around the platter" is presented in Table 4.1. A full presentation of the 20 movements and practice tips can be found in TCC references.* Tai Chi Chih is best learned from a certified instructor in a group setting. Once the movements are learned, the form can be performed alone or in group. Loose-fitting clothes and soft shoes or bare feet are the preferred attire.

Unlike other styles of tai chi, the entire TCC routine does not have to be learned or mastered to begin benefiting from practice. Stone (1994) suggests learning five or six movements and practicing nine repetitions from both the right and left side in the morning and evening. This will provide approximately 25–30 minutes of exercise daily—which meets the current recommendations for physical activity (Pate et al., 1995). Stone (1994) also suggests choosing movements that circulate the most chi. Circulation of chi can be noted by the

---

*Persons may call or write Good Karma Publishing at P.O. Box 511, Yates, ND 58538 (701-854-7459).

amount of tingling felt in the fingers and hands. Movements that might target specific physical limitations have not been identified. Focusing on the physical movement externally and the flow of chi internally will allow for full integration of mind and body—revealing both the meditative/relaxational and physiological benefits.

Measurement of Effectiveness

The desired outcomes, determined by assessment of the patient, dictate the criteria to use in evaluating effectiveness of tai chi and other movement therapy techniques. Some of the outcomes used for older adults were described in previous sections. Many of the physiologic measures of balance, strength, and cardiorespiratory function are well established. Measurement of psychological variables, especially those related to relaxation and mood, while equally established, may not be adaptable to some methods of movement therapy. Tai chi, in particular, with Eastern philosophy origins embedded in its teaching and practice may prove elusive to current measurement methods. Few nursing conceptual frameworks based on energy or chi exist to be applied. More qualitative work is needed to identify the specific concepts surrounding the mystery of tai chi.

USES

The *University of California, Berkeley Health Letter* promoted five potential uses for tai chi: (a) strengthening and toning the muscles of the lower body, (b) improving balance, (c) relaxation/meditation, (d) improving flexibility and posture, (e) improving cardiorespiratory fitness (Meditation in motion, 1994). Tai chi has also been promoted as a safe alternative to traditional exercise therapy in patients with rheumatoid arthritis (Kirsteins, Dietz, & Hwang, 1991).

Most references to the use of tai chi as a therapeutic intervention are found in the geriatric, physical and occupational therapy, and exercise literature. The emphasis on older adults in research with tai chi is especially prudent given the projected growth of this population. The uses of tai chi related to balance, strength, relaxation, and fitness in elders will be discussed in this section. Nursing's ability to impact all age groups across a wide continuum of settings gives the profession ample opportunity to study and utilize tai chi as a therapeutic intervention.

Balance, muscular strength, and aerobic power are three components of physical fitness that are important for preservation of function (Blair & Garcia, 1996). Reductions in strength and balance
secondary to disuse and aging contribute to loss of independence
and falls in elders (Smith, Difabio, & Gilligan, 1990). Horak (1987)
noted that control of balance involves the complex organization of
many related senses by the central nervous system and the musculoskeletal system. A minor impairment in just one of the complex functions that affect balance can lead to poor balance, balance disorders,
and, ultimately, to falls (Tinetti, Speechley, & Ginter, 1988). Balance
training (Wolf et al., 1996) and strength training (Wolfson et al.,
1996) are important uses of tai chi for elders.

The exact mechanisms by which tai chi improves balance and
strength have not been investigated. Tse and Bailey's (1992) explanation of balance improvements have been discussed earlier. The slow,
graceful, and coordinated total body movements of tai chi performed
at a lowered center of gravity are thought to contribute to improvements in strength (Wolfson et al., 1996). Enough evidence exists to
recommend tai chi as a method to improve and maintain strength
and balance in elders.

Relaxation techniques (e.g., meditation, biofeedback, yoga, imaging, and exercise) have been used extensively for a wide variety of
physiological and psychological disorders, including hypertension,
chemical addictions, and depression. Minimal references were found
to the use of activities that combine exercise strategies with cognitive
strategies, or use interventions in which the combination is inherent.
Tai chi is an intervention that has both a cognitive and exercise
component.

Jin (1989) used both beginner and veteran tai chi practitioners
and found significantly lower levels of tension, anger, and depression
after 60 minutes of tai chi. In a second study, tai chi was found to be
as effective as brisk walking in reducing mood disturbances caused by
mental stress (Jin, 1992). Other authors, however, found no significant mood improvements with tai chi (Brown et al., 1995; Schaller,
1996). Both studies used healthy nonclinical populations that may
not be responsive to training and may not show changes with current
psychometric tools (Cramer, Nieman, & Lee, 1991). Blood pressure—
thought to be responsive to both exercise and meditation—did not
change significantly after 10 weeks of tai chi training (Schaller, 1996).
The mechanisms for cognitive changes are currently unknown. Approaching tai chi with a calm mind and relaxed body, and the slow
rhythmic moments may play a role (Stone, 1994).

The classification of tai chi as a moderate-intensity activity combined with its safety characteristics make it an ideal aerobic activity for older adults (Brown et al., 1995). Many activities that are designed to improve or maintain cardiorespiratory function or fitness are not well suited for older adults due to other physiological changes related to aging. Low-impact, low-velocity, moderate-intensity exercises with positive training effects are preferred and should be pursued (Blair & Garcia, 1996). Lai and colleagues (1995) used tai chi to examine long-term trends in cardiorespiratory function in older adults. They reported that regular practice of tai chi reduces the rate of decline in cardiorespiratory function.

Precautions

The initiation of a moderate-intensity exercise program does not require physician screening for most adults (American College of Sports Medicine [ACSM], 1991). However, those with chronic diseases or risk factors for chronic diseases should consult their health care provider before beginning an exercise program (ACSM, 1991). The presence of some conditions (e.g., diabetes, hypertension) or risk factors (e.g., smoking, obesity) may call for exercise testing prior to engaging in even moderate intensity exercise.

Nurses recommending tai chi classes to their clients should be aware of the particular styles taught in their area. Caution should be used when exaggerated benefits are claimed in advertisements. Scrutiny of the instructor's credentials and specifically looking for instructors who have obtained certification through a formal training program is recommended. Downs' (1992) summary of recommendations for choosing a tai chi class is cited in Table 4.2. It is vital to discover what tai chi style is being taught. Some forms are longer and contain more complex movements. Complex styles may have higher intensity levels and may be too difficult for some clients to learn. It is important for

TABLE 4.2   Tips for Choosing a Tai Chi Class

1. If possible find a studio or organization which specializes in tai chi.
2. Find an experienced teacher (6–10 years of experience) who demonstrates and verbally explains the movements. Ask to observe a class before joining.
3. Find a class with less than 20 students.
4. Avoid purchasing any special clothing or equipment.

Note. From "Tai chi," by L. B. Downs, 1992, *Modern Maturity, 35,* pp. 60–64.

nurses to match the activity closely with the client's ability level and goals.

RESEARCH QUESTIONS

Nurses can gain much information about the use of tai chi and other movement therapies from research in geriatrics, physical therapy, and occupational therapy. However, research on the use of movement therapies within the context of nursing is needed. Some questions for future research include:

1. What are the characteristics of persons who choose alternative activities like tai chi as opposed to the characteristics of those who choose more traditional activities? How do these characteristics affect outcomes?
2. While the majority of research on tai chi has focused on healthy community dwelling elders, would it be an appropriate intervention in those with some degree of functional limitation?
3. What role can tai chi play in rehabilitation? What specific conditions may benefit from a tai chi intervention?
4. What are the key concepts that must be developed to establish a conceptual framework for research related to tai chi?

REFERENCES

American College of Sports Medicine. (1991). *Guidelines for exercise testing and prescription* (4th ed.). Philadelphia: Lea & Febiger.

Berg, R. (1995, February). Cerebral fitness. *Working Woman,* pp. 45–50.

Blair, S. N., & Garcia, M. E. (1996). Get up and move: A call to action for older men and women. *Journal of the American Geriatrics Society, 44,* 599–600.

Brown, D., Mucci, W. G., Hetzler, R. K., & Knowlton, R. G. (1989). Cardiovascular and ventilatory responses during formalized t'ai chi chuan exercise. *Research Quarterly for Exercise and Sports, 60,* 246–250.

Brown, D. R., Wang, Y., Ward, A., Ebbeling, C. B., Fortlage, L., & Puleo, E. (1995). Chronic psychological effects of exercise and exercise plus cognitive strategies. *Medicine and Science in Sports and Exercise, 27,* 765–775.

Cramer, S. R., Nieman, D. C., & Lee, J. W. (1991). The effects of moderate exercise training on psychological well-being and mood state in women. *Journal of Psychosomatic Research, 35,* 437–449.

Downs, L. B. (1992). Tai chi. *Modern Maturity, 35(4),* 60–64.

Goldberg, W., & Fitzpatrick J. (1980). Movement therapy with the aged. *Nursing Research, 29,* 339–346.

Horak, F. B. (1987). Clinical measurement of postural control in adults. *Physical Therapy, 67,* 1881–1885.

Jin, P. (1989). Changes in heart rate, noradrenalin, cortisol, and mood during tai chi. *Journal of Psychosomatic Research, 33,* 197–206.

Jin, P. (1992). Efficacy of tai chi, brisk walking, meditation, and reading in reducing mental and emotional stress. *Journal of Psychosomatic Research, 36,* 361–370.

Kirsteins, A. B., Dietz, F., & Hwang, S. M. (1991). Evaluating the safety and potential use of a weight-bearing exercise, tai chi chuan, for rheumatoid arthritis patients. *American Journal of Physical Medicine and Rehabilitation, 70,* 136–141.

Lai, J. S., Lan, C., Wong, M. K., & Teng, S. H. (1995). Two-year trends in cardiorespiratory function among older tai chi chuan practitioners and sedentary subjects. *Journal of the American Geriatrics Society, 43,* 1222–1227.

Liao, W. (1990). *T'ai chi classics.* Boston: Shambhala.

Man-Ch'ing, C. (1981). *T'ai chi ch'uan: A simplified method of calisthenics for health and self defense.* Berkeley, CA: North Atlantic Books.

Man-Ch'ing, C., & Smith, R.W. (1983). *T'ai-chi: The "supreme ultimate" exercise for health, sport, and self defense.* Rutland, VT: Tuttle.

Meditation in motion: Tai chi and beyond. (1994, February). *University of California, Berkeley Wellness Letter, 10,* p. 7.

Pate, R. R., Pratt, M., Blair, S. N., Haskell, W. L., Macera, C. A., Bouchard, C. (1995). Physical activity and public health: A recommendation from the Centers for Disease Control and Prevention and the American College of Sports Medicine. *Journal of the American Medical Association, 273,* 357–436.

Schaller, K. J. (1996). Tai chi chih: An exercise option for older adults. *Journal of Gerontological Nursing, 22*(10), 12–17.

Schneider, D., & Leung, R. (1991). Metabolic and cardiorespiratory responses to the performance of wing chun and tai chi chuan exercises. *International Journal of Sports Medicine, 12,* 319–323.

Smith, E. L., DiFabio, R. P., & Gilligan, C. (1990). Exercise intervention and physiologic function in the elderly. *Topics in Geriatric Rehabilitation, 6,* 57–68.

Stone, J. F. (1994). *T'ai chi chih: Joy thru movement.* Fort Yates, ND: Good Karma.

Tinetti, M. E., Speechley, M., & Ginter, S. F. (1988). Risk factors among elderly persons living in the community. *New England Journal of Medicine, 19,* 1701–1707.

Tse, S. K., & Bailey, D. M. (1992). Tai chi and postural control in the well elderly. *American Journal of Occupational Therapy, 46,* 295–300.

Wanning, T. (1993). Healing and the mind/body arts: massage, acupuncture, yoga, t'ai chi, and feldenkrais. *American Association of Occupational Health Nurses Journal, 41,* 349–351.

Wolf, S. L., Barnhart, H. X., Kutner, N. G., McNeeley, E., Coogler, C., Tingsen, X. (1996). Reducing frailty and falls in older persons: An investigation of tai chi and computerized balance training. *Journal of the American Geriatrics Society, 44,* 489–497.

Wolfson, L., Whipple, R., Derby, Judge, J., King, M., Amerman, P. (1996). Balance and strength training in older adults: Intervention gains and tai chi maintenance. *Journal of the American Geriatrics Society, 44,* 498–506.

5

THERAPEUTIC TOUCH

Ellen C. Egan

Touch has been used throughout the history of nursing to convey compassion, provide comfort, and ease pain. Touch is associated with so many basic nursing skills that Krieger (1975) calls touch the "imprimatur of nursing" (p. 74).

There are many definitions of touch in the nursing literature: a form of nonverbal communication (Barnett, 1972; McCorkle, 1974), an interaction (Weiss, 1979), an experience (Ujhely, 1979), and an encounter (Ujhely, 1979). And, of course, there are many uses of touch that are associated with nursing assessment and intervention techniques. From a review of research literature that excluded therapeutic touch, Weiss (1988) concluded that touch does not have a universal meaning, rather the meaning of touch may be context-dependent and person-specific. However, therapeutic touch, the use of touch with the intention to transfer energy to another, is a specific nursing intervention. It can be differentiated from other types of touch by the intention of the action or purpose for which it is used.

DEFINITION

Therapeutic touch (TT) is a process by which energy is transmitted from one person to another for the purpose of potentiating the healing process of one who is ill or injured. Krieger (1979) calls TT a healing meditation in that the primary act of the intervener is to "center" oneself and to maintain that center throughout the process. TT consists of four phases: (a) centering oneself, (b) assessing the client's energy field for differences in the quality of energy flow, (c) mobilizing areas in the client's energy field that are perceived as not flowing, and (d) directing energy through the hands to the client (Krieger, 1979, 1993).

Dolores Krieger (who coined the term *therapeutic touch*) and Dora Kunz began to teach the process to nurses in the early 1970s. Like many other nursing interventions, TT was practiced for some years before many research studies were conducted to measure its effects. Unlike most other nursing interventions, TT has attracted skepticism.

Wilson (1995) stated that TT is considered a controversial modality and presented a summary of criticisms. Critics have claimed that TT relies upon the untested axioms of energy field theory to explain its effects. They point out that some practitioners use TT discreetly (others openly) and use the term *touch* although physical touch is not a nec-essary component. The paucity of research supporting TT's claims of therapeutic value, as well as allegations concering the quality of some studies and the presence of inconsistent findings have all raised ob-jections. Finally, there is a debate regarding the appropriateness of the practice of therapeutic touch by Christian nurses.

The use of touch, or the therapeutic use of hands, has a long history. There are repeated references to it in Eastern, European, and religious literature (Krieger, 1979; Zefron, 1975). In these references the laying on of hands is thought to be used for healing or actually curing disease. Current TT, however, is different in that it is not done within a religious context, it does not bring about cures, and it does not require physical touch. Furthermore, unlike faith healing, the client does not need to have faith in TT for it to be effective.

SCIENTIFIC BASIS

The first basic assumption regarding TT is that a human being is an energy field which is in mutual simultaneous interaction with the environmental field that surrounds the body and that energy can be channelled intentionally from one person to another (Boguslawski, 1979, 1980; Krieger, 1993). It is also assumed that a human being is bilaterally symmetrical, that illness is an imbalance in an individual's energy field, and that human beings have natural abilities to trans-form and transcend their conditions of living (Krieger, 1993). Energy pattern imbalances are noted during assessment and are character-ized as blocks, congestion, or asymmetrical densities. The purpose of

TT, then, is to restore order and harmony of the energy pattern by intentional and specific interaction between the healer's energy field and the energy field of the client.

Two principles that accompany the process of TT are compassion and intentionality. Compassion is described as pure caring such that the person wants to help, but is without expectations for the outcome. Intentionality is the intent to help or heal and is the conscious direction of the energy to the patient with a deficit of energy. Compassion serves as the catalyst for the energy exchange process and intentionality serves as the means of transmitting energy (Fanslow, 1983).

Therapeutic touch has also been viewed as change which occurs in the human-environmental energy field patterning as the nurse assumes a meditative state of awareness, recognizes his or her own unitary nature and integrality with the environmental field, and focuses intent to help the patient (Meehan, 1990, 1993). This is based on Rogers' science of unitary human beings (Rogers, 1990).

Therapeutic touch has been described as a process of creating healing environments. The healing environment facilitates the person's response in the direction of healing and wholeness; the person doing TT creates the healing environment. One's consciousness is not separate and apart but integral with all consciousness. Through the intentional use of consciousness one can knowingly participate in this interconnectedness toward repatterning and healing for oneself and for others. There is a shift in the consciousness of the practitioner (centering) through which there can also be a shift in consciousness of the recipient (Quinn, 1992). Quinn's assumptions incorporate theoretical perspectives from Rogers' science of unitary human beings (Rogers, 1990) and Newman's (1994) theory of health as expanded consciousness.

Although there are differing views, it is assumed that energy is transmitted during the TT process. However, it is not clear how the energy compensates for an energy deficit and balances the energy patterns of the recipient or how recipients utilize the energy to enhance their self-healing processes.

There are probably more published descriptions and studies of TT than any other nursing intervention. The Nurse Healers-Professional Associates Cooperative 1995 Therapeutic Touch Bibliography includes over 200 citations of books, journal articles, and dissertation/thesis abstracts. At least 50 of these citations refer to different research studies. Selected research studies are reported below.

Krieger (1975) began the systematic study of the effects of TT on human subjects in the early 1970s. (Studies of the effect of TT on plants and animals occurred earlier.) She selected changes in hemoglobin level as a measurement of the effect of TT based on an assumed relationship between *prana,* an energy, and hemoglobin. In each of three studies, Krieger was able to demonstrate that the level of hemoglobin increased significantly in groups who were treated with TT.

Several researchers have studied the effects of TT in reducing anxiety or stress. It has been demonstrated that subjects who received physical contact TT (Heidt, 1981) and noncontact TT (Quinn, 1984) experienced a significantly greater decrease in state anxiety than control groups. The state anxiety level of institutionalized elderly subjects who received TT in the form of a back rub was found to be significantly lower than subjects who received a routine back rub without TT, but not lower than subjects who received a back rub from a nurse who purposefully blocked the TT exchange (Simington & Laing, 1993). Also the self-reported anxiety of inpatient psychiatric subjects was significantly lowered by TT (Gagne & Toye, 1994).

In a study of stress reduction of subjects who experienced a natural disaster, TT significantly lowered perceived stress (state anxiety). It was also found that the decrease in state anxiety was significantly correlated with the length of the TT session (Olson, Sneed, Bonadonna, Ratliff, & Dias, 1992). In another study, there was a greater (although not statistically significant) reduction of anxiety in a high-anxiety group than in a low- to moderate-anxiety group of healthy professional caregivers/students following TT (Olson & Sneed, 1995). The authors indicated that the number of subjects in each group was too small to demonstrate significance. (In this study TT was administered prior to the occurrence of a stressor—note the similarity to the results of the Randolph study reported below.)

In the following studies infants and children served as subjects. Stress behavior and transcutaneous oxygen pressure were used to measure stress associated with measuring infants' vital signs. Therapeutic touch was effective in reducing the behavioral stress of infants, but not physiological stress. An increase in stress with mock TT was an unexpected finding (Fedoruk, 1984). Kramer (1990) found a significantly greater reduction of stress (using relaxation scores based on measurements of pulse, skin temperature and galvanic skin response) of hospitalized children following TT than with casual touch. Therapeutic touch decreased the time needed to calm the children after a stressful experience.

In subjects experiencing anticipatory nausea and vomiting during chemotherapy, TT significantly improved positive affect and decreased symptom severity after chemotherapy, reduced symptom distress and severity before and after chemotherapy, and decreased disruption in normal activities (Sodergren, 1994). Using TT significantly increased relaxation, as measured by observations of relaxation behaviors and pulse rate, in persons with dementia who exhibited agitation behaviors. However, no decrease in agitation behaviors was produced (Snyder, Egan, & Burns, 1995).

The effect of TT in the alleviation of pain has also been investigated. In a study of the effect of TT on tension headache, a significantly greater reduction of pain was found in the TT group immediately following the treatment and 4 hours later (Keller & Bzdek, 1986). In another pain study, Meehan (1993) investigated the effect of TT on acute pain in postoperative patients using TT, a mimicked TT treatment, or the standard treatment (narcotic analgesic injection). There was a difference between the TT and mimicked TT groups, but these differences were not significant. The standard treatment was significantly more effective than TT. However, subjects who received TT waited a significantly longer time before requesting further analgesic medication as compared to those who received mimic TT.

Wirth (1990) and Wirth, Richardson, Eidelman, and O'Malley (1993) examined the effect of TT or no treatment on the rate of healing of full thickness dermal wounds (incisions made for the purpose of the study). There were significant reductions in wound size on days 8 and 16 following the incision in the first study and on days 5 and 10 in the replication study in the TT groups. These studies were carefully designed to control for the placebo effect.

No significant results were found in the following studies of the effects of TT on anxiety levels among hospitalized adults. In a study of elderly patients, no differences were found between a TT group and two mimic TT groups. Interestingly, all three groups had a slight increase in anxiety at the posttest measurement time (Parkes, 1985). In Hale's (1986) study no significant differences were found for any of the dependent variables of state anxiety, systolic and diastolic blood pressure, and pulse rate. Quinn (1989) found no significant differences in state anxiety, blood pressure and heart rate between the TT group and the control groups.

Randolph (1984) studied whether TT produces a relaxation response such that subjects would be less responsive to stressful stimuli. Experimental and control groups observed a film which served as a stressful stimulus. The experimental group received TT during the film and the control group subjects were touched in a similar manner without TT. No differences in skin conductance, electromyogram, or skin temperature were found between the two groups.

Quinn (1988) summarized eight research studies conducted to demonstrate the effects of TT on such variables as hemoglobin, anxiety, physiologic response to stressful stimuli, response to stress, postoperative pain, and tension headache pain. Subjects included hospitalized adults, neonates, cardiovascular patients, college students, postoperative adult patients, gerontological hospitalized patients and adults. The findings from these studies did not consistently support the effectiveness of TT in reducing anxiety and relieving pain.

Quinn provided an analysis and possible explanations for the inconsistent findings. Some of the explanations are summarized as follows:

1. Substantial deviations exist in the administration of TT and the lack of expertise of practitioners.
2. Research protocols have utilized only a 5-minute TT treatment, while clinical practitioners typically administer TT treatments of 15 minutes or longer.
3. The stress response would be considered a natural phenomenon and a protection from external threat; therefore, it is questionable that TT should cause the relaxation response in such a situation.
4. Very conservative tests of statistical significance and small samples had been used, so differences very close to being significant are not considered significant.

From a review of the TT research it can be concluded that the effectiveness of TT has been demonstrated, but there have been some inconsistent results. Quinn's critique (1988) as well as the thoughtful analyses of other investigators can be used to design studies that will facilitate the development of knowledge regarding the phenomenon of TT.

INTERVENTION

Technique

The process of TT consists of four steps: centering, assessment, unruffling, and transferring energy.

Centering. The first step of the process is centering. Centering is considered a meditative state in which one quiets oneself and directs attention inward. There are many ways of centering, but one of the simplest methods is to assume a comfortable sitting position, relax tension areas of the body, inhale deeply, exhale slowly, and mentally count "one" with each exhalation. Very quickly there is an experience of quiet, relaxation, and unity. Centering is maintained throughout the TT process and facilitates the remaining steps of the process with control and the ability to direct energies and attention. There is a sense of detachment that enhances sensitivity, while there is less personal involvement in the outcomes of therapy.

Assessment. After the therapist is centered the assessment process is begun. The purpose of the assessment process is to find differences in the quality of the energy flow of the client. Differences in the energy flow are detected by sensing heat, cold, tingling, congestion, pressure, emptiness, or other sensations. These sensations usually are asymmetrical, present on one side of the body but not on the other. Assessment is a scanning process. Both hands are used to establish a field and the palms are held 2 to 4 inches from the skin surface of the client. The scanning is started with assessment of the head and slowly progresses down the entire front and back of the client.

The practitioner makes mental notes of the sensations that are perceived during the scanning process. From the information obtained during assessment the practitioner identifies areas where the quality of the energy flow is different. If an area is sensed to be hot there can be an inflammatory process, pain, injury, or other pathological problem present in the underlying area. An area of coldness indicates a block in the flow of energy to the area. If the sensations are of emptiness this usually indicates a general lack of energy. Congestion or heavy areas indicate a situation of uneven or poor energy flow. Most clients will tell the practitioner what is troubling them, and this information can also be used in determining the nature of the treatment. The information from the assessment is synthesized and used to determine where, how, and what kind of energy will be directed to the client. Thus, the intervention plan is developed.

Unruffling the Field. Krieger (1979) equates the sensation of a congested energy field with the word *ruffled*. The sensation is one of pressure and overlapping layers of densities, like ruffles. When this is encountered, *unruffling* can be used to mobilize the flow of energy in these areas. The unruffling process is accomplished by moving the hands (palms facing the client) from the area where pressure was felt in a sweeping-away motion from the center to the periphery. This sweeping motion of the hands is continued down the body following the long bones.

The unruffled field, or mobile field, seems to enhance the transfer of energy from the practitioner and the client's field seems to be more receptive of energy. Wyatt and Dimmer (1988, p. 42) describe "balancing" (shifting energy from areas of congestion to areas of deficit) in order to smooth out the entire energy field after depleted areas of the field have been energized.

Transferring Energy.   The actual transferring of energy is brought about by the intention of doing so. In other words, by intending to transfer energy, energy will be transferred from the practitioner through the hands to the client. This seems the simplest part of the intervention and can be accomplished by most people who engage in the process. It does, however, necessitate having the genuine intention to help another. The complex part of the process is to know the form of energy to use, how to modulate energy, and where to apply the energy.

The form of energy is related to colors. Blue energy is a sedating kind of energy, yellow energy is stimulating and energizing, while green is harmonizing. Because of the different effects of the forms of energy, different forms are used for different conditions of the client. Blue energy is used to calm, relieve pain, and to reduce edema. Yellow energy is used to restore energy for someone fatigued or depleted of energy. Green energy is used to restore the harmony of the person. Energy forms can be modulated through visualization of the colors of the energy. For example, the practitioner would visualize or imagine light streaming through a blue stained glass window when wishing to transfer blue energy.

Where to apply energy is dependent upon the assessment. In some instances the energy is applied directly to a particular area—for example, an area where the client has pain. In some instances, such as when the client is fatigued, the energy is applied to one of the *chakras* located in the thoracic or solar plexus areas. (Chakras are special channels, or centers, within the energy field that serve as entry areas for energy from the environment.) Energy may also be applied in minimal amounts by keeping the hands in motion over particular areas or over the entire body using a motion similar to the sweeping motion of unruffling. Only minimal amounts of energy are appropriately used in the area of the head or with infants.

Usually it is desirable for the flow of energy through the extremities to be enhanced and for energy to be distributed. This has been called *grounding*, in that the energy flows through the extremities, hands or feet while the practitioner serves as a grounding rod. The flow of energy through an arm can be accomplished by placing one hand between the shoulder blades and the other hand palm to palm with the client. When the flow of energy is established the energy can be felt in the receiving palm. To facilitate the flow of energy, the hand that was placed on the palm of the client can be cupped and moved down the arm in the manner of pushing a pressure ridge down the arm and out of the hand. Energy can be distributed by using a sweeping motion of the hands from a particular area to surrounding areas. The unruffling motion can be used to distribute energy over the entire body.

Clients tend to draw energy. They will usually experience heat or warmth in the area where the energy is directed. A relaxation response exhibited by deeper breathing and a flushed appearance usually results. The treatment is stopped when the practitioner senses a cessation or decrease of sensations, a feeling of rebound of energy from the client, or cessation of reception by the client. The practitioner will also stop the treatment when it is thought enough energy has been given for a treatment.

Guidelines for the administration of TT are found in Table 5.1.

TABLE 5.1 Therapeutic Touch Guidelines

1. Have the client comfortably seated sideways on an armless chair or lying in bed. The client's arms and legs should be uncrossed with shoes removed, if treatment involves the feet.
2. Centering is achieved by the practitioner and maintained throughout the TT process.
3. Assessment is done using both hands to establish a field with the palms held 2 to 4 inches from the skin surface of the client. The assessment starts at the head and slowly progresses down the entire front and back of the client. Mental notes of the sensations perceived during assessment are used to establish the treatment plan.
4. Unruffling is done by moving the hands (palms facing the client) in a sweeping-away motion from the center to the periphery. This sweeping motion of the hands is continued down the body. Unruffled, the field enhances the transfer of energy.
5. Energy is transferred from the practitioner through the hands to the client. The form of energy to use, how to modulate energy, and where to apply the energy is based on the assessment. Unruffling is used at the end of the process to smooth the energy field.
6. Have the client rest for 5 to 10 minutes following the treatment.

USES

Therapeutic touch is used to help restore the balance of the energy field and to provide additional energy to be used in the recuperative and self-healing process of the client. Three notable consequences of TT are a generalized relaxation response, relief of pain, and accelerated healing. Research studies that measured the effectiveness of TT on these outcomes were described earlier.

Anecdotal reports of the use of TT have been described for various populations and conditions. For example, TT has been used in the practice of midwifery to alleviate the painful sensations of labor contractions, enhance relaxation, stimulate the baby immediately following birth and help stimulate contractions to facilitate the delivery of the placenta (Wolfson, 1984). Leduc (1987) used TT to calm fussy babies, improve respiratory distress and provide energy to babies.

Other populations that have benefitted from TT are the elderly, dying patients and rehabilitation patients. Therapeutic touch has been used to improve ambulation and mobility; to decrease pain, inflammation, and joint swelling, and spasticity. It has been used to elicit a sense of peace and calm in dying patients (Fanslow, 1984). With rehabilitation patients, TT has been used to improve speech in aphasic clients and to facilitate sleep and verbalization of feelings regarding the disability (Payne, 1989). TT has also been used to alleviate symptoms such as dyspnea, coughing, hiccups, diarrhea, cramping abdominal pain, constipation, fever, pain, and anxiety associated with AIDS (Newshan, 1989).

Measurement of Outcomes

Among the notable outcomes of TT are a relaxation response, relief of pain, and accelerated healing. A summary of the many different means used to measure these outcomes follows.

- Self-report measures of state anxiety include Spielberger's State/ Trait Anxiety Inventory (Gagne & Toye, 1994; Heidt, 1981; Olson & Sneed, 1995; Quinn, 1984, 1989; Simington & Laing, 1993), Profile of Mood States (Olson & Sneed, 1995), and visual analogue scales (Olson & Sneed, 1995).
- Measures that have been used to assess the physiological parameters of anxiety have included blood pressure (Quinn, 1989) and heart rate (Quinn, 1989).

- Measurement of the relaxation response have included skin conductance, muscle tension (electromyographic response), peripheral skin temperature (Olson et al., 1992; Randolph, 1984), blood pressure (Olson et al., 1992), heart rate (Olson et al., 1992; Snyder et al., 1995) and respiratory rate (Olson et al., 1992).
- Relaxation behaviors have been measured using a modified Luiselli Relaxation Checklist (Snyder et al., 1995).
- Visual analogue scales also have been used to measure psychological parameters of the perceived stress (Olson et al., 1992). Stress reduction has also been measured by pulse, peripheral skin temperature and galvanic skin response observations (Kramer, 1990).
- Relief of pain has been measured using Pain Visual Analogue Scales (Meehan, 1993) and the McGill-Melzack Pain Questionnaire (Keller & Bzdek, 1986).
- Accelerated healing (rate of re-epithelialization) has been measured by direct observation of wounds and the assessment of photographs of wounds (Wirth et al., 1993) and Direct Tracing of the wound (Wirth, 1990).

PRECAUTIONS IN USE

As a general rule the client will take the amount of energy that is needed and then will stop drawing from the energy source, however, in some instances precautions must be taken. Infants and children are very sensitive to treatments. Energy should be given slowly and gently in small amounts by an experienced practitioner (Boguslawski, 1979). Aged, extremely ill, or dying individuals may require modifications in treatment or gentle energy input. The head is also very sensitive and only cooling, sweeping motions are used in the head area. Patients with cancer are treated in such a way that energy is not concentrated in a particular area.

A final precaution is directed to the learner of TT. Although it is possible to learn to transfer energy in a short period of time, knowing when and how to use therapeutic touch requires mentorship and practice. TT is learned through an apprenticeship. In this learning process with a mentor, it may take one to two years to perfect a knowledgeable practice.

FURTHER RESEARCH

A few suggestions for research endeavors include:

1. empirical validation of the energy exchange process
2. determination of appropriate protocols for the administration of TT with varying conditions amenable to TT
3. differentiation of the placebo effect and therapeutic effect of TT
4. examination of the longitudinal effects of therapeutic touch
5. continued validation of the pain relief and accelerated healing effects of TT

REFERENCES

Barnett, K. (1972). A theoretical construct of the concepts of touch as they relate to nursing. *Nursing Research, 21,* 102–103.

Boguslawski, M. (1979). The use of therapeutic touch in nursing. *The Journal of Continuing Education in Nursing, 10*(4), 9–15.

Boguslawski, M. (1980). Therapeutic touch: A facilitator of pain relief. *Topics in Clinical Nursing, 2*(1), 27–37.

Fanslow, C. A. (1983). Therapeutic touch: A healing modality throughout life. *Topics in Clinical Nursing, 5*(2), 72–79.

Fanslow, C. A. (1984). Touch and the elderly. In C. C. Brown (Ed.), *The many facets of touch* (pp. 183–189). Skillman, NJ: Johnson & Johnson.

Fedoruk, R. B. (1984). Transfer of the relaxation response: Therapeutic touch as a method for reduction of stress in premature neonates. *Dissertation Abstracts International, 46,* 978B. (University Microfilms No. ADG85–09162)

Gagne, D., & Toye, R. C. (1994). The effects of therapeutic touch and relaxation therapy in reducing anxiety. *Archives of Psychiatric Nursing, 8,* 184–189.

Hale, E. H. (1986). A study of the relationship between therapeutic touch and the anxiety levels of hospitalized adults. *Dissertation Abstracts International, 47,* 1928B. (University Microfilms No. ADG86–18897)

Heidt, P. (1981). Effect of therapeutic touch on anxiety level of hospitalized patients. *Nursing Research, 30,* 32–37.

Keller, E., & Bzdek, V. (1986). Effects of therapeutic touch on tension headache pain. *Nursing Research , 35,* 101–106.

Kramer, N. A. (1990). Comparison of therapeutic touch and casual touch in stress reduction of hospitalized children. *Pediatric Nursing, 16,* 483–485.

Krieger, D. (1975). Therapeutic touch: The imprimatur of nursing. *American Journal of Nursing, 75,* 784–787.

Krieger, D. (1979). *The therapeutic touch: How to use your hands to help or heal.* Englewood Cliffs, NJ: Prentice-Hall.

Krieger, D. (1993). *Accepting your power to heal: The personal practice of therapeutic touch.* Santa Fe: Bear.

Leduc, E. (1987). Letter to the editor. *Neonatal network, 5*(6), 46–47.

McCorkle, R. (1974). Effects of touch on seriously ill patients. *Nursing Research, 23,* 125–132.

Meehan, T. C. (1990). The science of unitary human beings and theory-based practice: Therapeutic touch. In E. A. M. Barrett (Ed.), *Vision of Rogers' science-based nursing* (pp. 67–81). New York: National League for Nursing.

Meehan, T. C. (1993). Therapeutic touch and postoperative pain: A Rogerian research study. *Nursing Science Quarterly, 6*(2), 69–77.

Newman, M. A. (1994). *Health as expanding consciousness.* New York: National League for Nursing Press.

Newshan, M. A. (1989). Therapeutic touch for symptom control in persons with AIDS. *Holistic Nursing Practice, 3*(4), 45–51.

Olson, M., & Sneed, N. (1995). Anxiety and therapeutic touch. *Issues in Mental Health Nursing, 16,* 97–108.

Olson, M., Sneed, N., Bonadonna, R., Ratliff, J. & Dias, J. (1992). Therapeutic touch and post–Hurricane Hugo stress. *Journal of Holistic Nursing, 10,* 1120–1136.

Parkes, B. S. (1985). Therapeutic touch as an intervention to reduce anxiety in elderly hospitalized patients. *Dissertation Abstracts International, 47,* 573B. (University Microfilms No. 8609563)

Payne, M. B. (1989). The use of therapeutic touch with rehabilitation clients. *Rehabilitation Nursing, 14,* 69–72.

Quinn, J. F. (1984). Therapeutic touch as energy exchange: Testing the theory. *Advances in Nursing Science, 6*(2), 42–49.

Quinn, J. F. (1988). Building a body of knowledge: Research on therapeutic touch 1974–1986. *Journal of Holistic Nursing, 6*(1), 37–45.

Quinn, J. F. (1989). Therapeutic touch as energy exchange: Replication and extension. *Nursing Science Quarterly, 2*(2), 79–87.

Quinn, J. F. (1992). Holding sacred space: The nurse as healing environment. *Holistic Nursing Practice, 6*(4), 26–36.

Randolph, G. L. (1984). Therapeutic and physical touch: Physiological response to stressful stimuli. *Nursing Research, 33,* 33–36.

Rogers, M. E. (1990). Nursing: Science of unitary, irreducible, human beings: Update 1990. In E. A. M. Barrett (Ed.), *Vision of Rogers' science-based nursing* (pp. 5–11). New York: National League for Nursing.

Simington, J. A., & Laing, G. P. (1993). Effects of therapeutic touch on anxiety in the institutionalized elderly. *Clinical Nursing Research, 2,* 438–450.

Snyder, M., Egan, E. C., & Burns, K. R. (1995). Interventions for decreasing agitation behaviors in persons with dementia. *Journal of Gerontological Nursing, 21*(7), 34–40.

Sodergren, K. A. (1994). The effect of absorption and social closeness on responses to educational and relaxation therapies in patients with anticipatory nausea and vomiting during cancer chemotherapy. *Dissertation Abstracts International, 54*(12), 6137B. (University Microfilms No. 9413052)

Ujhely, G. B. (1979). Touch: Reflections and perceptions. *Nursing Forum, 18,* 18–33.

Weiss, S. J. (1979). The language of touch. *Nursing Research, 28,* 76–80.

Weiss, S. J. (1988). Touch. In J. J. Fitzpatrick, R. L. Taunton, & J. Q. Benoliel (Eds.), *Annual review of nursing research* (Vol. 6, pp. 3–27). New York: Springer.

Wilson, D. F. (1995). Therapeutic touch: Foundations and current knowledge. *Alternative Health Practitioner, 1,* 55–66.

Wirth, D. P. (1990). The effect of non-contact therapeutic touch on the healing rate of full thickness dermal wounds. *Subtle Energies, 1,* 1–20.

Wirth, D. P., Richardson, J. T., Eidelman, W. S., & O'Malley, A. C. (1993). Full thickness dermal wounds treated with non-contact therapeutic touch: a replication and extension. *Complementary Therapies in Medicine, 1,* 127–132.

Wolfson, I. S. (1984). Therapeutic touch and midwifery. In C. C. Brown (Ed.), *The many facets of touch* (pp. 166–172). Skillman, NJ: Johnson & Johnson.

Wyatt, G., & Dimmer, S. (1988). The balancing touch. *Nursing Times, 84*(21), 40–42.

Zefron, L. J. (1975). The history of the laying-on of hands in nursing. *Nursing Forum, 14,* 350–363.

6

MASSAGE

Mariah Snyder and WenYun Cheng

According to Ellis, Hill, and Campbell (1995), Hippocrates developed his "wheel of health essentials" in the fifth century B.C. and identified rubbing or massage as his favorite wheel spoke. Massage has been part of nursing's armamentarium for centuries. Back rubs were one of the first skills the authors learned as nursing students. Although little scientific evidence existed to support administering the back rub 3 times a day, we noted that patients seemed more comfortable and relaxed and slept better. Current nursing practice, however, rarely includes back rubs as a routine part of care. Reasons for the decreased use are not clear. It is ironic that at a time when the public is seeking out masseurs, nursing is relinquishing one of its traditional interventions. Few nurses have or are conducting research on massage and its impact on achieving positive patient outcomes (Dunn, Sleep, & Collett, 1995).

DEFINITION

Massage involves the manipulation of soft tissues for therapeutic purposes (Barr & Taslitz, 1970). Dunn et al. (1995) defined massage as the application of various systematic and usually rhythmic hand movements performed on the soft tissues of the body. These movements produce different effects depending on a number of factors, such as the type and speed of movements; the pressure exerted by the hands, fingers, or thumbs; and the area of the body treated.

A number of different types of massage exist: Swedish (a more vigorous massage with long, flowing strokes), Esalen (a meditative massage with a light touch, and a highly variable style), deep tissue or neuromuscular (an intense kneading of the body), sports massage (a vigorous massage to loosen and ease sore muscles), Shiatsu (a Japanese pressure-point technique to relieve stress), and reflexology (a deep foot massage stimulating all parts of the body). The varying types of massage incorporate different strokes and procedures. Commonly used techiques include effleurage (stroking), friction, pressure, petrissage (kneading), vibration, and percussion. In addition to their presence in multiple types of massage, these techniques have been applied to the entire body or to specific areas of the body such as the back, feet, or hands (Cochrane, 1993).

SCIENTIFIC BASIS

Massage has been identified as one of the interventions that promotes mind-body connection (Wells-Federman et al., 1995). Thus, it fits with nursing's holistic approach to health care.

Massage produces therapeutic effects on multiple body systems: integumentary, musculoskeletal, cardiovascular, lymphatic, and nervous. Manipulating the skin and underlying muscle makes the skin more supple. The addition of essential oils to massage contributes to improvement in skin function. Massage increases or enhances movement in the musculoskeletal system by reducing swelling, loosening and stretching contracted tendons, and aiding in the reduction of soft tissues adhesions. Friction to the skin and underlying tissues releases histamines which, in turn, produces vasodilation of vessels and enhances venous return. Use of massage improves the flow of lymph (Simpson, 1991); the improvement may be as high as 25% (Wakim, 1985).

Variable results have been found from the use of massage, particularly back massage (Corley, Ferriter, Zeh, & Gifford, 1995; Fraser & Kerr, 1993; Meek, 1993). In some instances, arousal rather than a relaxation response has occurred. Barr and Taslitz (1970) found that sympathetic arousal occurred during massage, but not during the control period, when back massage was administered to 10 female subjects. Reed and Held (1988) used sequential connective tissue massage (CTM) and suggested that CTM had no consistent immediate or long-term effects on the autonomic nervous system in healthy middle-aged and elderly subjects. When using a 6-minute back massage, Longworth (1982) found that the heart and electromyogram readings of female subjects increased from those present during the baseline period. However, the systolic and diastolic blood pressure readings decreased. Likewise, subjects' scores on an anxiety instrument indicated that they felt relaxed following the back massage. Others (Ferrell-Torry & Glick, 1993; Fraser & Kerr, 1993; Meek, 1993; Snyder, Egan, & Burns, 1995b) found that massage resulted in a decrease in physiological parameters (systolic and diastolic blood pressure, heart rate, and skin temperature), indicative of the relaxation response, in cancer patients, institutionalized elders, hospice clients, or dementia subjects.

To establish the safety of using back massage with patients who were critically ill, Tyler, Winslow, Clark, and White (1990) administered a 1-minute back rub. Findings included increases in the heart rate and decreases in the SVO_2; these gradually returned to the baseline by minute 4. However, the investigators noted that although these changes were statistically significant, the changes were not clinically significant, as the heart rate only increased by 4 beats per minute.

The results from the studies on use of massage do not provide conclusive physiological evidence to support that it produces relaxation. One factor that may contribute to the heart rate and other increases found is the short time massage was administered. Some authors suggest that massage may initially cause stimulation of the sympathetic nervous system before the relaxation response occurs (Ferrell-Torry & Glick, 1993; Tyler et al., 1990; Weiss, 1986). However, in the majority of studies reviewed, subjective indexes for relaxation (anxiety inventories and self-reports) suggested that subjects felt relaxed after the massage intervention.

Longworth (1982) suggested that the relaxation response occurs through the habituation to tactile stimuli and the inhibition of the muscle spindle by the passive stretch on the tendinous insertion of the muscles. Habituation occurs as the result of repetitive, monotonous stimuli. After a period of time has transpired the frontal lobe no longer perceives the stimuli originating from the muscles as being threatening and arousal disappears. Stretching the tendon insertions temporarily relaxes the muscle. Although support exists for administering massage for a period of time, the exact length has not been determined.

The impact of massage on the psychoneuroimmunological functions of the body are beginning to be explored. Groer and colleagues (1994) reported that administration of a 10–minute back massage stimulated the production of antibodies (salivary secretory immunoglobulin A, s-IgA). Anecdotal reports have suggested that massage has produced positive results in persons with AIDS. Further research is needed to explore the possible holistic results occurring from administration of massage.

INTERVENTION

As noted earlier, many types of massage exist, applicable to the entire body or to specific body areas. Back massage has been traditionally been a part of nursing interventions. Application of massage to either the hands or the feet is becoming more common in nursing. The techniques for massage of these two areas will be presented in this section.

The environment in which massage is administered and the oils used for massage add to the therapeutic effects produced. Room temperature is very important; the room must be warm enough so that the person is comfortable. Shivering would negate the effects of the massage. In addition, privacy needs to be ensured.

Adding aromatherapy and music to massage sessions may enhance the effectiveness of the massage intervention (Dunn et al., 1995). Chapter 11 details aromatherapy and the intervention of music is described in chapter 21.

Massage Strokes

Effleurage is slow, rhythmic stroking made with light skin contact. Effleurage may be applied with varying degrees of pressure depending on the part of the body and the outcome desired. The palmar surface of the hands is used for larger surfaces with the thumbs and fingers used for smaller areas. On large surfaces, long, gliding strokes about 10–20 inches in length are applied.

In *friction* movements, moderate, constant pressure to one area is made with the thumbs or fingers. The fingers may be held in one place or moved in a small circumscribed area. The *pressure stroke* is similar to the friction stroke; however, pressure strokes are made with the hands.

Petrissage, or kneading, involves lifting a large fold of skin and the underlying muscle and holding the tissue between the thumb and fingers. The tissues are pushed against the bone, then raised and squeezed in circular movements. Grasp of the tissues is alternately loosened and tightened. Tissues are supported by one hand while kneading is done with the other hand. Variations of kneading include pinching, rolling, wringing, and kneading with fists or fingers. Petrissage is limited to tissues having a significant muscle mass.

Vibration strokes can be administered with either the entire hand or with the fingers. Rapid, continuous strokes are used. Because administering vibration strokes requires much energy, mechanical vibrators are often used.

For *percussion* strokes, the wrist acts as a fulcrum for the hand with the hand hitting the tissue. Strokes are made with a rapid tempo over a large body area. Tapping and clapping are variants of percussion strokes.

Foot Massage

According to Joachim (1983), foot massage is an important, but neglected, nursing intervention. Conley (1996) used foot massage with elders with dementia to produce relaxation and promote comfort. To receive foot massage, the patient may be either recumbent or sitting in a chair. The entire foot and ankle areas are rubbed with oil. While holding the foot firmly, the nurse makes circular strokes around the ankle area and over the entire ventral area of the foot. A finger is used to trace a space between the tendons on the foot, starting at the toes and moving toward the ankle. A tapping, squeezing movement is used to massage the four sides of each toe. At the conclusion of massaging the individual toe, the tip of the toe is squeezed. A fist is used to make circular movements on the sole of the foot. Many patients enjoy the effects of a pounding motion made with the wrist on the sole proceeding from the toes to the ankle. The sides of the foot are massaged by moving the tissue between the index and third fingers. Firm, sweeping motions over the top and bottom of the foot are used to conclude the massage of the first foot before moving to the second foot.

The foot massage may be combined with foot care. Soaking the feet in a basin of water before massaging is found to be enjoyable. Using heated towels and covering the massaged foot with a warm towel is also pleasurable. It is important to use firm strokes when massaging the feet as light strokes may produce tickling. The nurse needs to be alert to the facial expressions of the patient, as some areas of the foot may be painful or highly sensitive to touch.

TABLE 6.1   Technique for Hand Massage

Each hand is massaged for 2-1/2 minutes. Do not massage if hand is injured, reddened, or swollen.

1. *Back of Hand*
   a. Short medium length straight strokes are done from the wrist to the finger tips; moderate pressure is used (effleurage).
   b. Large half circular stretching strokes are made from the center to the side of the hand using moderate pressure.
   c. Small circular strokes are made over the entire hand using light pressure (make small Os with the thumb).
   d. Featherlike straight strokes are made from the wrist to the finger tips using very light pressure.
2. *Palm of Hand*
   a. Short, medium length straight strokes are made from the wrist to the finger tips using moderate pressure (effleurage).
   b. Gentle milking and lifting of the tissue of the entire palm of the hand is done using moderate pressure.
   c. Small circular strokes are made over the entire palm using moderate pressure (making little Os with index finger).
   d. Large half circle stretching strokes are used from the center of the palm to the sides using moderate pressure.
3. *Fingers*
   a. Gently squeeze each finger from the base to the tip on both the sides and the front/back using light pressure.
   b. Gentle range of motion of finger.
   c. Gentle pressure on nail bed.
4. *Completion*
   a. Place client's hand on yours and cover it with your other hand. Gently draw your top hand toward you several times. Turn the client's hand over and gently draw your other hand toward you several times.

Hand Massage

A technique for implementing hand massage is presented in Table 6.1. The technique is easy to implement with many populations including: elders (Cho, 1995), elders with dementia (Snyder, Egan, & Burns, 1995a, 1995b), and children with asthma (LaVelle, 1995). The time noted in the technique for administering massage is 2-1/2 minutes per hand. In an initial study, Snyder and colleagues (1995b) administered hand massage for 5 minutes to each hand. In a subsequent study, when hand massage was administered for 2-1/2 minutes (Snyder et al., 1995a), the level of relaxation found was not as great as that found in the first study. Subsequently, Burns, Egan, and Teshima (1995) found no differences in the relaxation achieved when massage was administered for 10 versus 5 minutes.

Measurement of Effectiveness

Both physiological and psychological outcomes have been used to measure the effectiveness of massage. Indexes of relaxation (heart rate, blood pressure, skin temperature, and muscle tension) have been used in many studies. Anxiety inventories and visual analogue scales to measure pain have been used to determine the efficacy of massage. It is important that both short- and long-term effects be measured.

USES

The pleasant experience of the massage and aromatherapy allows relationships to develop between receiver and giver. Nurses need to be aware that massage can help to release emotions and should be prepared to be adaptable when the subject feels comfortable talking through personal issues during the massage. Multisensory massage can enhance the pleasure effect for people with profound and multiple learning disabilities. Sometimes, a client may like to return the experience and massage the nurse's hands. This is actively encouraged in interactive massage where improvement in relationships and decrease in stress is sought (Sanderson, Harrison, & Price, 1991).

A list of the numerous conditions for which massage has been used is found in Table 6.2. Use of massage to produce relaxation and reduce pain will be discussed below.

Relaxation

Many persons go to a massage practitioner to have their stress ameliorated. In addition to use of massage with patients, nurses can use massage with colleagues and patient families. Nurses in many settings can use the various types of massage to produce relaxation.

The majority of studies that have been conducted on the use of massage have included measurements of the relaxation response. Lloyd (1995) and Trevelyan (1989) suggested that nurses could give quick

TABLE 6.2   Uses of Massage

Promote relaxation
    Decrease aggressive behaviors (Snyder et al., 1995a, 1995b)
    Produce sleep (Bauer & Dracup, 1987; Field et al., 1996)
    Lessen fatigue (Fakouri & Jones, 1987; Longworth, 1982)
    Lessen pain (Ferrell-Torry & Glick,1993; Weinrich & Weinrich, 1990)
Reduce edema (Cyriax, 1980)
Improve mobility (Wakim, 1985)
Decrease need for episiotomy (Mynaugh, 1991; Stiles, 1980)
Increase communication (Bauer & Dracup, 1987; Conley, 1996; Fraser & Kerr, 1993; Simpson, 1991)
Increase sense of well-being (Simpson,1991; Wells-Federman et al., 1995)
Lessen depression (Field et al., 1996)
Lessen anxiety (Dunn et al., 1995; Fraser & Kerr, 1993).

massages to colleagues to promote relaxation. A short massage given to family members often enables the family to more effectively cope with the stress of the hospitalization of a loved one. Massage also assists patient and families alike to communicate more openly and facilitate closure (Ellis et al., 1995).

Pain

Several factors may contribute to the efficacy of massage in the management of pain. Massage improves circulation which will reduce edema and pressure on adjoining tissues and nerves. Increased blood flow hastens the removal of fluid and toxic metabolic waste products and decreases ischemia. Massage helps to modify the myofascial and muscle tension types of pain and possibly other forms of cancer pain by reducing muscle spasms and tension, particularly of large muscle groups (Ferrell-Torry & Glick, 1993). Day, Mason, and Chesrown (1987) hypothesized that massage stimulates the production of endogenous opiates that in turn modulate the pain experienced.

Weinrich and Weinrich (1990) administered a 10-minute back massage to persons with cancer. The results of their study indicated that males experienced a significant decrease in pain immediately after massage was administered. Meek (1993) found that slow stroke back massage administered to hospice patients produced relaxation; she recommended use of back massage to promote the comfort of hospice patients. Ferrell-Torry & Glick (1993) suggested administering 30 minutes of therapeutic massage on two consecutive evenings to promote relaxation and to alleviate the perception of pain and anxiety in hospitalized cancer patients.

Precautions

The nurse should obtain the permission of the patient before administering massage, as some people do not like to be touched. Although some persons may be sensitive to touch, increasing the gentleness of the strokes may overcome their discomfort. Good assessments of patients prior to administering massage are needed. Care is needed when areas of the body are reddened, bruised, or have skin rashes.

Patients with breathing problems, arthritic conditions, and abdominal surgery will have difficulty maintaining the prone position. A foot massage is an alternative to consider for these patients.

Several investigators tried to determine if back rubs produced deleterious effects in specific populations, such as persons who have had a myocardial infarct (Bauer & Dracup, 1987; Tyler et al., 1990). Bauer and Dracup concluded that massage does not need to be restricted in patients with cardiac conditions.

RESEARCH QUESTIONS

As noted earlier, minimal research has been done on the use of massage. This is particularly true for use of the techniques for hand and foot massage. Studies that use adequate sample sizes, control for confounding variables, and incorporate rigorous testing of reliability and validity of instruments measuring psychophysiological parameters are needed. The following are a few of the specific areas in which further research is needed:

1. Snyder et al. (1995a) reported an increase in aggressive behaviors in males with dementia after the administration of hand massage but a decrease in the female subjects. Weinrich & Weinrich (1990) found the opposite results in their study. Van der Riet (1995) noted that males students found massage to be more heavily laden with implicit sexual meanings than did female students. Thus, explorations about the impact that gender has on the results obtained from use of massage are needed. Both the

gender of the client and of the person administering massage need to be examined.

2. Burns et al. (1995) found no difference in relaxation between 5- and 10-minute administration of hand massage. No consistency in results were found when varying times were used for administering back massage. Some have suggested that a sufficient time is needed to obtain the relaxation response. However, additional data are needed to guide nurses in the length of time to administer massage.

3. The impact that massage has on pyschoneuroimmunologcial functions would make significant contributions to its use with many health conditions such as AIDs and cancer.

REFERENCES

Barr, J., & Taslitz, N. (1970). The influence of back massage on autonomic functions. *Journal of Physical Therapy, 50,* 1679–1689.

Bauer, W. C., & Dracup, K. A. (1987). Physiologic effects of back massage in patients with acute myocardial infarction. *Focus on Critical Care Nursing, 14*(6), 42–46.

Burns, K. R., Egan, E. C., & Teshima, M. (1995, April). *Testing hand massage protocols for persons with dementia.* Paper presented at the meeting of the Midwest Nursing Research Society Conference, Kansas City, MO.

Cho, K. (1995). Use of hand massage to increase relaxation in Korean-American elders. Unpublished paper.

Cochrane, F. S. (1993). Psychological effects of massage. International *Journal of Alternative and Complementary Medicine, 11*(9), 21–24.

Conley, D. M. (1996, August 30). *Biobehavioral responses of individuals with dementia to tactile stimulation (foot massage) intervention.* Presentation at Gerontological Nursing Interventions Research Conference, Iowa City, Iowa.

Corley, M. C., Ferriter, J., Zeh, J., & Gifford, C. (1995). Physiological and psychological effects of back rubs. *Applied Nursing Research, 8,* 39–43.

Cyriax, J. (1980). Clinical application of massage. In J. Rogoff (Ed.), *Manipulation, traction, and massage* (pp. 152–169). Baltimore: Williams and Wilkins.

Day, J. A., Mason, R. R., & Chesrown, S. E. (1987). Effect of massage on serum level of B-endorphin and B-lipotropin in healthy adults. *Physical Therapy, 67,* 926–930.

Dunn, C., Sleep, J., & Collett, D. (1995). Sensing an improvement: An experimental study to evaluate the use of aromatherapy, massage, and periods of rest in an intensive care unit. *Journal of Advanced Nursing, 21,* 34–40.

Ellis, V., Hill, J., & Campbell, H. (1995). Hospice techniques: Strengthening the family unit through the healing power of massage. *The American Journal of Hospice & Palliative Care, 12*(5), 19–21.

Fakouri, C., & Jones, P. (1987). Relaxation RX: Slow stroke back rub. *Journal of Gerontological Nursing, 13*(2), 32–35.

Ferrell-Torry, A. T., & Glick, O. J. (1993). The use of therapeutic massage as a nursing intervention to modify anxiety and the perception of cancer pain. *Cancer Nursing, 16,* 93–101.

Field, T., Grizzle, N., Scafidi, F., & Schanberg, S. (1996). Massage and relaxation therapies' effects on depressed adolescent mothers. *Adolescence, 31,* 903–911.

Fraser, J., & Kerr, J. R. (1993). Psychophysiological effects of back massage on elderly institutionalized patients. *Journal of Advanced Nursing, 18,* 238–245.

Groer, M., Mozingo, J., Droppleman, P., Davis, M., Jolley, M., Boynton, M., Davis, K., & Kay, S. (1994). Measures of salivary immunoglobulin A and state anxiety after a nursing back rub. *Applied Nursing Research, 7*(1), 2–6.

Joachim, G. (1983). How to give a good foot massage. *Geriatric Nursing, 4*(1), 28–29.

LaVelle, E. C. (1995). Use of music and massage with children with asthma. Unpublished paper.

Lloyd, K. (1995). The power to colleagues and clients with a two-minute massage. *The Lamp, 51*(22), 30.

Longworth, J. C. (1982). Psychophysiological effects of slow back massage in normotensive females. *Advances in Nursing Science, 4*(4), 44–61.

Meek, S. S. (1993). Effects of slow back massage on relaxation in hospice patients. *Image: Journal of Nursing Scholarship, 25,* 17–21.

Mynaugh, P. A. (1991). A randomized study of two methods of teaching perineal massage: effects on practice rates, episiotomy rates, and lacerations. *Birth, 18*(3), 153–159.

Reed, B., & Held, J. (1988). Effects of sequential connective tissue massage autonomic nervous system of middle-aged and elderly adults. *Physical Therapy, 68*(8), 1231–1234.

Sanderson, H., Harrison, J., & Price, S. S. (1991). *Aromatherapy and massage for people with learning difficulties.* Birmingham: Hands On.

Simpson, J. (1991, July). Massage: Positive strokes in palliative care. *New Zealand Nursing Journal, 84*(6), pp. 15–17.

Snyder, M., Egan, E.C., & Burns, K.R. (1995a). Efficacy of hand massage in decreasing agitation behaviors associated with care activities in persons with dementia. *Geriatric Nursing, 16*(2), 60–63.

Snyder, M., Egan, E. C., & Burns, K. R. (1995b). Interventions for decreasing agitation behaviors in persons with dementia. *Journal of Gerontological Nursing, 21*(7), 34–40.

Stiles, D. (1980). Techniques for reducing the need for an episiotomy. *Issues in Health Care of Women, 2,* 105–111.

Trevelyan, J. (1989). Relaxing with massage. *Nursing Times, 85*(39), 26.

Tyler, D. O., Winslow, E. H., Clark, A. P., & White, K. M. (1990). Effects of a 1-minute back rub on mixed venous oxygen saturation and heart rate in critically ill patients. *Heart & Lung, 19,* 562–565.

van der Riet, P.(1995). Massage and sexuality in nursing. *Nursing Inquiry, 2,* 149–156.

Wakim, K. (1985). Physiologic effects of massage. In J. Basmajian (Ed.), *Manipulation, traction, and massage* (pp. 256–262). Baltimore: Williams and Wilkins.

Weinrich, S. P., & Weinrich, M. C. (1990). The effect of massage on pain in cancer patients. *Applied Nursing Research, 3,* 140–145.

Weiss, S. J. (1986). Psychophysiologic effects of caregiver touch on incidence of cardiac dysrhythmias. *Heart Lung, 15,* 495–505.

Wells-Federman, C. L., Stuart, E. M., Deckro, J. P., Mandle, C. L., Baim, M., & Medich, C. (1995). The mind-body connection: The psychophysiology of many traditional nursing interventions. *Clinical Nurse Specialist, 9*(1), 59–66.

7

Biofeedback

Marion Good

DEFINITION

Biofeedback, an intervention of relatively recent origin, is based on a holistic perspective in which psyche and soma are not separated. The goal of biofeedback is increased control over one's functioning. Biofeedback is defined by Williams, Nigl, & Savine (1981) as

> The technique of using equipment (usually electronic) to reveal to human beings some of their internal physiological events, normal and abnormal, in the form of visual and auditory signals in order to teach them to manipulate these otherwise involuntary or unfelt events by manipulating the displayed signals. This technique inserts a person's volition into the gap of an open feedback loop, hence the artificial name of biofeedback.

The holistic philosophy behind biofeedback and its focus on helping persons gain more control over their functioning makes the intervention an appropriate one for nurses to use.

Biofeedback has been used to control functions related to all areas of the nervous system: brain activity and somatic and autonomic nervous system (ANS) responses. These responses are monitored and feedback is provided to the patient concerning the degree of control achieved so the person can eventually control the response without feedback.

SCIENTIFIC BASIS

Biofeedback originated from research in the fields of psychophysiology, learning theory, and behavioral theory. For centuries it was believed that responses such as heart rate and respiration were outside the individual's control. In the 1960s scientists found that the ANS had an afferent system as well as a motor system, and control of its functions was possible with instrumentation and conditioning. Katkin and Goldband (1980) selected a skills acquisition model as the basis for teaching biofeedback. Following this model, persons determine the relationship between their voluntary muscle or cognitive/affective activities and ANS functioning. They learn skills to control muscular and cognitive activities, which can then be reinforced to control ANS responses. The biofeedback instrument has a visual and/or auditory display that informs persons whether or not the control has been achieved; thus, learning is reinforced.

Providing behavioral strategies to modify physiological activity is an integral part of using biofeedback (Nakagawa-Kogan, 1994). Biofeedback can be used with relaxation strategies to control ANS responses that affect brain waves, peripheral vascular activity, heart rate, blood glucose, and skin conductance. Biofeedback combined with exercise can strengthen muscles weakened by conditions such as chronic pulmonary disease, knee surgery, or age, and can recruit auxiliary motor nerves in hemiplegia. In combination with positioning and biomechanics, biofeedback can reduce injury from repetitive activities such as typing.

INTERVENTION

Nurses are ideal professionals to provide biofeedback because of their knowledge of physiology, psychology, and health/illness states. However, nurses need to acquire special information and skills to use biofeedback. Classes and workshops are available in many locations, and it is recommended that nurses using biofeedback become certified.* Although state practice acts differ, the Nurses Network of AAPB is working toward nationwide acceptance of autonomous nursing biofeedback practice and inclusion of biofeedback principles in basic

---

*The Association for Applied Psychophysiology and Biofeedback (AAPB) is an excellent resource for information and certification and can be contacted at 10200 W. 44th Ave., Wheat Ridge, CO 80033 (303-422-8436).

nursing education programs (Smart, 1990). This chapter provides an overview of biofeedback, the health conditions in which it is useful, and a protocol that can be used by nurses trained in biofeedback techniques.

Techniques

A biofeedback unit consists of a sensor that monitors the patient's physiological activity, and a transducer that converts what is measured into an electronic visual or auditory signal to the patient. Frequently measured physiological parameters include muscle depolarization monitored by electromyogram (EMG) and peripheral temperature.

Biofeedback provides information about changes in a physiological parameter when behavioral treatments, such as relaxation or strengthening exercises, are used for a health problem. For example, a relaxation tape helps persons relax muscles to reduce blood pressure while the EMG biofeedback instrument informs the learner of progress. Peripheral temperature feedback is also used with relaxation: as muscles relax, circulation improves and the fingers and toes get warmer. When exercises are used to strengthen perineal muscles in preventing urinary incontinence, success in contracting the correct muscles may be monitored by a pressure sensor inserted into the vagina. In health conditions exacerbated by stress, biofeedback is often combined with stress management counseling.

Biofeedback is most frequently used in an office or clinic setting. Brown (1977) advocated using between seven and twelve 30-minute training sessions. The number of sessions should be decided upon by the therapist and patient during the initial session prior to beginning training. If the patient has not achieved mastery or control of a function at the end of the agreed upon number of sessions, the reasons and the need for further sessions should be discussed.

The first session is devoted to assessing the patient, choosing the appropriate mode of feedback, discussing the roles of the nurse and patient, and obtaining baseline measurements. Measuring several parameters helps in getting valid baseline data. Because success will be determined by changes from baseline, it is essential that these be accurate and reflect the true status of the parameter being used. The first session will be longer than subsequent ones, perhaps lasting 1–2 hours. Behavioral exercises are provided. Understanding the content of this session is preliminary to using the equipment.

The therapist plays a key role in the success of biofeedback. It is helpful for the nurse to have advanced training in relaxation, imagery, and stress management counseling. Because practice of the behavioral techniques is vital, the nurse who succeeds in motivating patients to practice at home will have patients who achieve their goals.

The final sessions focus on integration of the learning into the person's life. The patient is connected to the machine but does not receive feedback while practicing the technique; the nurse monitors the degree of control achieved. Descriptions of stressful situations are provided, and the person is asked to practice the procedure as if in that situation. Final measurements are taken. Follow-up sessions at 1 month and 6 months are advocated.

Example: Technique for Biofeedback-Assisted Relaxation.   Table 7.1 outlines a protocol for using biofeedback with cognitive-behavioral interventions for relaxation and stress management. This technique could be used for hypertension, anxiety, asthma, irritable bowel syndrome, headache, or chronic pain because muscle relaxation improves these conditions. The protocol should be tailored to the patient, condition, and type of feedback.

Various types of relaxation exercises such as autogenic phrases or systematic relaxation (see chapter 1 of this volume) may be used. To increase patient awareness of the relaxed state, progressive muscle relaxation may be helpful. Imagery (chapter 9) may relax patients by distraction and reduction of negative or stressful thoughts. Hypnosis and self-hypnosis (chapter 10) produce an alternative state of mind. Music (chapter 21) relaxes and distracts and may be used with relaxation or imagery.

It is important to keep the requirements for home practice simple, interesting, and meaningful. Boredom with the same relaxation tape, failure to find a convenient time to practice, and lack of noticeable improvements may decrease adherence to home practice. Providing a new relaxation technique can revive interest. To integrate new skills into daily life, patients can progress to mini-relaxation and use of cues (thoughts, positions, or activities) to signal relaxation. Other intervention protocols are found in the literature (Coxe, 1994; King, 1992; Schwartz & Associates, 1995).

Although some patients have multiple symptoms requiring treatment, training should only address one symptom at a time. Other symptoms can be treated sequentially after mastery of the first one is attained. The patient decides which symptom will be treated first.

TABLE 7.1 Biofeedback Protocol

1. Before first session
   A. Determine health problem for which biofeedback treatment is sought.
   B. Ask for physician's name so care can be coordinated.
   C. Give information on location, time commitment, and cost.
   D. Request a 2-week patient log of medications and the frequency and severity of the health problem (e.g., the number, intensity, and time of headaches).
   E. Answer questions.
2. First session
   A. Interview patient for a health history with attention given to the specific health condition.
   B. Assess abilities for carrying out current medical regimen and behavioral intervention.
   C. Discuss rationale for using biofeedback, type of feedback, and behavioral intervention.
   D. Explain that the role of the nurse is to provide ten 50-minute sessions once a week, using the biofeedback instrument to supply physiological information.
   E. Explain that the patient is the major factor in the successful use of biofeedback; that it is important to continue to keep a log of the health problem and also to include home practice sessions. The patient should consult the physician if health problems occur.
   F. Explain the procedure. If using frontal muscle tension feedback, apply 3 sensors to the forehead after cleaning the skin with soap and water and applying gel. Set the biofeedback machine and operate according to instructions.
   G. Obtain baseline EMG readings of frontal muscle tension for 5 minutes while the patient sits quietly with closed eyes.
   H. Instruct the patient to practice taped relaxation instructions for 20 minutes while the EMG sensors are on the forehead. Ask the patient to watch the biofeedback display for information on the decreasing level of muscle tension.
   I. Review 2-week record of the health problem and set mutually determined goals.
   J. Give a tape and instructions for practicing relaxation at home. Provide a log to record practice and responses. Discuss timing, frequency, length, and setting for practice.
   K. Discuss self-care for any possible side effects to the behavioral intervention.
3. Subsequent sessions
   A. Open session with a 20-minute review of the health problem log, stressors and ways used for coping in past week; provide counseling for adaptive coping.

(Continued)

TABLE 7.1   (continued)

B. Apply sensors and earphones and let the patient practice relaxation for 20 minutes while watching the display. Quietly leave room after patient masters the technique.

C. Vary relaxation techniques to maintain interest and increase skill.

D. Give instructions for incremental integration of relaxation into daily life. For example, add 30–second mini-relaxation exercises for busy times of the day.

4. Final session

A. Conduct session as above; obtain final EMG readings.

B. Discuss plan for ongoing practice and management of stress after end of treatment.

Measurement of Effectiveness

Table 7.2 lists feedback parameters that reflect mastery of the behavioral intervention or control of the health problem. Frequently used parameters include heart rate, muscle tension, peripheral temperature, and blood pressure. Monitoring via EMG demonstrates changes more quickly than by temperature or galvanic skin response, but the choice may depend on the appropriateness to the health condition. Temperature feedback is used in peripheral vascular problems; health care outcomes may be fewer episodes of painful vasoconstriction. Electromyogram feedback and temperature feedback are used in persons

TABLE 7.2   Conditions and Populations in Which Biofeedback has been Used

Anxiety (Scandrett, Bean, Breedan, & Powell, 1986)

Children (Olness & Kohen, 1996)

Chronic pain (Spense, Sharpe, Newton-John, & Champion, 1995; Strong, Cramond, & Maas, 1989)

Chronic pulmonary disease (Delk, Gevertz, Hicks, Carden, & Rucker, 1994)

Diabetes mellitus (McGrady, Bailey, & Good, 1992)

Headaches (Engle & Rapoff, 1990)

Heart disease (Dracup, Woo, & Stevenson, 1993; Nakagawa-Kogan, Garber, Jarrett, Egan, & Hendershot, 1994)

Hypertension (Blanchard et al. 1989; McGrady, 1994; Nagagawa-Kogan et al. 1988)

Irritable bowel (Radnitz & Blanchard, 1989)

Older adults (Arena, Hannah, Bruno, & Meador, 1991; Burns et al. 1993)

Raynaud's disease (Surwit & Jordan, 1987; Schwartz & Kelly, 1995).

Urinary incontinence (Beckman, 1995; Coxe, 1994)

with diabetes mellitus, tension headache, and chronic pain. Outcomes may include decreased glycoslated hemoglobin, headaches, or pain.

USES

Populations/Conditions

Biofeedback has been used in the treatment of many medical and psychological problems. For example, a review of research on the use of biofeedback in Raynaud's disease indicated evidence that biofeedback is often efficacious in treating this condition (Surwit & Jordan 1987). Biofeedback-assisted relaxation has been more successful in the treatment of tension headache than migraine headache (Andrasik & Blanchard, 1987; Blanchard & Andrasik, 1987). Patients with advanced heart failure using biofeedback can voluntarily decrease vascular resistance, thus increasing cardiac output (Dracup, Woo, & Stevenson, 1993; Moser, Stevenson, Woo, & Dracup, 1992). Persons with cystic fibrosis used biofeedback with pursed lip breathing to improve forced expiratory volume (Delk, Gevertz, Hicks, Carden, & Rucker, 1994). Other conditions and populations treated with biofeedback are described in Table 7.2.

Hypertension. When Westerners noted that yogis and shamans were able to lower their blood pressure by meditating and relaxing, they began to study the use of biofeedback to lower blood pressure. A review of studies of biofeedback for hypertension (Glasgow & Engel, 1987) noted that systolic reductions of 4 to 22 mm Hg and diastolic decreases of 1 to 15 mm Hg were achieved and maintained for periods of 6 to 48 months. Such reductions might allow reduction in dosages of antihypertensive medications. Recently, research has focused on the effects of biofeedback-assisted relaxation on blood pressure and immune factors, and has examined the physical and psychological predictors of those who reduced their blood pressure (Blanchard et al., 1989; McGrady, 1994; Nakagawa-Kogan et al., 1988).

Chronic Pain. Biofeedback combined with relaxation, imagery, music, or hypnosis can be used for cancer or back pain, as a complementary therapy to medication. Such use can teach patients control over their pain and may reduce the side effects of analgesic medication.

Jacox et al. (1994) reported that well-designed quasi-experimental studies show the efficacy of biofeedback in reducing chronic pain.

Urinary Incontinence. Urinary incontinence is a major problem in an aging population. It causes embarrassing and restrictive problems and is a major reason for institutionalization. Interventions to manage incontinence would significantly reduce health care costs. The Urinary Incontinence Guideline Panel (1992) reports 54% to 95% improvement in incontinence when the combination of biofeedback and behavioral treatments is used. The panel suggests that therapists become familiar with the anatomic and physiological basis for different forms of bladder dysfunction and learn strengthening exercises and special measurement methods. The goal is to optimize use of striated pelvic floor muscles to control bladder function (Tries & Eisman, 1995).

Diabetes Mellitus. Research has shown that biofeedback-assisted relaxation has been useful in reducing blood glucose in both insulin dependent and non–insulin dependent diabetes mellitus (McGrady, Bailey, & Good, 1991; Surwit & Feinglos, 1983). It is suggested that this intervention be used with persons who are adherent to their diabetic regimen, yet present stress-related symptoms that seem to affect their glycemic control. Biofeedback has reduced average blood glucose, glycoslated hemoglobin, and fasting values (McGrady, Graham, & Bailey, 1996).

Children and Older Adults. Olness and Kohen (1996) describe many conditions in children—such as migraine, hypertension, and fecal incontinence—in which biofeedback combined with hypnotherapy teaches children to change their thoughts, so they can cause changes in their body. The authors describe special biofeedback equipment and techniques that appeal to children. Biofeedback has also been successfully used with older adults (Middaugh et al., 1991). Modifications in biofeedback sessions may be needed for older adults to increase comprehension and retention (Arena et al., 1991). Because of sensory changes in elders, visual feedback should be large enough for them to see and auditory feedback loud enough to hear.

Precautions

Biofeedback should be used cautiously, if at all, for persons with depression psychosis, seizures, and hyperactive conditions. Persons with rigid personalities may be unwilling to change their mode of functioning (Williams et al., 1981). However, negative reactions may be related to relaxation rather than biofeedback, and may be avoided by patient education and type of relaxation used (Schwartz & Schwartz, 1995).

Biofeedback-assisted relaxation is expected to lower blood pressure, heart and respiratory rates. Excessive decreases should be avoided in patients with cardiac conditions, hemodynamic instability, or multiple illnesses. Use of relaxation therapies might also result in a need for reduced medication in diabetes mellitus, hypertension, and asthma. This should be discussed with patients and physicians; responses should be carefully monitored.

For example, relaxation exercises in persons with diabetes can beneficially reduce blood glucose, but hypoglycemic reactions may occur if adjustments in insulin or diet are not made. McGrady and Bailey (1995), suggest a team approach that includes the physician, a certified diabetic educator, a certified biofeedback practitioner, and the patient. Patients should be taught to manage hypoglycemia because reactions can occur at a single relaxation session, or after the program lowers blood glucose over time. The nurse should also keep simple carbohydrates, glucagon and a blood glucose monitor in the office and provide expertise to administer them. Home practice can be scheduled to avoid times of low blood glucose (McGrady & Bailey, 1995).

Electric shock is a hazard when any electrical equipment is used. Dangerous levels of current flow may arise from equipment malfunction or operator error (Katkin & Goldband, 1980). The AAPB publishes a list of companies whose products meet their safety code.

Although biofeedback is noninvasive, cost effective, and very promising in the treatment of many conditions, it is not a miracle intervention. It requires that the therapist be knowledgeable about the health problem, intervention, and medication effects, and have a sincere interest in the patient outcome. Considerable patient time, attention, and motivation are needed for success. To control the condition, ongoing use of the behavioral technique may be needed after biofeedback sessions end. This should be made very clear before training is initiated.

RESEARCH QUESTIONS

There is great need for controlled clinical trials to determine the effectiveness of biofeedback in treating physiological and psychological conditions (Hatch, Fisher, & Rugh, 1995). Nurses employing bio-feedback can address the following questions:

1. What are the self-care characteristics of persons who benefit most from biofeedback?
2. Does autogenic training with peripheral temperature feedback improve diabetic foot ulcers?
3. What is the effect of biofeedback-assisted relaxation on chronic back pain?
4. Do persons who lower their blood pressure with biofeedback/relaxation continue home practice and maintain the lower level when the sessions are completed?
5. Does biofeedback plus medication result in better health outcomes than medication alone?
6. Does a biofeedback-assisted intervention reduce the amount of medication needed and side effects of medications?

REFERENCES

Andrasik, F., & Blanchard E. B. (1987). The biofeedback treatment of tension headache. In J. Hatch, J. Fisher, & J. Rugh (Eds.), *Biofeedback: Studies in clinical efficacy* (pp. 281–321). New York: Plenum.

Arena, J. G., Hannah, S. L., Bruno, G. M., & Meador, K. J. (1991). Electromyographic biofeedback training for tension headache in the elderly: A prospective study. *Biofeedback and Self Regulation 16*, 379–390.

Beckman, N. J. (1995). An overview of urinary incontinence in adults: Assessments and behavioral interventions. *Clinical Nurse Specialist 9*, 241–247.

Blanchard, E. B., & Andrasik, F. (1987). Biofeedback for vascular headache. In J. Hatch, J. Fisher, & J. Rugh (Eds.), *Biofeedback: Studies in clinical efficacy* (pp. 1–48). New York: Plenum.

Blanchard, E. B., McCoy, G. C., Berger, M., Musso, A., Pallmeyer, T. P., Gerardi, R., Gerardi, M. A., & Pangburn, L. (1989). A controlled comparison of thermal biofeedback and relaxation training in the treatment of essential hypertension, IV: Prediction of short-term clinical outcome. *Behavior Therapy, 20*, 405–415.

Brown, B. (1977). *Stress and the art of biofeedback*. New York: Bantam.

Burns, P., Pranikoff, K., Nochajski, T., Hadley, E., Levy, K., & Ory, M. (1993) . A comparison of effectiveness of biofeedback and pelvic muscle exercise treatment of stress incontinence in older community-dwelling women. *Journal of Gerontology: Medical Sciences, 48,* M167–M174.

Coxe, J. (1994). Assessment for biofeedback and behavioral therapy for urinary incontinence. *Urologic Nursing, 14,* 82–84.

Delk, K. K., Gevertz, R., Hicks, D. A., Carden, F., & Rucker, R. (1994). The effects of biofeedback assisted breathing retraining on lung function in patients with cystic fibrosis. *Chest, 105*(2), 23–28.

Dracup, K., Woo, M., & Stevenson, L. (1993). Use of BF in patients with advanced heart failure to reduce systemic vascular resistance. *AACN Clinical Issues in Critical Care, 3,* 30.

Engle, J. M., & Rapoff, M. A. (1990). Biofeedback-assisted relaxation training for adult and pediatric disorders. *Occupational Therapy Journal of Research, 10,* 283–299.

Glasgow, M. S., & Engel, B. T. (1987). Clinical issues in biofeedback and relaxation therapy for hypertension: Review and recommendations. In J. P. Hatch, J. G. Fisher, & J.D. Rugh (Eds.), *Biofeedback: Studies in clinical efficacy* (pp. 81–121). New York: Plenum.

Hatch, J. P., Fisher, J. G., & Rugh, J. D. (1987). Biofeedback: Studies in clinical efficacy. New York: Plenum.

Jacox, A., Carr, D. B., Payne, R. et al. (1994). *Management of Cancer Pain Clinical Practice Guideline No. 9* (AHCPR Publication No. 94–0592). Rockville, MD: Agency for Health Care Policy and Research, Public Health Service, U.S. Department of Health and Human Services.

Katkin, E., & Goldband, S. (1980). Biofeedback. In F. Kanfer & A. Goldstein (Eds.). *Helping people change* (pp. 537–558). New York: Pergamon.

King, T. I. (1992). The use of electromyographic biofeedback in treating a client with tension headaches. *American Journal of Occupational Therapy, 46,* 839–842.

McGrady, A. (1994). Effects of group relaxation training and thermal biofeedback on blood pressure and related physiological and psychological variables in essential hypertension. *Biofeedback and Self-Regulation, 19,* 51–66.

McGrady, A., & Bailey, B. K. (1995). Biofeedback-assisted relaxation and diabetes mellitus. In M. S. Schwartz & Associates (Eds.), *Biofeedback: A practitioner's guide* (2nd ed., pp. 471–489). New York: Guilford.

McGrady, A., Bailey, B. K., & Good, M. (1992). Biofeedback-assisted relaxation in insulin dependent diabetes mellitus: A controlled study. *Diabetes Care, 14,* 185–189.

McGrady, A., Graham, G., & Bailey, B. (1996). Biofeedback-assisted relaxation in insulin dependent diabetes: A replication and extension study. *Annals of Behavioral Medicine, 18(3),* 47–51.

Middaugh, J., Woods, S. E., Kee, W. G., Harden, R., & Peters, J. R. (1991).

Biofeedback-assisted relaxation training for the aging chronic pain patient. *Biofeedback and Self Regulation, 16,* 361–363.

Moser, D., Stevenson, L., Woo, M., & Dracup, K. (1992). Voluntary control of regional blood flow with biofeedback in advanced heart failure patients. *Heart and Lung, 21*(3), 292.

Nakagawa-Kogan, H. (1994). Self-management training: Potential for primary care. *Nurse Practitioner Forum, 5,* 77–84.

Nakagawa-Kogan, H., Garbar, A., Jarrett, M., Egan, K. J., & Hendershot, S. (1988). Self-management of hypertension: Predictors of success in diastolic blood pressure reduction. *Research in Nursing and Health, 11,* 105–115.

Olness, K., & Kohen, D. P. (1996). *Hypnosis and hypnotherapy with children* (3rd ed.). New York: Guilford.

Radnitz, C. L., & Blanchard E. B. (1988). Bowel sound biofeedback as a treatment for irritable bowel syndrome. *Biofeedback and Self-Regulation, 13,* 169–179.

Scandrett, S. L., Bean, J. L., Breedan, S., & Powell, S. (1986). A comparative study of biofeedback and progressive relaxation in anxious patients. *Issues in Mental Health Nursing, 8,* 255–271.

Schwartz, M. S., & Associates. (1995). *Biofeedback: A practitioner's guide* (2nd ed). New York: Guilford.

Schwartz, M. S., & Kelly, M. F. (1995). Raynaud's disease: Selected issues and considerations in using biofeedback therapies. In M. S. Schwartz & Associates (1995). *Biofeedback: A practitioner's guide* (2nd ed., pp. 429–444). New York: Guilford.

Schwartz, M. S., & Schwartz, N. M.(1995). Problems with relaxation and biofeedback: Assisted relaxation and guidelines for management. In M. S. Schwartz & Associates (Eds.), *Biofeedback: A practitioner's guide* (2nd ed., pp. 288–300). New York: Guilford.

Spence, S. H., Sharpe, L., Newton-John, T., & Champion, D. (1995). Effect of EMG biofeedback compared to applied relaxation training with chronic upper extremity cumulative trauma disorders. *Pain, 63,* 199–206.

Strong J., Cramond, T., & Maas, F. (1989). Effectiveness of relaxation techniques with patients who have chronic low back pain. *Occupational Therapy Journal of Research, 1,* 184–192.

Surwit, R. S., & Feinglos, M. N. (1983). The effects of relaxation on glucose tolerance in non–insulin dependent diabetes mellitus. *Diabetes Care, 6,* 176–179.

Surwit, R. S., & Jordan, J. S. (1987). Behavioral treatments for Raynaud's syndrome. In J. Hatch, J. Fisher, & J. Rugh (Eds.), *Biofeedback: Studies in clinical efficacy* (pp. 255–279). New York: Plenum.

Tries, J., & Eisman, E. (1995). Urinary incontinence: Evaluation and biofeedback treatment. In M. S. Schwartz & Associates (Eds.), *Biofeedback: A practitioner's guide* (2nd ed., pp. 597–632), New York: Guilford.

Urinary Incontinence Guideline Panel (1992). *Urinary incontinence in adults: Clinical practice guideline* (AHCPR Pub. No. 92–0038). Rockville, MD: Agency for Health Care Policy and Research, Public Health Service, U.S. Department of Health and Human Services.

Williams, M., Nigl, A., & Savine, D. (1981). *A textbook of biological feedback.* New York: Human Sciences.

8

Application of Heat and Cold

Sharon Ridgeway, Donna Brauer, Jacqueline Corso, Jessie S. Daniels and Mary Steffes

The sight of a nurse applying a cool washcloth to the forehead of a person in pain is a commonly portrayed image of the profession. Cold has been used throughout time as a mode of treatment. Hippocrates prescribed cold drinks to alleviate fever, while Savonarola treated constipation by having persons walk on cold, wet marble floors (Lehmann & de Lateur, 1982). Heat has also been used to relieve pain since humans first experienced the therapeutic effects of the sun (Licht, 1982). New uses for heat and cold are continually being explored.

Heat and cold have a long tradition in nursing. Florence Nightingale (1859/1992) advocated the use of hot bottles, warm bricks, and warm flannels for the prevention of chilling. The first textbooks on nursing fundamentals included procedures for the therapeutic use of heat and cold (Hampton, 1893; Vannier & Thompson, 1929). Mobily, Herr, and Nicholson (1994) found that heat or cold application was one of five cutaneous stimulation interventions which advanced practice nurses utilized most frequently for pain management. Therapeutic heat and cold applications are listed as interventions for the nursing diagnosis of pain (Carpenito, 1995) and classified by the Iowa Intervention project as nursing modalities for the promotion of physical comfort (McCloskey & Bulechek, 1996).

Heat and cold treatment modalities are not unique to nursing: Physical therapy and sports medicine also make extensive use of them. Research findings from these disciplines provide guidance for the use of heat and/or cold in nursing practice. This chapter will provide an overview of these two modalities in nursing, review the outcomes research with a focus on the last decade, describe an intervention technique, and suggest areas in which further research is needed.

HEAT

Definition and Scientific Basis

Heat is energy associated with the motion of atoms or molecules and is capable of being transmitted to the tissues by conduction, convection, radiation, and conversion. Solids (heating pads), liquids (water and wax), and gases (steam) at temperatures between 40°C and 45°C for 5 to 30 minutes can produce therapeutic effects in tissues (Lehmann, 1990).

Heating modalities used in therapy may be divided into those that heat superficial tissues (e.g., hot packs), which nurses typically use, and those that heat deeper structures (e.g., ultrasound). The therapeutic application of heat (thermotherapy) affects (a) the smooth muscle of blood vessels, (b) peripheral nerve activity, (c) muscle spindle response, (d) extensibility of collagen, (e) total body heat loss, and (f) blood and synovial fluid viscosity.

The general response to superficial heat applications is vasodilation with subsequent resolution of inflammatory infiltration, edema, and exudates. The vasodilation may be due to an axon reflex, the release of chemical mediators secondary to temperature elevation, and local spinal cord reflexes (Michlovitz, 1996). Additionally, other untreated areas of the body experience a dilatory consensual response which is less intense.

Application of superficial heat increases the firing threshold of peripheral nerves producing analgesia proximal to the application. Thermal stimulation may also provide a counterirritation, thereby activating the large diameter fibers, which may close the gate to pain impulses transmitted by the smaller fibers (McCaffery & Wolff, 1992; Tepperman & Devlin, 1983).

Skin stimulation by superficial heat may decrease gamma motor neuron activity and muscle spindle response with a subsequent reduction in striated muscle spasm (Lehmann, 1990; Michlovitz, 1996). Application of cold produces the same effect, however the effect of warming is greater than that of cooling (Lehmann, 1990).

Surface heating increases extensibility of collagen by altering its structure. When combined with exercise or stretching, tissue extensibility leads to increased ease of joint motion (Lehmann, 1990; Michlovitz, 1996).

Intervention

Many modalities are used in thermotherapy to effect physiological outcomes: hot packs, hot water bottles, commercial aquathermia pads with water flowing through them, electric heating pads, paraffin wax, whirlpools, warming blankets, and moist heating packs. The nurse needs to consider application parameters when selecting an appropriate modality.

Increased thicknesses of toweling reduce the amount of heat the body receives. Heat is conducted more rapidly through wet towels than dry cloths. Transfer of heat from hot packs to deep muscles is usually not significant because fat acts as an insulator. Care should be taken to reduce the space between the hot pack and the skin as air is a poor conductor of heat (Lehmann, 1990).

Physiological outcomes. Superficial applications of heat are prescribed to decrease muscle spasm, to improve joint movements, decrease abdominal and menstrual cramps, resolve superficial thrombophlebitis, and help heal localized infections of the skin (Lehmann, 1990). Psychologically, heat may be better tolerated than cold.

Nursing research provides intervention-specific outcomes for reduction of inflammation, infiltration, and exudates (Hastings-Tolsma, Yucha, Tompkins, Robson, & Szevereny, 1993), relief of nipple soreness (Buchko et al., 1993), and postanesthesia rewarming (Ciufo, Dice, & Coles, 1995; Krenzischek, Frank, & Kelly, 1995; Lennon, Hosking, Conover, & Perkins, 1990; Summers, Dudgeon, Byram, & Zingsheim, 1990). Nursing investigations did not substantiate the efficacy of heat applications in the relief of postpartum perineal discomfort (Rhode & Barger, 1990). Research within other disciplines provide intervention-specific outcomes for decreased pain (Curkovic, Vitulic, Babic-Naglic, & Durrigl, 1993), muscle spasms (Fountain, Gersten, & Senger, 1960), and joint stiffness (Backlund & Tiselius, 1967). Table 8.1 provides details of these research studies.

Precautions In Use

Side effects of heat application include burns, metabolic depletion in areas of deficient arterial supply, and increases in waste metabolites,

TABLE 8.1   Thermotherapy: Research Studies

Outcomes Effected	Physiological Basis	Specifics of Treatment	Citation
Reduced inflammation, infiltration, & exudates	Acceleration of inflammatory response	Aquathermia pad at 43 °C to IV extravasation site	Hastings-Tolsma, et al., 1993.
Decreased pain	Gate theory. Decrease in nerve activity	1. Limb immersion in 38 °C warm water bath for 10 min. 2. Apply 38 °C warm water compresses QID to nipples after breast feeding.	1. Curkovic et al., 1993. 2. Buchko, et al., 1993.
Decreased muscle spasms	Reduced muscle spindle response	Hot packs to posterior neck muscles or the hamstrings for 20 minutes in patients with cervical osteoarthritis and neck or hamstring spasms secondary to poliomyelitis.	Fountain et al., 1960
Decreased joint stiffness	Increased extensibility of collagen	Hand immersion into 43 °C water for 10 min.	Backlund et al., 1967.
Postanesthesia rewarming and decreased postanesthesia shivering	Convective heat transfer	Forced-air warming blanket applied postoperatively.	Lennon et al., 1990; Summers et al., 1990; Ciufo et al., 1995; Krenzischek et al., 1995.

which may become pathogenic in persons with impaired venous or lymphatic removal. Inflammation, effusion, swelling, and consensual dilatation may be desirable or undesirable side effects. Decreased blood pressure and increased heart rate secondary to vasodilation may be an adverse side effect. A decrease in muscle strength and endurance may occur after heat applications of greater than 43°C (Michlovitz, 1996).

Carefully assess for photosensitivity and sensitivity to heat because urticaria develop in persons who are sensitive to heat or light (Willis & Epstein, 1974). Heat exacerbates symptoms in people with multiple sclerosis, so extensive use of heat with this population is not recommended. Exacerbation of the acute inflammatory processes associated with rheumatoid arthritis may occur. Heat is contraindicated in persons with hemorrhagic diathesis and after trauma because application of heat increases blood flow to the area and may aggravate bleeding (Lehmann, 1990). Caution is needed in using heat with persons who have decreased levels of responsiveness or impaired sensation (e.g., elders, infants, children, those with paraplegia). They will be unable to sense the heat or communicate pain that may be an indicator of tissue damage. Heat is contraindicated in areas that have inadequate blood supply, decreased sensation, or excoriative extravasation of IV fluids.

COLD

Definition and Scientific Basis

Cold is the removal of energy from an object (heat extraction). The principal modes of energy transfer for therapeutic use of cold are conduction, convection, and evaporation (Michlovitz, 1996). Therapeutic effects in tissues occur at temperatures between 10°C and 18°C. Therapeutic duration is 10 to 15 minutes for skin and superficial nerves and 30 to 45 minutes for muscles or deep nerves (Lehmann, 1982; Waylonis, 1967). The therapeutic application of cold (cryotherapy) affects (a) smooth muscles of blood vessels, (b) peripheral activity, (c) muscle spindle response, and (d) total body temperature.

The general response to superficial cold application is a decrease in tissue metabolism which results in an increase in smooth muscle tone as well as a reflex excitation of sympathetic adrenergic fibers leading to vasoconstriction, an increase in blood viscosity, and a decrease in vasodilator metabolites. If the temperature of the tissue is less than 10°C or if vasoconstriction is longer than 15 minutes, a reactive vasodilation occurs which is termed the *hunting response* (Lewis, 1930). A neurotransmitter is released which results in arterial vasodilation until the temperature is elevated above 10°C, at which time a cycle of vasoconstriction occurs.

At temperatures of 15°C, the conduction velocity and synaptic activity of peripheral nerves is delayed, especially in those neurons with small diameter myelinated fibers. Peripheral nerves of rats stop conducting impulses at 4°C (Li, 1958). Additionally, stimulation of cold receptors may activate the large diameter fibers, which may close the gate to pain impulses transmitted by smaller fibers (McCaffery & Wolff, 1992; Tepperman & Devlin, 1983).

Lowering the temperature of the muscle may decrease gamma motor neuron activity and reduce muscle spindle response. The net effect is a reduction in striated muscle spasm (Lehmann, 1982; Michlovitz, 1996).

Intervention

Many modalities are used in cryotherapy to effect physiological outcomes: chipped ice in a bag, gel packs (a plastic pouch containing cold-retaining gel), chemical ice envelope, ice baths, refrigerant-inflated bladders, ice water, vapocoolants, ice massage, and cold packs (Halkovich, Personius, Clamann, & Newton, 1981; Lehmann & de Lateur, 1982; Michlovitz, 1996). A contrast bath (a warm whirlpool bath alternated with a cool bath) is another modality, however it is not well researched (Michlovitz, 1996; Lehmann, 1990). Research findings have been inconclusive on the most effective cold modality.

In comparing the effectiveness of chipped ice, frozen gel, chemical ice envelopes, and refrigerant-inflated bladders, McMaster, Liddle, and Waugh (1978) found that chipped ice was the most efficient means, with frozen gel a close second. Local freezing sprays produce only superficial cooling and therefore are not effective in the treatment of tissue trauma. Ice massage (rubbing the skin with ice) is advocated by Bugaj (1975), as it more quickly produces greater temperature reduction. Ice massage causes less patient discomfort than other forms of cryotherapy.

The manner in which ice is applied affects the degree of tissue cooling. LaVelle & Snyder (1985) tested the amount of cold that penetrated various barriers (ace bandage, dry washcloth, no barrier, damp washcloth, and padded ace bandage) placed over an ankle. The greatest reduction in skin temperature occurred with the use of chipped ice in a baggie that was placed over a damp washcloth; skin temperature after 30 minutes was 9.9°C.

Amount of subcutaneous fat influences the time required to achieve a specific tissue temperature. Lehmann and de Lateur (1982) reported that in subjects with less than 1 cm of subcutaneous fat there is a significant reduction in muscle temperature after 10 minutes of application of cold. However, if the person has more than 2 cm of subcutaneous fat, only a minimal change in temperature occurs after 10 minutes.

Physiological Outcomes.   Superficial cold applications are prescribed to reduce bleeding and edema formation in mechanical trauma, reduce the inflammatory reaction, relieve pain, provide sedation, reduce muscle spasms, and reduce total body temperature. Nursing research provides intervention-specific outcomes for trauma minimization (Pinkerton & Beard, 1961), decreased pain (Barclay & Martin, 1983; Ramler & Roberts, 1986, Roberts, 1995), sedation (Ross et al., 1988), and reduced total body temperature (Harker & Gibson, 1995;). Research within other disciplines provide intervention-specific outcomes for trauma minimization (Cote, Prentice, Hooker, & Shields, 1988), decreased pain (Curkovic et al., 1993), and decreased muscle spasm (Miglietta, 1973; Price, Lehmann, Boswell-Bessette, Burleigh, & de Lateur, 1993). (See Table 8.2 for details regarding the research studies.) Additionally, Newman (1985) studied cool sponging for fever reduction and found it to be ineffective.

Precautions

The side effects of cold therapy include an increase in frost nip, frost bite, joint stiffness, reactive hyperthermia, a delayed return to baseline temperature in the cooled area, and a transient increase in systolic and diastolic blood pressure. Immediately following trauma, cold applications over long periods of time result in increased edema. Cold applied for one to two hours directly over a superficial nerve may cause nerve damage. Additionally, cold retards tissue healing (Lehmann, 1982; Michlovitz, 1996).

Contraindications for cryotherapies include specific sensitivities to cold, such as cold urticaria. Cold is absolutely contraindicated in cryoglobulinemia, Raynaud's phenomenon, and paroxysmal cold hemoglobulinemia. According to Lehmann (1990), cold should not be used for persons with periarteritis nodosa or lupus erythematosus. Those clients with vascular insufficiency (arterial), altered consciousness, diabetes, peripheral neuropathies, and psychologic aversion to cold should refrain from using cryotherapies. Cold applications are contraindicated for areas with regenerating peripheral nerves, areas that are anesthetized, and open wounds.

GUIDELINES FOR ONE TECHNIQUE FOR THE APPLICATION OF HEAT AND COLD

Nurses apply hot and cold packs frequently in their practice. Table 8.3 presents techniques for the application of hot and cold packs.

TABLE 8.2　Cryotherapy: Research Studies

Outcomes Effected	Physiological Basis	Specifics of Treatment	Citation
Trauma minimization	Reduced inflammatory response & vasometabolite production Vasoconstriction	1. Injured ankle immersed in 10 °C–15 °C water for 20 min. minimized edema 2. Perineal ice pack 24–48 hours after delivery resulted in a reduction of edema and swelling.	1. Cote et al., 1988 2. Pinkerton et al., 1961
Decreased pain	Gate theory. Decreased nerve activity. Decreased muscle spasm. Increased endorphins	1. Ice massage to the arthritic joint for 1-3 min. increased the pain threshold 20-30 min. after treatment 2. Sitz baths (ice added to cool water or 15.6 °C–18.3 °C) taken 24 to 48 hours after delivery resulted in less pain than warm sitz baths. 3. Simultaneous cold cabbage leaf application on one breast & chilled gel-pack on other breast resulted in breast engorgement pain relief in both breasts.	1. Curkovic et al., 1993. 2. Barclay et al., 1993. Ramler et al., 1986 3. Roberts, 1995
Sedation	Increased endorphins	Application of cold wet sheet packs (similar to swaddling an infant) to hospitalized psychiatric patients	Ross et al., 1988
Decreased muscle spasm	Decreased spindle activity. Decreased muscle contractility	1. Calf muscle cryotherapy (water and ice mixture in a plastic bag wrapped in a cloth towel applied for 40 min.) reduced spasticity 2. Triceps surae muscle cryotherapy (7 °C for 30 min.) abolished clonus	Price et al., 1993
Decreased body	Heat transfer	Evaporative cooling (water spray & fan) is superior to cool water immersion in the treatment of heat stroke.	Harker et al., 1995 (review)

TABLE 8.3   Technique for the Application of Hot and Cold Packs

Application of a hot pack	Application of a cold pack
1. Collect: washcloths, water proof pad, bath towel, basin or water from faucet.	1. Collect: washcloths, water proof pad, bath towel, basin or water from faucet, chipped ice placed in in a plastic bag with air removed and secured with a twist tie.
2. Wash hands.	2. Wash hands.
3. Inspect and palpate area.	3. Inspect and palpate area.
4. Fill basin with 45 °C water or use water from faucet.	4. Fill basin with 18 °C water or use water from faucet.
5. Place wash cloths in basin or under faucet.	5. Place wash cloths in basin or under faucet.
6. Place wet wash cloths in dry bath towel.	6. Place wet wash cloths in dry bath towel.
7. Wring out wash cloths by twisting bath towel (to remove excess water without burning yourself).	7. Wring out wash cloths by twisting bath towel (to remove excess water).
8. Carry towel containing wash cloths to bedside (to retain heat in wash cloths).	8. Carry towel containing wash cloths to bedside (to retain cold in wash cloths).
9. Assess temperature of wash cloths and place wash cloths on affected area.	9. Assess temperature of wash cloths and place wash cloths on affected area.
10. Assess client's perception of temperature of wash cloth.	10. Apply ice bag to the washcloth barrier and assess client's perception of the temperature of the pack.
11. Apply waterproof pad and secure if necessary.	11. Apply waterproof pad and secure if necessary.
12. Assess skin color after 5 minutes and remove in 20 minutes.	12. Assess skin color after 5 minutes and remove after 30 to 45 minutes.
13. Assess for outcomes and adverse effects.	13. Assess for outcomes and adverse effects.

FURTHER RESEARCH

Nurses have used heat and cold treatments for years. A review of the literature within the last decade indicated an increase in related research, but significantly more research is needed to provide a scientific basis for the use of these treatment modalities and to more clearly delineate the conditions for which each would be most appropriate. Some of the questions that need to be answered are:

1. Are there conditions in which a combination of the two modalities are indicated?
2. What are the application parameters for heat and cold, e.g. frequency, duration, client populations or conditions?
3. How can cold applications be made comfortable so that persons will continue to use them?
4. Is there a reflex phenomenon in heat application which is similar to the hunting response in cold application?

REFERENCES

Backlund, L., & Tiselius, P. (1967). Objective measurement of joint stiffness in rheumatoid arthritis. *Acta Rheumatology Scandanavia, 13,* 275–288.

Barclay, L., & Martin, N. (1983). A sensitive area: Care of the episiotomy in the postpartum period. *Australian Journal of Advanced Nursing, 1,* 12–19.

Buchko, B. L., Pugh, L. C., Bishop, B. A., Cochran, J. F., Smith, L. R., & Lerew, O. J. (1993). Comfort measures in breast feeding primiparous women. *Journal of Obstetric, Gynecologic, and Neonatal Nursing, 17*(3), 203–209.

Bujag, R. (1975). The cooling, analgesic, and rewarming effects of ice massage on localized skin. *Physical Therapy, 55,* 11–19.

Carpenito, L. J. (1995). *Nursing diagnosis: Application to clinical practice.* Philadelphia: Lippincott.

Ciufo, D., Dice, S., & Coles, C. (1995). Rewarming hypothermic postanesthesia patients: A comparison between a water coil warming blanket and forced-air warming blanket. *Journal of Postanesthesia Nursing, 10*(3), 155–158.

Cote, D. J., Prentice, W. E., Hooker, D. N., & Shields, E. W. (1988). Comparison of three treatment procedures for minimizing ankle sprain swelling. *Physical Therapy, 68,* 1072–1076.

Curkovic, B., Vitulic, V., Babic-Naglic, D., & Durrigl, T. (1993). The influence of heat and cold on the pain threshold in rheumatoid arthritis. *Zeitschrift fur Rheumatology, 52,* 289–291.

Fountain, F. P., Gersten, J. W., & Senger, O. (1960). Decrease in muscle spasm produced by ultrasound, hot packs, and infrared radiation. *Archives of Physical Medicine and Rehabilitation, 41(7),* 293–298.

Halkovich, L., Personius, W., Clamann, M., & Newton, R. (1981). Effect of fluromethane spray on hip flexion. *Physical Medicine, 61,* 185–189.

Hampton, I. (1893). *Nursing, its principles and practice for hospitals and private use.* Cleveland: Koechert.

Harker, J., & Gibson, P. (1995). Heat-stroke: A review of rapid cooling techniques. *Intensive and Critical Care Nursing, 11,* 198–202.

Hastings-Tolsma, M. T., Yucha, C. B., Tompkins, J., Robson, L., & Szevereny, N. (1993). Effect of warm and cold applications on the resolution of IV infiltrations. *Research in Nursing and Health, 16,* 171–178.

Krenzischek, D. A., Frank, S. M., & Kelly, S. (1995). Forced-air warming versus routine thermal care and core temperature measurement sites. *Journal of Postanesthesia Nursing, 20(2),* 69–78.

LaVelle, B. E., & Snyder, M. (1985). Differential conduction of cold through barriers. *Journal of Advanced Nursing, 10,* 55–61.

Lehmann, J. (ed.). (1982). *Therapeutic heat and cold* (3rd ed.). Baltimore: Williams & Wilkins.

Lehmann, J. (Ed.). (1990). *Therapeutic heat and cold* (4th ed.). Baltimore: Williams & Wilkins.

Lehmann, J., & de Lateur, B. (1982). Therapeutic heat. In J. Lehmann (Ed.), *Therapeutic heat and cold* (pp. 404–562). Baltimore: Williams & Wilkins.

Lennon, R. L., Hosking, M. P., Conover, M., & Perkins, W. J. (1990). Evaluation of a forced-air warming system for warming hypothermic patients. *Anaesthesia Analgesia, 70,* 424–427.

Lewis, T. (1930). Observations upon the reactions of vessels of the human skin to cold. *Heart, 15,* 177–208.

Li, C. L. (1958). Effect of cooling on neuromuscular transmission in the rat. *American Journal of Physiology, 194,* 464–470.

Licht, S. (1982). History of therapeutic heat and cold. In J. Lehmann (Ed.), *Therapeutic heat and cold* (pp. 1–34). Baltimore: Williams & Wilkins.

McCaffery, M., & Wolff, M. (1992). Pain relief using cutaneous modalities, positioning, and movement. *Hospice Journal, 8(1/2),* 121–153.

McCloskey, J. C., & Bulechek, G. M. (Ed.). (1996). *Nursing interventions classification (NIC).* St. Louis: Mosby.

McMaster, W., Liddle, S., & Waugh, T. (1978). Laboratory evaluation of various cold therapy and modalities. *The American Journal of Sports, 6,* 291–293.

Michlovitz, S. L. (1996). *Thermal agents in rehabilitation.* Philadelphia: Davis Company.

Miglietta, O. (1973). Action of cold on spasticity. *American Journal of Physical Medicine, 52,* 198–205.

Mobily, P. R., Herr, K. A., & Nicholson, A. C. (1994). Validation of cutaneous stimulation interventions for pain management. *International Journal of Nursing Studies, 31*(6), 533–544.

Newman, J. (1985). Evaluation of sponging to reduce body temperature in febrile children. *Canadian Medical Association Journal, 132,* 641–642.

Nightingale, F. (1992). *Notes on nursing.* Philadelphia: Lippincott. (Original work published 1859)

Pinkerton, J. H., & Beard, R. W. (1961). Ice packs after episiotomy. *British Medical Journal, 1,* 1536–1537.

Price, R., Lehmann, J. F., Boswell-Bessette, S., Burleigh, A., & de Lateur, B. J. (1993). Influence of cryotherapy on spasticity at the human ankle. *Archives of Physical Medicine and Rehabilitation, 74,* 300–304.

Ramler, D., & Roberts, J. (1986). A comparison of cold and warm sitz baths for relief of postpartum perineal pain. *Journal of Obstetrical, Gynecological, & Neonatal Nursing, 15* (6), 471–474.

Rhode, M. A., & Barger, K. (1990). Perineal care: Then and now. *Journal of Nurse-Midwifery, 35*(4), 220–230.

Roberts, K. L. (1995). A comparison of chilled cabbage leaves and chilled gelpaks in reducing breast engorgement. *Journal of Human Lactation, 11*(1), 17–20.

Ross, D. R., Lewin, R., Gold, K., Ghuman, H. S., Rosenblum, B., Salzberg, S., & Brooks, A. M. (1988). The psychiatric uses of cold wet sheet packs. *American Journal of Psychiatry, 145*(2), 242–245.

Summers, S., Dudgeon, N., Byram, K., Zingsheim, K. (1990). The effects of two warming methods on core and surface temperatures, hemoglobin oxygen saturation, blood pressure, and perceived comfort of hypothermic postanesthesia patients. *Journal of Postanesthesia Nursing, 5,* 354–364.

Tepperman, P. S., & Devlin, M. D. (1983). Therapeutic heat and cold. *Postgraduate Medicine, 73*(1), 69–76.

Vannier, M. L., & Thompson, B. A. (1929). *Nursing procedures: A manual used in the teaching of the principles and practice of nursing in the Associated Hospitals in the University of Minnesota School of Nursing.* Minneapolis: University of Minnesota Press.

Willis, I., & Epstein, J. (1974). Solar vs. heat-induced urticaria. *Archives of Dermatology, 110,* 389–392.

Waylonis, G. W. (1967). The physiologic effects of ice massage. *Archives of Physical Medicine and Rehabilitation, 48,* 37–42.

9

Imagery

Janice Post-White

Imagery is a mind-body intervention in which the body affects the mind and the mind affects the body. This bidirectional relationship, first proposed a century ago by William James, the father of American psychology, reverses the 17th century Cartesian belief in separation of mind and body. During the past 30 years, there has been a powerful scientific movement to explore the mind's ability to influence the body.

There are several rationales proposed for this recent interest in mind-body interventions, particularly imagery. The rise in chronic illnesses, the exposure of Western medicine to other cultures' healing systems, consumer involvement in personal health practices, and costs of technology-driven health care have spurred the growth of adjunctive client-centered interventions. Environmental and emotional stresses of current society have been implicated in contributing to the increased incidence of chronic illness, resulting in the belief that reducing these stresses can result in better health of our population.

Imagery can be used to help reduce or manage stressors in daily life in a more effective way to prevent illness or to help the individual manage or cope with the effects of illness. The proposed physiologic and immunologic effects of mind-body interventions are predominantly thought to result from reducing stress responses. Imagery has been successfully used and tested in alleviating acute and chronic pain, reducing nausea and vomiting associated with cancer chemotherapy, reducing allergic responses, lowering high blood pressure, controlling irregular heartbeats, relieving gastrointestinal symptoms, and speeding healing after injury. In addition to these effects resulting from lowering sympathetic nervous system responses, imagery also contributes to psychological and spiritual well-being by helping the individual find meaning and insight.

DEFINITION

Imagery is the mental representation of an object, place, event, or situation. Deep physical and mental relaxation is necessary to allow subconscious thoughts and emotions to surface into conscious awareness, where they can be acknowledged and interpreted. An example of a deeply relaxed state is the hypnogogic phase just prior to sleep. Imagery may be receptive, with the individual perceiving messages from the body, or it may be active, with the individual cognitively evoking thoughts or ideas. Active imagery can be outcome-or end-state-oriented, in which case the individual envisions a goal, such as being healthy and well; or it can be process-oriented, in which case the mechanism of the desired effect is imagined, such as envisioning a strong immune system fighting a viral infection or tumor.

Images employ all six senses—visual, aural, tactile, olfactory, proprioceptive, and kinesthetic. Although imagery is often referred to as "visualization," imagery includes imagining through any sense and not just being able to "see something" in the mind's eye. While inducing imagery, the individual often imagines seeing, hearing, smelling, tasting, and/or touching something in the image. The term *self-hypnosis* is often used synonymously with imagery. While both interventions rely on an altered state of consciousness, they differ in that hypnosis is the induction of a particular state of mind, while imagery is used to achieve a desired outcome, such as a behavior change (Rossman, 1993; Olness, 1993).

SCIENTIFIC BASIS

Although the scientific basis for how imagery and other mind-body interventions influence physiologic responses is in its infancy, there is evidence that there are biochemical connections between the brain and the body and that mind-body interventions, such as imagery, can alleviate or control specific disorders. The three purposes of imagery are to (a) induce physiologic changes, (b) heighten psychological insight, and (c) enhance emotional awareness (Rossman, 1993). There is evidence that imagery influences physiological and immunological responses through the autonomic nervous system, provides psychological insight by overcoming logical linear thinking with the ability to see the bigger picture and to restructure the meaning of a situation, and increases emotional awareness by accessing subconscious feeling states of the limbic system through relaxation. Achterberg (1985) and Leuner (1984) suggest that the imagery itself does not produce the favorable results, but that the individual's attitude, belief in his or her ability, and emotional response to the imagery explain the outcomes.

Evidence for the effects of the mind on the immune system surfaced in the 1970s when Robert Ader discovered that white rats could suppress their immune system T-cells through a single association of saccharin water laced with cyclophosphamide, a powerful alkylating chemotherapeutic agent that causes profound nausea and immune suppression. Subsequent exposures to saccharin water alone resulted in similar immune suppression and conditioned nausea. Extensive research by Ader and Nicholas Cohen (1981) confirmed that the immune system can be conditioned by expectations and beliefs. These findings provided the impetus for future research in psychoneuroimmunology, a field of study that measures relationships among the mind, the neuroendocrine system, and the immune system.

Many of the benefits of imagery are a direct result of stress reduction. The effects of stress on the immune system are mediated through neuroendocrine and sympathetic nervous system pathways (Blalock, Harbour-McMenamin, & Smith 1985; Ader, Felten, & Cohen, 1991). Increases in pulse rate, respiratory rate, muscle tension, blood glucose, and adrenalin secretion are all attributable to an increase in sympathetic activity of the autonomic nervous system in response to stress (Selye, 1978). Deep relaxation counters the effects of stress by activating the parasympathetic nervous system, resulting in decreases in heart rate, respiratory rate and volume, oxygen consumption, blood pressure, skeletal muscle tension, and gastric acidity and motility and increases in peripheral blood flow, the production of slow alpha brain waves, and activity of natural killer cells (Benson, 1975).

Relaxation also makes the mind more receptive to new information (Benson, 1993). Deep relaxation is necessary for imagery because it reduces muscle tension, enhances the production of images, and triggers the unconscious, which stimulates emotions in the limbic system. Breathing during imagery uses abdominal (versus chest) muscles, which comprise the solar plexus center, or *chakra* (Sodergren, 1992). This center is immediately above the navel and regulates power and emotion and overcoming the effects of stress. Regular practice of the relaxation response seems to block the ability of stress hormones to influence the brain and body. This response resembles the effect of alpha and beta blockers, which act by blocking the action of noradrenaline (Benson, 1993).

Emotional states also trigger directly physiological responses through the amygdala, a neuropeptide-rich area in the limbic system. The amygdala responds to emotions by innervating brainstem catecholaminergic cells that communicate with the hypothalamus (Gray, 1991). Serotonin and dopamine are two neurotransmitters that increase in production with stress and activate hypothalamic activity (Black, 1995). In response to negative emotional states, the hypothalamus secretes corticotropin-releasing hormone (CRH), which directly suppresses NK cytotoxicity (Irwin, Vale, & Britton, 1987) and inhibits IL-2 production by T-cells (Gillis, Crabtree, & Smith, 1979). CRH also signals the release of adrenocorticotropin-releasing hormone (ACTH) from the pituitary, norepinephrine and epinephrine from peripheral sympathetic nerve terminals, and immunosuppressive cortisol from the adrenal gland. The ACTH responds by directly interfering with macrophage-mediated tumoricidal activity and interferon gamma (Heijnen, Kavelaars, & Ballieux, 1991). Through this psychoneuroimmunologic pathway, negative emotional states create a stress type immune response. Ongoing or chronic negative emotions may be the most harmful to cellular immune function and may impair the immune system's ability to ward off viruses and tumor cells. Imagery can be used to reduce tension associated with stress responses, access unconscious thoughts and emotions that have meaning for the individual, identify internal resources and strengths, and reinforce positive emotions and coping.

Positron emission tomography (PET) has been used to demonstrate that the same parts of the cerebral cortex are activated whether people imagine something or actually experience it (Rossman, 1993). Visual images activate the optic cortex, imagined listening to music arouses the auditory cortex, and conjuring up tactile sensations stimulates the sensory cortex. Vivid imagery sends messages to the lower brain centers, including the limbic system, which is the emotional center of the brain. From there, the message is relayed to the endocrine system and the autonomic nervous system. If individuals can use imagery to understand and control their patterns of thinking, to access and more deeply experience emotion, to find meaning in events and situations, and to control sympathetic nervous system stress responses, they have a powerful tool to use in the promotion of health.

INTERVENTION

Techniques

Imagery may be practiced independently, with a coach or teacher, or with a videotape or audiotape. The least expensive way to learn imagery is through an audiotape. However, there are innumerable tapes available, and selecting one to match the needs of the individual is often time consuming and expensive. The images that work for one individual may not be appropriate (or powerful) for others. The most effective imagery intervention is one that is specific to the individual's personality, to their preferences for relaxation and specific settings, and to the desired outcomes. For example, a 54-year-old woman with metastatic breast cancer had trouble identifying with a "Pac-Man" type image of devouring suggested by the media. Her idea for a more powerful image came to her as she watched her Siberian husky dogs devour their breakfast. Future images involved imagining large (friendly) dogs scouring her body for tumor cells. Others may find this image too aggressive, however, and may prefer to imagine healing light or water washing through their body removing any stray tumor cells.

When working with clients who have never practiced imagery, it can be helpful to use an audiotape to teach them relaxation methods. Some individuals feel self-conscious relaxing in front of others and may prefer to practice in privacy. In these situations, audiotapes may be preferable, at least until they learn how to relax quickly and easily. Generating images, on the other hand, often requires assistance from others. Some individuals have naturally high hypnotic abilities; these individuals tend to have active imaginations and visual preferences. Others, however, will struggle to "see something" and will need guidance in using the other five senses to have a satisfying and effective imagery. Like any skill, imagery is learned more rapidly with guidance and is perfected with practice. Independent of the method of intervention, the nurse should assist with the interpretation or processing of the images and emotional responses.

Teaching someone imagery requires knowledge of various techniques and practice. Practicing imagery oneself is extremely helpful in guiding others. Recognition and assessment of individual preferences for settings, situations, and relaxation techniques can reduce time and frustration with learning imagery. For example, while starting an intravenous line in a 45-year-old man with poor venous access, it was suggested that the individual take three deep abdominal breaths and imagine being somewhere he would rather be. He quickly responded with the desire to be in a motorboat on the ocean. Although the nurse's strong preference was to be sailing instead of moving by technological means, she could still focus the imagery on imagining the breeze across one's face, the spray of salty sea water, the heat of the sun beating down, and the joy of controlling the boat's speed and direction. The imagery helped both the client and the nurse relax so that the line was inserted with relative ease and minimal pain. With reduced muscle tension, the client's peripheral veins may have been dilated and more accessible and the perception of pain less. And the nurse was probably more confident in managing the technical skill as well as the client's response.

Guidelines for Imagery.   Imagery techniques vary considerably based on the client's needs, preferences of the coach, and specific goals of the imagery. Imagery sessions should last 15–30 minutes and should be repeated daily to obtain changes in physiology or behavior. One of the most important elements of general imagery is that it be pleasant. An example of the steps of a general imagery session is outlined in Table 9.1.

The time needed to achieve a relaxed state will vary, depending on the conduciveness of environment, comfort level of client and coach (physical and emotional), and experience of client. Frequent imagery practice reduces the time needed to obtain a relaxed state. The level of interaction between the client and coach also varies by individual preference. Some people are very comfortable responding verbally within the context of the imagery session, such as describing the setting or indicating when they feel very relaxed. Others focus better by concentrating on their images and conversing about the experience afterwards.

Deciding whether to include music in the background or not is best left up to the individual. Some people concentrate better in total silence; others prefer soft music to facilitate relaxation. If music is selected, the tempo should be moderate and mimic the heart rate of 60 beats per minute. Music is thought to trigger emotional responses by directly influencing the limbic system, and can be used adjunctively with imagery to increase awareness of emotions and influence neurohormone responses (Lane, 1994).

Scenes commonly used to induce relaxation include sitting on a hillside watching a sunset, lying in a meadow watching the clouds float by, sitting on a warm beach watching the seagulls fly over the sea, sitting by a fire on a snowy evening, and floating through water or through space. The scene used should be one that the client has

TABLE 9.1   General Guided Imagery Technique

A. Achieving a relaxed state
   1. Find a comfortable sitting or reclining position (not laying down).
   2. Uncross any extremities.
   3. Close your eyes or focus on one spot or object in the room.
   4. Focus on breathing with abdominal muscles; with each breath say to yourself "in" and "out"
   5. Feel your body becoming heavy and warm—from the top of your head to the tips of your fingers and toes.
   6. If your thoughts roam, bring your mind back to thinking of your breathing and your relaxed body.
B. Specific suggestions for imagery
   1. In your mind, go to a place you enjoy and feel good.
   2. What do you see—hear—taste—smell—and feel?
   3. Take a few deep breaths and enjoy being there.
   4. Now imagine yourself the way you want to be . . . (describe the desired goal specifically)
   5. Imagine what steps you will need to take to be the way you want to be.
   6. Practice these steps now—in this place where you feel good.
   7. What is the first thing you are doing to help you be the way you want to be?
   8. What will you do next?
   9. When you reach your goal of the way you want to be, feel yourself, touch yourself, embrace yourself, listen to the sounds surrounding you. . . .
C. Summarize process and reinforce practice
   1. Remember that you can return to this place, this feeling, this way of being . . . anytime you want.
   2. You can feel this way again by focusing on your breathing, relaxing, and imagining yourself in your special place.
   3. Come back to this place and envision yourself the way you want to be every day.
D. Return to present
   1. When you are ready you may return to the room we are in.
   2. You will feel relaxed and refreshed and be ready to resume your activities.
   3. You may open your eyes and tell me about your experience when you are ready.

actually experienced previously and found to be relaxing. The setting may change with each imagery session as the individual tries to find a place that provides the greatest level of comfort and relaxation.

The images that appear may be very concrete and visual or they may be more of a feeling state and difficult to describe. For example,

TABLE 9.2   Conditions for Which Imagery has been Tested

Conditions	Selected Sources
Psychotherapy	
Conflict resolution	Margolis (1982); Korn (1983);
Phobias/Anxiety	Shorr (1983); Leuner (1984);
Depression	Schultz (1984); Thompson & Coppens, 1994
Behavioral Change	
Cardiac rehabilitation	Ornish, Scherwitz, & Doody, (1983)
Weight control	Sheikh (1983); Barber (1984)
Smoking cessation	Sheikh (1983); Barber (1984)
Physical	
Warts	Sinclair-Geiben & Chalmers (1959); Surman, Gottlieb, Hackett, & Silverberg (1973)
Psoriasis	Zachariae, Oyster, Bjerring, & Kragballe (1996);
Cancer	Achterberg, Lawless, Simonton, & Simonton (1977); Spiegel, Bloom, Kraemer, & Gottheil (989); Fawzy (1990)
Immune system	Zachariae et al. (1994); Gruber et al. (1993); Kiecolt-Glaser et al. (1985); Achterberg & Lawlis (1984)
Childbirth/post partum care	Rossi (1986); Rees (1995)
Surgery recovery	Manyande et al. (1995)
Critical care	Tiernan (1994)
Symptom Management	
Nausea and vomiting	Frank (1985); Burish & Jenkins (1992); Troesch, Rodehaver, Delaney, & Yanes (1993)
Pain	Ilacqua (1994); Spira & Spiegel (1992); Syrjala, Cummings, & Donaldson (1992); Walco, Varni, & Ilowite (1992)
Migraine headaches	Olness, Culbert, & Uden (1989); Ilacqua (1994)
Weight gain	Dixon (1984)

clients directed to produce an image of their inner guide by their side may envision an angel, a godlike figure, a mother figure, or may just sense a presence or feel a breeze rustle by. Concrete visual images are not any more effective than abstract ones obtained through the other senses. Similarly, physiological representations of illness are not desired. Instead of teaching clients exactly what their cancer or immune cells look like, it is more powerful for the individual to image a symbolic representation of their immune system fighting viruses or cancer cells.

Sometimes clients are unable to visualize or experience anything describable. Suggestions can be offered, such as closing eyes and counting the number of windows at home or visualizing a popular flower, such as a rose. Practicing imaging something very familiar will help them practice imagery with greater confidence of perceived success. However, pressuring a client to visualize something when he or she is unable to will create anxiety. In these situations, using general relaxation imagery of a comfortable place may be preferable. Even though imagery provides energy through relaxation, it takes initial energy to practice, particularly when first learning this skill.

USES

Conditions/Populations

Although imagery originally was used for psychotherapy, it now is considered standard intervention in many clinical applications. Table 9.2 lists conditions for which imagery has been used and tested as an effective intervention. Imagery is used for many other conditions; however, most reports of effectiveness are anecdotal. Considering that the three main purposes of imagery are to change physiological outcomes, increase emotional awareness, and enhance psychological insight, imagery can be helpful in modifying many physical conditions, emotional states, or behaviors. Two conditions in which imagery has been found to be helpful are pain and cancer. Evidence for effectiveness of imagery in these conditions will be discussed here.

Pain. Whether pain is from cancer or other illness, side effects of treatment, injury, or physical stress on the body, emotional factors contribute to pain perception, and psychological interventions such as imagery can help make the pain more manageable. Stress, anxiety, and fatigue decrease the threshold for pain, making the pain more intense. Imagery can break this cycle of pain-tension-worry-anxiety-pain. Relaxation with imagery decreases pain directly by reducing muscle tension and related spasms and indirectly by lowering anxiety and improving sleep, which influence pain perception. Imagery also is a distraction strategy; vivid, detailed images using all senses tend to work best for pain control. In addition, cognitive reappraisal/restructuring used with imagery can increase a sense of control and power over the ability to reframe the meaning of pain. Interestingly, several studies indicate that the perception of pain and suffering is reduced with imagery, but that physiologic correlates are not (Spira & Spiegel, 1992; Zachariae & Bjerring, 1994).

Imagery is especially helpful in muscle tension related pain, such as some headaches or muscle spasms. Relaxation with or without imagery has been used to reduce migraine headache pain and low back pain. Imagery also eases pain associated with dental procedures, childbirth, and surgery. While highly hypnotizable persons benefit more readily than others, practically all patients can learn to better manage their pain and pain-related stresses through simple imagery exercises (Spira & Spiegel, 1992).

Distraction imagery is most useful for severe pain that is exhausting. Suggestions for drawing attention completely from the physical pain include floating or other pleasant sensation, recalling a pleasant past experience or feeling, or distracting oneself from the pain source by rubbing fingers together or squeezing and releasing hands. The focus with moderate pain is to alter the interpretation or perception of pain. Metaphors for pain can be used to dissociate from the pain and gain control (initially over the metaphor used), thereby reducing the intensity of the pain. Another alternative is to identify pleasant sensations with the metaphor. Associations with hot or cold temperature also can be used, with the individual concentrating on raising and lowering the intensity/level and associating pleasant sensations with different temperatures.

Focusing and transferring analgesia are most effective for mild pain. Several techniques can be used, such as imagining the area being injected with novocaine, being wooden, or being painted a color that numbs the area. It is helpful to numb an unaffected area first, such as a hand-in-glove anesthesia, and then transfer that numbness to the affected (painful) area (Levitan, 1992). Although elements of relaxation, vividness, and distraction were important to pain reduction, Zachariae and Bjerring (1994) found that focused analgesia was the most effective in reducing acute pain, particularly in subjects with high hypnotizability ratings.

In a randomized pretest-posttest study of 67 hospitalized patients with cancer pain, imagery combined with progressive muscle relaxation reduced pain sensation, intensity, and severity, and lowered nonopioid PRN breakthrough analgesia use (Sloman, 1995). There were no differences between the subjects who used audiotapes or those whose imagery was guided by a nurse. Similarly, in two clinical trials of bone marrow transplant patients, Syrjala and colleagues measured reduced levels of mucositis-related pain in the imagery/hypnosis group (Syrjala, Cummings, & Donaldson, 1992; Syrjala, Donaldson, Davis, Kippes, & Carr, 1995). Twice weekly imagery sessions were augmented with daily audiotape sessions. Imagery included progressive muscle relaxation, deep relaxation, transference of sensations, and individualized imagery. Other studies measuring the effect of imagery on pain suggest that short-term imagery (6–8 weeks) can improve the ability to cope with migraine pain, although it did not change frequency or medication use (Ilacqua, 1994), and can significantly reduce pain and dysfunction associated with juvenile rheumatoid arthritis (Walco, Varni, & Ilowite, 1992).

In a study conducted by Benson, chronic pain patients who meditated had fewer health care costs (Caudill, Schnable, Zuttermeister, Benson, & Friedman, 1991). Recent recommendations of a National Institutes of Health technology assessment panel were that behavioral therapies for chronic cancer pain be accepted as standard treatment and reimbursed similarly to medical treatments (Eastman, 1995). Imagery is cost-effective and easily integrated into care provided by nurses, social workers, and psychologists.

Cancer and the Immune System.   The immune system is a focal point of images related to cancer. Specific images are often used to target natural killer or T-cells, both of which kill tumor cells or viruses. Although the cellular immune system is thought to help control cancer, it is not known whether images of active immune cells actually change immune function or whether changes in immune function actually change tumor burden or clinical outcome. However, several changes in immune or neurohormone levels have been correlated with tumor progression or remission. Increases in natural killer cytoxicity, interleukin-2, increased immunoglobulins, and increased T-cell responsiveness were measured (Gruber, Hall, Hersh, & Dubois, 1988; Gruber et al., 1993) in response to imagery. In contrast, in 30 healthy subjects, Zachariae and colleagues (1994) demonstrated a *decrease* in natural killer cell activity and lymphocyte proliferative responsiveness immediately after imagery/relaxation intervention. Subjects who were highly hypnotizable (*N*=15) had greater decreases in T-cell and NK-cell response than subjects whose hypnotizability ratings were low. The discrepancy in responses to imagery may be explained by differences in immune response to acute and chronic stress or to the meaning attached to the imagery itself.

Although immune response was not measured, a landmark study by Spiegel and colleagues showed that a year of weekly supportive group therapy sessions with self-hypnosis taught for pain control extended survival in women with metastatic breast cancer (Spiegel, Bloom, Kraemer, & Gottheil, 1989). Women randomly assigned to the intervention group lived an average of 19 months longer than women in the control group. In a study of patients with early-stage melanoma, Fawzy and colleagues measured delayed (6-month) increases in natural killer cell function in response to a cognitive-behavioral-educational intervention (Fawzy et al., 1990). However, it is difficult to tease out the effects of imagery alone in these studies.

Two related studies of women with breast cancer were conducted in an attempt to differentiate the effects of imagery from the effects of support group interventions. In one study of 73 women (Post-White et al., 1997) imagery participants had greater interleukin-2, T helper cell levels (CD4), and IL-2 receptors (CD4/25) than support group participants or controls, but there were no differences on immune measures in another study of 47 women (Richardson et al., 1997). There were no significant effects in either study on natural killer cell function. In both studies, the imagery and support intervention groups had better coping responses and more positive psychological states than the control groups, suggesting that both imagery and support play a role in mediating psychoneuroimmune outcomes in breast cancer.

Imagery also can be used to control symptoms in cancer, such as nausea, anticipatory vomiting, learned food aversions, and pruritis. Metaphors, dissociation, control of switches to shut off symptoms, and cooling waterfall images can be used to reduce symptoms and related anxiety or anticipation. In addition, positive suggestions throughout the day to imagine the body as healing itself and knowing how to heal gives permission for healing to occur (Levitan, 1992).

A dilemma of research in this field is lack of consistency in defining the intervention and variability in measures of outcomes, particularly immune function. Differentiating between expected immunological functions and acute and chronic stress states will be important to determining clinical significance of immune results.

Measurement of Outcomes

Measurable outcomes of imagery have included physiological and immunological changes, perception of psychological benefit, and changes in emotional responses, such as lower anxiety and depression and improved coping. Recent emphasis also has been on measuring morbidity and survival, cost effectiveness, and quality-of-life outcomes.

The outcomes measured should reflect the client situation and the rationale and framework for using imagery. If imagery is used to facilitate relaxation and progression during the birthing experience, outcomes might include level of pain, medications used, perceived helpfulness, and progression of labor. If imagery is used for symptom management of clients undergoing chemotherapy for cancer, expected outcomes might include reduced nausea, vomiting, and fatigue and enhanced body image and quality of life.

Immune outcomes, such as T-cell or natural killer cell response are sometimes measured to determine cellular immune response to a virus or tumor. Measuring the numbers of immune cells by flow cytometry provides information on how many cells are circulating at the time, while measuring cytotoxicity provides information on the ability of T-cells or natural killer cells to actually kill tumor cells in vitro. Although it is often assumed that the immune system will respond automatically to guided imagery, measuring the effects of guided imagery on immune responses is elusive, expensive, and not always reliable. Individual variability in physiologic and emotional responses also confound measurement of immune or physiological responses to guided imagery. It is recommended that clinical indexes of illness be measured with immune changes to facilitate interpretation of immune outcomes in relation to relevant clinical outcomes.

The psychological benefits of imagery include a sense of participation in healing, an increased awareness of emotions, a discovery of meaning of the event or illness, strengthened self-esteem, identification of resources, and a positive change in attitude and behavior (Post-White & Johnson, 1991). Measuring coping responses, emotional states, body image, spirituality, and behavior changes can capture some of the emotional and psychological benefits of imagery. Even if guided imagery does not have documented physiological or clinical effects, the emotional benefits make it a valuable part of care. The most consistent outcome, although elusive to measurement, is the perceived benefit.

One of the most difficult conclusions to draw is whether the outcomes are the result solely of imagery or of a combination of interventions. For example, learning and practicing imagery often change other health-related behaviors, such as getting more sleep, eating a healthier diet, stopping smoking, or exercising regularly. Perhaps the dedication of 20 minutes each day to escape from normal activities is the beneficial component of imagery. The therapist's attention and compassion also may be an intervention, independent of the imagery. Although these practices are synergistically beneficial for the individual, they confound the testing of results and interpretation of cause-and-effect relationships between intervention and outcome. It is important to remember that changes do not appear immediately. Long-term psychological and physiological changes may take several weeks or months and may appear gradually, making them difficult to recognize (Benson, 1993).

Several tools are available to measure the vividness of imagery or the ability to enter into a hypnogogic trance in which imagery is facilitated. Approximately five percent of the general population is considered highly hypnotizable (Hall, 1984). These individuals recall pictures more accurately, generate more complex images, have higher dream recall frequency in the waking state, and make fewer eye movements in imagery than poor visualizers. Tools to measure vividness or characteristics of imagery ability include the Betts Questionnaire upon Mental Imagery (Sheehan, 1967), Marks's Vividness of Visual Imagery (Marks, 1973), and the Harvard Group Scale of Hypnotic Susceptibility (Shor & Orne, 1962). The Image CA is a 14–item tool that specifically rates the individual's ability to visualize his or her cancer cells, white blood cells, and treatment (Achterberg & Lawlis, 1984). A higher score reflects stronger imagery and perception of immune function.

PRECAUTIONS IN USE

The physical and emotional risks of mind-body techniques are virtually nonexistent as long as they are not used in place of conventional medicine (Goleman & Gurin, 1993). Some individuals experience airway constriction or difficulty breathing when they focus on breathing techniques. Using another centering method, such as focusing on an object in the room or repeating a mantra, can reduce this distressing response and still induce relaxation.

The intended use of imagery should guide the nurses' judgment in using imagery to achieve outcomes in practice. Nurses can learn imagery techniques to help clients manage side effects or undesirable symptoms, such as pain, nausea, or vomiting; facilitate relaxation, sleep, or anxiety reduction; and encourage awareness of personal preferences and emotional responses. Using imagery as a technique in psychotherapy should be restricted to trained psychologists, psychotherapists, or psychiatrists. Clients with underlying psychiatric disorders or clinical depression also should receive help from trained psychotherapists.

There are minimal direct costs associated with guided imagery unless tapes and recorders are used. Indirect costs include professional time to train clients in imagery techniques. If imagery is used for biofeedback or psychotherapy, significant costs can be incurred for professional services. Although some medical insurance plans cover partial costs of mind-body interventions, interventions used for medical purposes (e.g., increased circulation in Raynaud's disease) are more likely to be covered than imagery used for coping or improved mood states.

FURTHER RESEARCH

Despite documented relationships between the mind and the body, many of the intervention trials testing the effectiveness of guided imagery and other mind-body interventions lack the scientific rigor of randomized controlled clinical trials. Research has progressed from anecdotal reports and case studies, predominant in the 1970s, to demonstrated effects over time in small groups of clients, to a relatively few studies comparing effects between groups of clients exposed or not exposed to the intervention. Current research focuses on demonstrating that mind-body interventions are more effective than placebo or no intervention in producing outcomes in larger samples. Few of these studies are longitudinal, however.

The key question that remains to be answered is whether psychoneuroimmune responses to imagery actually influence clinical outcomes and quality of life. Determining personal preferences for types of complementary interventions also is important to intervening and demonstrating significant clinical effects. Measuring clinical outcomes relevant to quality of life and health/illness states is critical to demonstrating cost effectiveness and the efficacy of imagery as an intervention useful in practice.

Questions regarding imagery that will advance the broader goals of mind-body intervention research include:

1. Is imagery more effective than relaxation alone in producing stress-reducing outcomes?

2. Does the type of imagery (general or specific) produce different psychoneuroimmune responses? Does imaging the immune system in cancer actually influence immune response?
3. Are there certain characteristics of individuals that determine their ability to respond to imagery and produce desired outcomes? Are introverted or internally oriented persons more open to learning imagery and therefore better able to influence outcomes? Are there certain individuals or conditions for whom imagery should not be recommended?
4. What are the long-term effects of imagery? Can imagery reduce stress, enhance well-being, create healthier lifestyles, and reduce illness in individuals over time?

REFERENCES

Achterberg, J., & Lawlis, G. F. (1984). *Imagery and disease: Diagnostic tools?* Champaign, IL: Institute for Personality and Ability Testing.

Achterberg, J. (1985). *Imagery in healing: Shamanism and modern medicine.* Boston: Shambhala.

Achterberg, J., Lawlis, R., Simonton, S. M., & Simonton, O. C. (1977). Psychological factors and blood chemistries as disease outcome predictors for cancer patients. *Multivariate Experimental Clinical Research, 3,* 107–122.

Ader, R., & Cohen, N. (1981). Conditioned immunopharmacologic responses. In R. Ader (Ed.), *Psychoneuroimmunology* (pp. 281–319). New York: Academic.

Ader, R. Felten, D. L., & Cohen, N. (1991). *Psychoneuroimmunology* (2nd ed.). San Diego: Academic.

Barber, T. X. (1984). Changing unchangeable bodily processes by hypnotic suggestions: A new look at hypnosis, cognitions, imagining, and the mind-body problems. In A. A. Sheikh (Ed.), *Imagination and healing* (pp. 69–127). Amityville, NY: Baywood.

Benson, H. (1975). *The relaxation response.* New York: William Morrow.

Benson, H. (1993). The relaxation response. In D. Goleman and J. Gurin (Eds.), *Mind/body medicine* (pp. 233–258). Yonkers, NY: Consumers Union.

Black, P. H. (1995). Psychoneuroimmunology: Brain and immunity. *Scientific American Science and Medicine, 2*(6), 16–25.

Blalock, J. E., Harbour-McMenamin, P., & Smith, E. M. (1985). Peptide hormones shared by the neuroendocrine and immunologic systems. *Journal of Immunology, 132,* 1067–1070.

Burish, T.G., & Jenkins, R.A. (1992). Effectiveness of biofeedback and relaxation training in reducing the side effects of cancer chemotherapy. *Health Psychology, 11*(1), 17–23.

Caudill, M., Schnable, R., Zuttermeister, P., Benson, H., & Friedman, R. (1991). Decreased clinic use by chronic pain patients: Response to behavioral medicine intervention. *Journal of Chronic Pain, 7,* 305–310.

Dixon, J. (1984). Effect of nursing interventions on nutritional and performance status in cancer patients. *Nursing Research, 33,* 330–335.

Eastman, P. (1995). Panel endorses behavioral therapy for cancer pain. *Journal of the National Cancer Institute, 87,* 1666–1667.

Fawzy, F. I., Kemeny, M. E., Fawzy, N. W., Elashoff, M. D., Cousins, N., Fahey, J. L. (1990). A structured psychiatric intervention for cancer patients. II: Changes over time in immunological measures. *Archives of General Psychiatry, 47,* 729–735.

Frank, J. (1985). The effect of music therapy and guided imagery on chemotherapy induced nausea and vomiting. *Oncology Nursing Forum, 12,* 47–52.

Gillis, S., Crabtree, C. R., & Smith, K. A. (1979). Glucocorticoid-induced inhibition of T cell growth factor production. I: The effect on mitogen-induced lymphocyte proliferation. *Journal of Immunology, 123,* 1624–1631.

Goleman, D. J., & Gurin, J. (1993). *Mind/body medicine.* Yonkers, NY: Consumers Union.

Gray, T. S. (1991). Amygdala: Role in autonomic and neuroendocrine responses to stress. In J. A. McCubbin, P. G. Kaufman, & C. B. Nemeroff (Eds.), *Stress, neuropeptides, and systemic disease* (pp. 37–55). San Diego, CA: Academic.

Gruber, B. L., Hall, N. R., Hersh, S. P., & Dubois, P. (1988). Immune system and psychologic changes in metastatic cancer patients while using ritualized relaxation and guided imagery: A pilot study. *Scandinavian Journal of Behavioral Therapy, 17,* 25–46.

Gruber, B. L., Hersh, S. P., Hall, N. R., Waletzky, L. R., Kunz, J. F., Carpenter, J. K., Kverno, K. S., & Weiss, S. M. (1993). Immunological responses of breast cancer patients to behavioral interventions. *Biofeedback and Self Regulation, 18*(1), 1–22.

Hall, H. R. (1984). Imagery and cancer. In A. A. Sheikh (Ed.), *Imagination and healing* (pp. 159–169). Amityville, NY: Baywood.

Heijnen, C. J., Kavelaars, A. & Ballieux, R. E. (1991). Proopiomelanocortin-derived peptides in the modulation of immune function. In R. Ader, D. L. Felten, & N. Cohen (Eds.), *Psychoneuroimmunology* (2nd ed., pp. 429–446). San Diego, CA: Academic.

Ilacqua, G. E. (1994). Migraine headaches: Coping efficacy of guided imagery training. *Headache, 34*(2), 99–102.

Irwin, M., Vale, W., & Britton, K. (1987). Central corticotropin releasing factor suppresses natural killer cytotoxicity. *Brain, Behavior, and Immunity, 1,* 81–87.

Kiecolt-Glaser, J. K., Glaser, R., Williger, D., Stout, J., Messick, G., Sheppard, S., Ricker, D., Romisher, S. C., Briner, W., Bonnell, G., & Donnerberg, R. (1985). Psychosocial enhancement of immunocompetence in a geriatric population. *Health Psychology, 4,* 25–41.

Kiecolt-Glaser, J.K., & Glaser, R. (1992). Psychoneuroimmunology: Can psychological interventions modulate immunity? *Journal of Consulting and Clinical Psychology, 60*(4), 1–7.

Korn, E. R. (1983). The use of altered states of consciousness and imagery in physical and pain rehabilitation. *Journal of Mental Imagery, 7,* 25–34.

Lane, D. (1994). Effects of music therapy on immune function of hospitalized patients. *Quality of Life: A Nursing Challenge, 3*(4), 74–80.

Leuner, H. (1984). *Guided affective imagery.* New York: Thiemme-Stratton.

Levitan, A. A. (1992). The use of hypnosis with cancer patients. *Psychiatric Medicine, 10*(1), 119–131.

Manyande, A., Berg, S., Gettins, D., Stanford, S.C., Mazhero, S., Marks, D.F., & Salmon, P. (1995). Preoperative rehearsal of active coping imagery influences subjective and hormonal responses to abdominal surgery. *Psychosomatic Medicine, 57*(2), 177–182.

Margolis, C. G. (1982). Hypnotic imagery with cancer patients. *American Journal of Clinical Hypnosis, 25*(2–3), 128–134.

Marks, D. F. (1973). Visual imagery differences in the recall of pictures. *British Journal of Psychology, 64,* 17–24.

Olness, K. (1993). Hypnosis: The power of attention. In D. Goleman & J. Gurin (Eds.), *Mind/Body Medicine* (pp. 277–290). Yonkers, NY: Consumers Union of United States, Inc.

Olness, K., Culbert, T., & Uden, D. (1989). Self-regulation of salivary immunoglobulin A by children. *Pediatrics, 83,* 66–71.

Ornish, D., Scherwitz, L. W., Doody, R. D. (1983). Effects of stress management training and dietary changes in treating ischemic heart disease. *JAMA, 249,* 54–59.

Post-White, J., & Johnson, M. (1991). Complementary nursing therapies in clinical oncology practice: Relaxation and imagery. *Dimensions in Oncology Nursing, 5*(2), 15–20.

Post-White, J., Schroeder, L., Hannahan, A., Johnston, M. K., Salscheider, N., & Grandt, N. (1997). Psychoimmune response to imagery and support in breast cancer survivors. Manuscript submitted for publication.

Rees, B.L. (1995). Effect of relaxation with guided imagery on anxiety, depression, and self-esteem in primaparas. *Journal of Holistic Nursing,* *13*(3), 255–267.

Richardson, M. A., Post-White, J., Grimm, E. A., Moye, L. A., Singletary, S. E., & Justice, B. (1997). Coping, life attitudes, and immune responses to imagery and group support after breast cancer. *Alternative Therapies, 3*(5), 62–70.

Rossi, E. L. (1986). *The psychobiology of mind-body healing: New concepts of therapeutic hypnosis.* New York: Norton.

Rossman, M. (1993). Imagery: Learning to use the mind's eye. In D. Goleman & J. Gurin (Eds.), *Mind/body medicine* (pp 291–300). Yonkers, NY: Consumers Union.

Schultz, K. D. (1984). The use of imagery in alleviating depression. In A. A. Sheikh (Ed.), *Imagination and healing* (pp. 129–157). Farmingdale, NY: Baywood.

Schulz, K. H., & Schulz, H. (1992). Overview of psychoneuroimmunologic stress-and intervention studies in humans with emphasis on the uses of immunological parameters. *Psycho-Oncology, 1,* 51–70.

Selye, H. (1978). *The stress of life.* New York: McGraw Hill.

Sheehan, P. W. (1967). A shortened form of Betts Questionnaire upon Mental Imagery. *Journal of Clinical Psychology, 23,* 386–389.

Sheikh, A. A. (1983). *Imagery: Current theory, research, and application.* New York: Wiley.

Shor, R. E., & Orne, E. C. (1962). Norms on the Harvard Group Scale of Hypnotic Susceptibility. *International Journal of Clinical and Experimental Hypnosis, 11,* 39–47.

Shorr, J. E. (1983). *Psychotherapy through imagery.* New York: Thieme-Stratton.

Sinclair-Geiben, A. H. C., & Chalmers, D. (1959). Evaluation of treatment of warts by hypnosis. *Lancet, 2,* 480–482.

Sloman, R. (1995). Relaxation and the relief of cancer pain. *Nursing Clinics of North America, 30*(4), 697–709.

Sodergren, K. (1992). Guided imagery. In M. Snyder (Ed.), *Independent nursing interventions* (2nd ed., pp. 95–109). Albany, NY: Delmar.

Spiegel, D., Bloom, J. R., Kraemer, H. C., & Gottheil, E. (1989). Effect of psychosocial treatment on survival of patients with metastatic breast cancer. *Lancet, 2,* 888–891.

Spira, J. L., & Spiegel, D. (1992). Hypnosis and related techniques in pain management. *Hospice Journal, 8*(1–2), 89–119.

Stevens, M. M., Pozza, L. D., Cavelletto, B., Cooper, M. G., & Kilham, H. A. (1994). Pain and symptom control in paediatric palliative care. *Cancer surveys, 21,* 211–231.

Surman, O. S., Gottlieb, S. K., Hackett, T. P., & Silverberg, E. L. (1973).

Hypnosis in the treatment of warts. *Archives of General Psychiatry, 28,* 439–441.

Syrjala, K. L., Cummings, C., & Donaldson, G. W. (1992). Hypnosis or cognitive behavioral training for the reduction of pain and nausea during cancer treatment: A controlled clinical trial. *Pain, 48,* 137–146.

Syrjala, K. L., Donaldson, G. W., Davis, M. W., Kippes, M. E., & Carr, J. E. (1995). Relaxation and imagery and cognitive-behavioral training reduce pain during cancer treatment: A controlled clinical trial. *Pain, 63,* 189–198.

Thompson, M.B., & Coppens, N.M. (1994). The effects of guided imagery on anxiety levels and movement of clients undergoing magnetic resonance imaging. *Holistic Nursing Practice, 8*(2), 59–69.

Tiernan, P. J. (1994). Independent nursing interventions: Relaxation and guided imagery in critical care. *Critical Care Nurse, 14*(5), 47–51.

Troesch, L.M., Rodehaver, C.B., Delaney, E.A., & Yanes, B. (1993). The influence of guided imagery on chemotherapy-related nausea and vomiting. *Oncology Nursing Forum, 20*(8), 1179–1185.

Walco, G. A., Varni, J. W., & Ilowite, N. T. (1992). Cognitive-behavioral pain management in children with juvenile rheumatoid arthritis. *Pediatrics, 89*(6), 1075–1079.

Zachariae, R., & Bjerring, P. (1994). Laser-induced pain-related brain potentials and sensory pain ratings in high and low hypnotizable subjects during hypnotic suggestions of relaxation, dissociated imagery, focused analgesia, and placebo. *International Journal of Clinical and Experimental Hypnosis, 42*(1), 56–80.

Zachariae, R., Hansen, J.B., Andersen, M., Jinquan, T., Petersen, K.S., Simonsen, C., Zachariae, C., & Thestrup-Pedersen, K. (1994). Changes in cellular immune function after immune specific guided imagery and relaxation in high and low hypnotizable healthy subjects. *Psychotherapy and Psychosomatics, 61*(1–2), 74–92.

Zachariae, R., Oster, H., Bjerring, P., & Kragballe, K. (1996). Effects of psychologic intervention on psoriasis: A preliminary report. *Journal of American Academy of Dermatology, 34,* 1008–1015.

10

Meditation

Mary Jo Kreitzer

Meditation is a self-directed practice for relaxing the body and calming the mind that has been used by people in many cultures since ancient times. The practice of meditation is frequently viewed as a religious practice, although its health benefits have been long recognized. Meditation is a recommended intervention for stress reduction, anxiety and anxiety-related disorders, for expanding awareness, and for improvement in well-being.

The resurgence in interest in meditation has drawn largely from Eastern religious practices, particularly those of India, China, and Japan. Records substantiate the use of meditation by Hindus in India as early as 1500 BC. Taoists in China and Buddhists in India included meditation as an integral part of their religious life. Zen Buddhism in Japan developed a special form of meditation called *zazen,* is a sitting meditation in which a quiet awareness is maintained of whatever is presently happening.

Meditation has also been an important aspect of the Western world and Judaeo-Christian tradition. Christian monks and hermits went to the desert to meditate and meditation remains a key element of monastic life. Christian contemplation, centering prayer, and praying the rosary or repeating the "Hail Mary" are forms of meditation. West (1979) noted the use of meditation in the American Indian culture, the Kung Zhu/twasi of Africa, and the Eskimos of North America. In the United States, the most common forms of meditation are sedentary, though there is an increasing interest in many moving meditations such as the Chinese martial art of Tai Chi, the Japanese martial art of Aikido, and walking meditation in Zen Buddhism. Although specific meditative practices vary considerably, the outcomes are very similar for all techniques.

This chapter will provide an overview of mediation in general and will highlight the meditative approaches of *transcendental meditation (TM), centering prayer,* the relaxation response, and mindfulness meditation in more detail.

DEFINITION

Many definitions of meditation can be identified in the literature. West (1979) defined meditation as an exercise in which the individual focuses attention or awareness in order to dwell upon a single object. The definition proposed by Goleman and Schwartz (1976) is similar in that attention is focused on a single percept. They defined meditation as:

> The systematic and continued focusing of the attention on a single target percept—for example, a mantra or sound—or persistently holding a specific attentional set toward all percepts or mental contents as they spontaneously arise in the field of awareness. (p. 457)

Welwood's definition (1979) is broader than the previous two; he viewed meditation as a technique that allows a person to investigate the process of his or her consciousness and experiences and to discover the more basic underlying qualities of one's existence as an animate reality. Intense concentration blocks other stimuli, allowing the person to become more aware of self.

Everly and Rosenfeld (1981) divided meditation techniques into four forms: mental repetition, physical repetition, problem concentration, and visual concentration. In mental repetition the person concentrates on a word or phrase, commonly called a mantra. Concentration on breathing is frequently the focus in physical repetition techniques; however, dance or other body movements can be the object of concentration. Jogging also allows for concentrating on a physical activity, repetitive breathing, and the sound of one's feet hitting the ground. In *samatha* Buddhist meditation, the person watches or concentrates on the breath entering and flowing from the tip of the nostrils. In problem contemplation techniques, an attempt is made to solve a problem that contains paradoxical components. Zen terms this problem the *koan.* Visual concentration techniques are akin to imagery.

Borysenko (1988) defines meditation simply as any activity that keeps the attention pleasantly anchored in the present moment. It is the way we learn to access the relaxation response.

SCIENTIFIC BASIS

An understanding of the scientific basis for meditation is emerging. In 1979, West noted that there were few theoretical explanations for meditation's effectiveness. Various explanations for its seeming effectiveness had been proposed, including adaptive regression (Shafii, 1973) and desensitization, as meditating allows the person to deal with unfinished psychic material (Tart, 1971). Another possible hypothesis for the effectiveness of meditation was that it was a way of learning to experience without categorizing or predetermining (Goleman, 1977). Everly and Rosenfeld (1981) suggested that the role of the focal device used in meditation is to allow the intuitive, non–ego-centered mode of thought processing to dominate consciousness in place of the normally dominant analytic, ego-centered style. When the left (rational, analytic) hemisphere of the brain is silenced, the intuitive mode produces extraordinary awareness. This state is frequently called *nirvana*. A positive mood, an experience of unity, an alteration in time-space relationships, an enhanced sense of reality and meaning, and an acceptance of things that seem paradoxical are experienced in this superconscious state. A serious meditator may progress through a continuum from the beginning meditation to this superconscious state.

In a report to the National Institutes of Health (1992) on alternative medical systems and practices in the United States, research on meditation was summarized as one of several mind-body interventions. In describing how and why meditation may work, Walton, director of the Neurochemistry Laboratory, Maharishi International University, was quoted as saying:

> The frequently striking results of [studies of transcendental meditation] have not been widely discussed in the medical literature, purportedly because there is no reasonable mechanism which could explain such a spectrum of health effects from a simple mental technology . . . Only in the last year has the stress connection emerged with the degree of clarity it now has. The . . . bottom line is the proposed vicious circle linking chronic stress, serotonin metabolism, and hippocampal regulation of the hypothalmic-pituitary-adrenocortical (HPA) axis. (p. 16)

A similar theory has been advanced by Everly and Benson (1989), who suggest that mediation is effective with a wide variety of conditions that may be called "disorders of arousal" in which the limbic system of the brain has become overstimulated. It is possible that relaxation and meditation work by "retuning" the nervous system by damping the production of adrenergic catecholamines which stimulate limbic activity. Everly and Benson further suggest that excessive limbic activity may also account for the association of chronic stress and increased susceptibility to infection.

INTERVENTION

While there are a wide variety of meditation techniques described in the literature (Carrington, 1984; Goleman, 1977; LeShan, 1974; Lichstein, 1988), the following four techniques will be described: transcendental meditation, centering prayer, relaxation response, and mindfulness meditation.

Techniques

Transcendental Meditation.   Transcendental meditation (TM), a much-publicized technique, was developed and introduced into the United States in the early 1960s by Indian leader Maharishi Mahesh Yogi. It is estimated that there are now well over two million practitioners. The concept of TM is relatively simple. Students are given a mantra (a word or sound) to repeat silently over and over again while sitting in a comfortable position. The mantra is selected not for its meaning but strictly for its sound. It is the understanding that this sound alone attracts the mind and leads it effortlessly and naturally to a slightly subtler level of the thinking process. If thoughts other than the mantra come to mind, the student is asked to notice them and return to the mantra. It is suggested that practitioners meditate for 20 minutes in the morning and again in the evening. TM is easily learned and is practiced by people of every age, education, culture, and religion. It is not a philosophy and does not require specific beliefs or changes in behavior or lifestyle (Russel, 1976).

Centering Prayer.   Centering prayer, while similar to TM in several respects, is Christianity-based and is designed to reduce the obstacles to contemplative prayer and union with God. Thomas Keating (1995), the founder of the centering prayer movement, describes centering prayer as a discipline designed to withdraw our attention from the ordinary flow of thoughts. The understanding is that people tend to identify with their thoughts, the debris that floats along the surface of the river, rather than being in touch with the river itself, the source from which these mental objects are emerging. Keating suggests that like boats or debris floating along the surface of a river, our thoughts and feelings must be resting on something. They are resting, he avers, on the inner stream of consciousness, which is our participation in God's being. As with TM, people are encouraged to find a comfortable position, to close their eyes and, in the case of centering prayer, to focus on a sacred word. Keating notes that 20 to 30 minutes is the minimum amount of time necessary for most people to establish interior silence and to get beyond their superficial thoughts.

Relaxation Response. The relaxation response incorporates four elements that are common in many of the other relaxation techniques. These elements are a quiet environment, a mental device, a passive attitude, and a comfortable position.

A quiet environment, which is an element of Benson's technique (1975), eliminates outside stimuli and allows the person to concentrate on the mental device. Some persons prefer a church or chapel for meditating, but such a place is usually not readily accessible. Playing music while meditating is not advocated because it may draw the person's attention away from the internal processes. Persons should select the place they wish to use for meditation and continue to use that place. This eliminates adjusting to new surroundings and stimuli each time a person meditates.

Use of a mental device helps to shift the mind from logical, externally oriented thought to inner rumination. The purpose of the mental device is to preoccupy oneself with an emotionally neutral, repetitive, and monotonous stimulus (Lichstein, 1988). Unlike TM, in which the teacher gives the student a mantra, Benson's technique requires each person to select the mental device that will be used whenever the person meditates. It may be a sound, word, or phrase that is repeated silently or aloud. Persons may choose to use a phrase or portion of a religious prayer or psalm. Fixation on an object also is sometimes used as the mental device.

Benson (1975) stresses that a passive attitude is the most important element in eliciting the physiological response resulting from meditation. Persons should be aware that distracting thoughts and images may occur. These should not be a cause of worry, but rather, a "let it happen" attitude should be assumed. When distractions do occur, the person is to simply return to use of the mental device. Repetition of the mental device or focusing attention on one's breathing helps in overcoming distractions. Distracting thoughts do not indicate that a person is not performing the technique correctly, but rather that renewed attention to the mental device is required. Even experienced meditators encounter distractions. Preparing oneself for meditation by relaxing the body helps reduce distractions. Progressive muscle relaxation and breathing techniques may be used to help achieve relaxation.

A comfortable position contributes to overall relaxation. Sitting in a chair that gives support to the body and yet allows for comfort is ideal. Sleep may result if the person tries to meditate in a recumbent position. Benson (1975) hypothesizes that the uncomfortable positions such as kneeling or sitting cross legged that are advocated in some techniques are intended to keep the person from falling asleep.

Mindfulness Meditation.   Mindfulness, awareness, or insight meditation are Western names used interchangeably to describe the Buddhist practice of *vipassana* meditation. The goal of this meditative practice is to increase insight by becoming a detached observer of the stream of changing thoughts, feelings, drives and visions until their nature and origin is recognized. The process includes eliciting the relaxation response, centering on breath, and then focusing attention freely from one perception to the next. In this form of meditation, no thought or sensation is considered an intrusion. When they drift into consciousness, they become the focus of attention (Kutz et al., 1985).

An extension of the practice of mindfulness meditation is what Borysenko (1988, p. 91) calls "meditation in action." It involves a "be here now" approach that allows life to unfold without the limitation of prejudgment. Using this approach, mindfulness exercises are carried out during normal, daily activities. It requires being open to an awareness of the moment as it is and to what the moment could hold. It produces a relaxed state of attentiveness to both the inner world of thoughts and feelings and the outer world of actions and perceptions. Borysenko notes that mindfulness requires a change in attitude: joy is not sought in finishing an activity, but rather in doing it.

GUIDELINES FOR MEDITATION

Borysenko (1988) describes a simple process of meditation that incorporates many of the concepts previously described and that can be used to teach meditation to patients:

1. Choose a quiet place where you will not be disturbed by other people or by the telephone.
2. Sit in a comfortable position with back straight and arms and legs uncrossed, unless you choose to sit cross-legged on a floor.
3. Close your eyes.
4. Relax your muscles sequentially from head to feet.
5. Focus on your breathing, noticing how the breath goes in and out, without trying to control it in any way.
6. Repeat your focus word silently in time with your breathing.

Coaching advises meditators not to worry about how they are doing. It is helpful to maintain a passive attitude and permit relaxation to occur at its own pace. When distracting thoughts occur, he counsels, try to ignore them by not dwelling on them and return to repeating chosen word. Success at meditation usually takes practice—at least once a day for 10 to 20 minutes.

Benson (1975) suggests that people wait for 2 hours after any meal before meditating, as the digestive processes seem to interfere with the elicitation of the relaxation response. He also emphasizes the importance of fitting the technique to the individual and making modifications as necessary. Therefore, before any teaching is initiated, an assessment of the individual is needed to determine what might be the most appropriate technique to use for a particular person or a specific condition. This requires that a nurse have knowledge about specific meditation techniques.

Mastery of meditation techniques result from daily or twice daily practice. LeShan (1974) commented that learning to meditate is hard work. Few authors provide information on the number of formal teaching sessions necessary for learning a technique although six or seven teaching sessions were recommended by Credidio (1982). According to Lehrer, Schoicket, Carrington, and Woolfolk (1980), 4 to 5 weeks of daily practice are needed before significant psychophysiologic changes are noted. Puente (1981) found that individuals who had meditated for a year and a half had the same physiological arousal levels as those who had meditated for more than five years.

USES

There is a substantial body of research supporting the use of meditation for a wide variety of conditions. Table 10.1 lists conditions for

TABLE 10.1   Conditions In Which Meditation Has Been Used

Anxiety (Miller, Fletcher, & Kabat-Zinn, 1995)
Asthma (Wilson, Honsberger, Chinn, & Novey, 1975)
Chronic pain (Kabat-Zinn, 1982; Kabat-Zinn, Lipworth, & Burney, 1985)
Coronary artery disease (Zamarra, Schneider, Besseghini, Robinson, &
    Salerno, 1996)
Coronary care units (Guzzetta, 1989; Melville, 1987)
Diagnostic procedures (Frenn, Fehring, & Kartes, 1986)
Desensitization for phobias (Goldfried, 1971)
Drug abuse (Benson & Wallace, 1972; Shafii, Lovely, & Jaffe, 1975)
Headache (Benson, Klemchuk, & Graham, 1974a)
Health promotion (Kolkmeier, 1988)
Hypertension (Benson, Rosner, Marzetta, & Klemchuk, 1974b; Blackwell et al.,
    1976; Schneider et al., 1995)
Insomnia (Woolfolk, Carr-Kaffashan, & McNulty, 1976)
Menstrual discomfort (Loevsky, 1978)
Posttraumatic stress disorder (Brooks & Scarano, 1985)
Psychotherapy (Bogart, 1991; Kutz et al., 1985)

which meditation has been used. Use of meditation for patients with chronic pain, hypertension, anxiety associated with coronary care units, and insomnia will be discussed.

In addition to being a low cost intervention with demonstrated efficacy, there is some data that suggest that meditative practices may also impact overall use of health care services. In a study comparing 2,000 people who meditated with a group of nonmeditators of comparable age, gender, and profession, it was found that over a 5-year period, use of medical services (visits to the doctor and hospitalizations) by the group who meditated was 30%–87% less than the group of non-meditators (Orme-Johnson, 1987). The difference was greatest for individuals over forty years of age.

Conditions and Populations

Chronic Pain.   Use of meditation for patients experiencing chronic pain has been well documented experientially and empirically. John Kabat-Zinn and colleagues (1985) in a study of mindfulness meditation with patients experiencing chronic pain found that statistically significant reductions were observed in measures of present-moment pain, negative body image, inhibition of activity by pain, mood disturbances, and psychological symptomatology including anxiety and depression. Additionally, drug utilization decreased and overall increases in activity levels and feelings of self-esteem were reported. In a follow-up 15 months after meditation training, improvements for all measures were maintained except for present-moment pain. The majority of participants in the study further reported high compliance with the meditation practice as part of their daily lives.

Hypertension. Benson (1975) explored the effectiveness of the relaxation response with persons who had hypertension because of the decreases in blood pressure experienced by persons who had practiced TM. Statistically significant changes between the experimental and control groups were found in his initial study. Mean systolic pressures decreased from 146 to 137 mm Hg, and mean diastolic pressures from 93.5 to 88.9 mm Hg in subjects who were taught and who practiced Benson's technique. Blood pressure was not measured immediately after the person had meditated, but rather readings were taken at random times throughout the day. It is hypothesized that meditation counteracts the sympathetic responses of the flight-fight reaction to stressors. Other studies (Benson, Rosner, et al., 1974; Blackwell et al., 1976; Pollock, Weber, Case, & Laragh, 1977) likewise found decreases in blood pressure in persons who regularly meditated. However, in the Blackwell and Pollock studies, only short-term (3-month) effects occurred. West (1980) attributes this to placebo effects showing diminishing returns with the passage of time. Alternatively, influence of the instructor may have prompted the persons to practice initially, and as the distance from this lengthened, the motivation to practice decreased. Benson (1975) stated that the relaxation response in and of itself will probably not be sufficient to lower severe or moderately high blood pressure, but its continued use will promote fewer or reduced doses of antihypertensive medications. Practice of meditation could potentially help to prevent the occurrence of hypertension.

Anxiety Associated with Coronary Care. A number of articles and several studies have explored the use of meditation with patients in coronary care units or those undergoing procedures related to coronary conditions (Frenn et al., 1986; Guzzetta, 1989; Melville, 1987; Moreno, 1987). Guzzetta studied the effects that music and the relaxation response had on various parameters of patients in coronary care units who had a myocardial infarct. Apical heart rates were lowered and peripheral temperatures were raised in subjects in these two groups as compared to subject in a control group. Patients in these two groups also had fewer complications. Although Frenn and colleagues did not find significant differences in parameters measured between the group taught the relaxation response and the control group in persons undergoing a cardiac catheterization, more subjects who practiced the relaxation response had lower respiratory rates, blood pressure, and scores on the state anxiety measure than did subjects in the control group. Thus, there is some evidence to support the use of relaxation response as an intervention for patients who may have increased anxiety because of the diagnosis of cardiac pathology or the fear of undergoing diagnostic procedures.

Insomnia.   Persons with high levels of stress frequently have difficulty getting to sleep or progressing through the normal sleep cycles. Interventions that seek to reduce stress levels should, therefore, improve sleep. Woolfolk and colleagues (1976) compared the effectiveness of meditation with progressive relaxation on decreasing insomnia. Significant improvement was found in both groups as compared to a control group. A follow-up at 6 months revealed that improvement persists over time. Many elderly experience difficulties with sleep. This is also a population for whom sleeping medications may cause dangerous untoward effects. Meditation may be an excellent alternative to medications for insomnia in the elderly.

Measurement of Outcomes

The purpose for which meditation is used will dictate the parameters to be used in evaluating its effectiveness. Commonly used measures include heart rate, blood pressure, respiratory rate, oxygen consumption, skin conductance, EEG and EMG recordings, scores on anxiety scales, and subjective reports. Benson (1975) reported that subjects practicing the relaxation response were calmer, more receptive to ideas, more patient, committed to daily exercise, less likely to use alcohol, and were happier overall. Although Credidio (1982) found no changes on the scores of the Eysenck Personality Inventory between persons taught meditation and persons in the control group, subjective reports indicated a positive reaction to the use of meditation. Because subjective reporting is a predictor of whether or not a person will continue to practice an intervention, how the person feels about the effects of meditation is important.

To document the efficacy of meditation, nurses in clinical areas can use blood pressure readings, heart rate, and respiratory rate as indicators of the effectiveness of meditation. Measures should not only be taken before and immediately after the practice of meditation, but also at other times during the day, with records kept to determine if changes occur over time. Because the person is resting while meditating, it would be expected that the readings would be lower after practice. It is also important that continued follow-up be done to determine if the effect persists over time.

PRECAUTIONS IN USE

Meditation is not a benign intervention. The nurse must be aware of side effects of the intervention, persons for whom it should not be used, and assessments to be made as the person practices meditation. Careful monitoring of reactions to medications is necessary, as doses may need to be altered. Everly and Rosenfeld (1981) noted problems of overdosage in the use of insulin, sedatives, and cardiovascular medications in persons who meditated. Because of the effect meditation can have on the cardiovascular system, the blood pressure should be checked before the person begins to meditate. It if is below 90 mm Hg, meditation should not be practiced. Patients should be instructed not to meditate if light-headedness or dizziness is felt. Also, the person should not stand immediately after meditating because a hypotensive state is frequently found.

Benson (1975) notes that hallucinations can occur if the person meditates for several hours at a time. Loss of contact with reality is a possibility and continued assessment is needed to determine if this is occurring. Lazarus (1976) reported cases of attempted suicide, schizophrenia, and severe depression after the continued practice of meditation. While meditation should perhaps not be prescribed for some people, the characteristics of people who would be harmed by meditation are unclear.

FURTHER RESEARCH

While nurses are increasingly using meditation within their practice, the research base within nursing for use of meditation is sparse. Much of the current research is being conducted by interdisciplinary teams. Because meditation holds great promise as a therapeutic nursing intervention, nurses should be encouraged to contribute to the research being conducted through either nursing investigations or interdisciplinary research. Questions and areas that merit further investigation include:

1. What are the characteristics of people who benefit from meditation? Do people who continue to practice meditation differ significantly from those who abandon it?
2. Longitudinal studies are needed to determine the long-term effects of meditation; the majority of studies have looked only at its immediate effects.
3. How generalizable are the effects of meditation? Does its use affect other areas of the person's life than those for which it was taught? If the person is taught meditation as a means for decreasing hypertension, is there also an improvement in sleep and/or other areas?
4. People vary in their motive for engaging in a meditative practice. Some use meditation as a spiritual discipline while others are primarily seeking health benefits. Do health outcomes differ based on a person's motivation?
5. How does meditation differ from other forms of self-regulation, such as hypnosis, relaxation, and guided imagery, in process and outcome?

REFERENCES

Benson, H. (1975). *The relaxation response.* New York: Avon.

Benson, H., Klemchuk, H., & Graham, J. (1974). The usefulness of the relaxation response in the therapy of headache. *Headache,14,* 49–52.

Benson, H., Rosner, B., Marzetta, B., & Klemchuk, H. (1974). Decreased blood pressure in pharmacologically treated hypertensive patients who regularly elicited the relaxation response. *Lancet, i,* 289–291.

Benson, H., & Wallace, R. (1972). Decreased drug abuse with transcendental meditation: A study of 1,862 subjects. In C. Arafontis (Ed)., *Drug abuse: Proceedings of the international conference* (pp. 369–376). Philadelphia: Lea & Febiger.

Blackwell, B., Henenson, I., Bloomfield, S., Magenheim, H., Gartide, P., Nidich, S., Robinson, A., & Zigler, R. (1976). Transcendental meditation in hypertension, individual response patterns. *Lancet, i,* 223–226.

Bogart, G. (1991). The use of meditation in psychotherapy: A review of the literature. *American Journal of Psychotherapy, 45,* 383–412.

Borysenko, J. (1988). *Minding the body, mending the mind.* New York: Bantam.

Brooks, J. S., & Scarano, T. (1985). Transcendental meditation in the treatment of post-Vietnam adjustment. *Journal of Counseling and Development, 64,* 212–215.

Carrington, P. (1984). Modern forms of meditation. In R. Woolfolk & P. Lehrer (Eds.), *Principles and practice of stress management* (pp. 108–141). New York: Guilford.

Credidio, S. (1982). Comparative effectiveness of patterned biofeedback vs. meditation training on EMG and skin temperature changes. *Behavior Research and Therapy, 20,* 233–241.

Everly, B. & Benson, H. (1989). Disorders of arousal and the relocation response: speculations on the nature and treatment of stress-related diseases. *International Journal of Psychosomatic, 36,* 15–21.

Everly, G., & Rosenfeld, R. (1981). *The nature and treatment of the stress responses.* New York: Plenum.

Frenn, M., Fehring, R., & Kartes, S. (1986). Reducing the stress of cardiac catheterization by teaching relaxation. *Dimensions of Critical Care Nursing, 5,* 108–116.

Goldfried, M. (1971). Systematic desensitization as training in self control. *Journal of Consulting and Clinical Psychology, 39,* 228–234.

Goleman, D. (1977). *The varieties of the meditative experience.* New York: Dutton.

Goleman, D., & Schwartz, G. (1976). Meditation as an intervention in stress reactivity. *Journal of Consulting and Clinical Psychology, 44,* 456–466.

Guzzetta, C.E. (1989). Effects of relaxation and music therapy on patients in a coronary care unit with presumptive acute myocardial infarct. *Heart & Lung, 18,* 609–616.

Kabat-Zinn, J. (1982). An outpatient program in behavioral medicine for chronic pain based on the practice. *General Hospital Psychiatry, 4,* 33–47.

Kabat-Zinn, J., Lipworth, L. & Burney, R. (1985). The clinical use of mindfulness meditation for the self-regulation of chronic pain. *Journal of Behavioral Medicine, 8*(2), 163–190.

Keating, T. (1995). *Open mind open heart.* New York: Continuum.

Kolkmeier, L. G. (1988). Relaxation: Opening the door to change. In B. Dossey, L. Keegan, C. Guzzetta, & L. Kolkmeier (Eds.), *Holistic nursing—a handbook for practice* (pp. 195–222). Rockville, MD: Aspen.

Kutz, I., Leserman, J., Dorrington, C., Morrison, C., Borysenko, J. & Benson, H. (1985). Meditation as an adjunct to psychotherapy. *Psychotherapy and Psychosomatics, 43*(4), 209–218.

Lazarus, A. (1976). Psychiatric problems precipitated by transcendental meditation. *Psychological Report, 39,* 601–602.

Lehrer, P., Schoicket, S., Carrington, P., and Woolfolk, R. (1980). Psy-

chophsiological and cognitive responses to stressful stimuli in subjects practicing progressive relaxation and clinically standardized
meditation. *Behavior Research and Therapy,18*, 293–303.

LeShan, L. (1974). *How to meditate.* Boston: Little, Brown.

Lichstein, K. L. (1988). *Clinical relaxation strategies.* New York: Wiley.

Loevsky, J. (1978). Menstruation: Alternatives to pharmacological therapy
for menstrual distress. *Journal of Nurse-Midwifery, 23,* 34–44.

Melville, S.B. (1987). Relaxation techniques in acute myocardial infarction: the theoretic rationale. *Focus on Critical Care, 14*(1), 9–11.

Miller, J. J., Fletcher, K. & Kabat-Zinn, J. (1995). Three-year follow-up and
clinical implications of a mindfulness meditation-based stress reduction intervention in the treatment of anxiety disorders. *General Hospital Psychiatry, 17,* 192–200.

Moreno, C. K. (1987). Concepts of stress management in cardiac rehabilitation. *Focus on Critical Care, 14*(5), 13–19.

National Institutes of Health. (1992). *Alternative medicine: Expanding medical horizons.* Washington, DC: US Government Printing Office.

Orme-Johnson, D. W. (1987). Medical care litigation and the transcendental meditation program. *Psychosomatic Medicine, 49,* 493–507.

Pollock, A., Weber, M., Case, D., & Laragh, J. (1977). Limitations of
transcendental meditation in the treatment of essential hypertension.
Lancet, i, 71–73.

Puente, A. (1981). Psychophysiological investigations on transcendental
meditation. *Biofeedback and Self-Regulation, 6,* 327–342.

Russel, P. (1976). *The TM technique.* Boston: Routledge and Kegan.

Schneider, R. H., Staggers, F., Alexander, C. W., Sheppard, W., Rainforth,
M., Kondwani, K., Smith, S. & King, C. G. (1995). A randomized
controlled trial of stress reduction for hypertension in older African-
Americans. *Hypertension 26,* 820–827.

Shafii, M. (1973). Adaptive and therapeutic aspects of meditation. *International Journal of Psychoanalysis and Psychotherapy, 2,* 431–443.

Shafii, M., Lovely, R., & Jaffe, R. (1975). Meditation and the prevention
of alcohol abuse. *American Journal of Psychiatry, 132,* 942–945.

Tart, C. (1971). A psychologist's experiences with transcendental meditation. *Journal of Transpersonal Psychology, 3,* 135–143.

Welwood, J. (1979). *The meeting of the ways: Explorations in East/West psychology.* New York: Schocken.

West, M. (1979). The psychosomatics of meditation. *Journal of Psychosomatic Medicine, 24,* 265–273.

West, M. (1980). Meditation. *British Journal of Psychiatry, 135,* 457–467.

Wilson, A. F., Honsberger, R. W., Chin, R. T. & Novey, H. S. (1975).
Transcendental meditation and asthma. *Respiration, 32,* 74–80.

Woolfolk, R., Carr-Kaffashan, L., & McNulty, T. (1976). Meditation training as a treatment for insomnia. *Behavior Therapy, 7,* 350–365.

Zamarra, J. W., Schneider, R. H., Besseghini, I., Robinson, D. K. & Salerno, J. W. (1996). Usefulness of the transcendental meditation program in the treatment of patients with coronary artery disease. *American Journal of Cardiology, 77,* 867.

11

AROMATHERAPY

Kirsten James

The use of aromatic oils has a long standing history in a number of different cultures, although the literature indicates that exact dates of origin are difficult to pinpoint. Some authors suggest that Australian aborigines used native plants for medicinal purposes as far back as 40,000 years ago (Alcorn, cited in Mackreth, 1995; Stevensen, 1995). Most authors, however, describe historical links to ancient Egyptian, Greek and Eastern (both Chinese and Indian) civilizations, as far back as 4,500 BC. Tisserand (1994), in his well-known book, *The Art of Aroma Therapy*, provides an extensive historical bibliography which dates back to *The Yellow Emperor's Classic of Internal Medicine*, circa 2650 BC.

The Arab physician Avicenna (AD 980–1037) is credited with the invention of the distillation process, enabling the extraction of essential oils and aromatic waters to be more efficient and refined. However, an archaeological discovery in 1975 of the Indus Valley civilization in Pakistan revealed perfume containers and perfectly preserved distillation apparatus suggesting that this process could be over 4,000 years old (Lawless, 1992).

The use of oils in religious ceremonies and rituals, including embalming and purifying, is well cited, as are other functions including fumigating, cleansing, healing, and beautifying (Lawless, 1992; Price, 1991; Tisserand, 1994). The Crusaders are credited with bringing the perfumes of Arabia back to Europe.

There was an apparent recognition of the antiseptic and bactericidal properties of certain oils, as well as an awareness of their positive effects on the immune system during the European plagues of the Middle Ages, and it is interesting to note today that many of our household cleaning and disinfecting products are scented with the fragrance of such oils, for example pine, lemon, eucalyptus and tea tree.

The term *aromatherapie* was coined by a French chemist, Gattefosse, who explored the therapeutic possibilities of essential oils while working in his family's perfumery in the 1920s. His work was further advanced by another Frenchman, Dr. Valnet, who became interested in the healing properties of essential oils following his successful treatment of specific medicinal and psychiatric conditions; his results were published in *Aromatherapie* in 1964 (Tisserand, 1994).

The holistic use of essential oils, however, is credited to Madame Maury, a French biochemist who introduced them to beauty therapy, where they became commonly used in skin preparations and massage. She aimed to revitalize her clients and chose oils to personally suit their temperament and particular health problem (Lawless, 1992; Price, 1991).

Today we see aromatic oils used as natural flavorings in foods, as perfumes in skin care and other beauty products, and in cleaning products. Clove, peppermint, and spearmint provide the refreshing and stimulating effects of toothpastes; eucalyptus is a component of medicinal inhalations and liniments; and teatree and lavender are found in antiseptic creams.

DEFINITION

Aromatherapy can be simply defined as the therapeutic use of aromatic substances derived from plants (Vickers, 1996). Essential oils are fragrant volatile liquids and are obtained from the tiny glands in the fruits or berries (e.g., juniper), petals (e.g., rose), leaves (e.g., geranium) and wood (e.g., sandalwood). These

> essences are like the blood of a person. . . . Like blood they die (lose their life force) if they are not properly preserved. Like blood they incorporate the characteristics of the body (plant) from which they come. They are like the personality, or spirit of the plant. (Tisserand, 1994, p. 8)

Aromatherapy can be used to treat a variety of physical conditions, but can also affect the mind and emotions (Davis, 1988; Stevensen, 1995; Tisserand, 1994; Worwood, 1992). Tisserand (1994) explains that because the essence is the most ethereal and subtle part of the plant, it has a more pronounced effect on the mind and emotions than herbal medicine.

The essential oil yield of a plant varies. For example, it takes 2 kg (4.4 lbs) of rose petals to produce 1 g (2.2 oz) of essential rose oil (Tisserand, 1994; White & Day, 1994). It is also important to note that the quality and chemical content of the oil is influenced by where it is grown. Soil quality, altitude and climate are determinants, and suppliers of quality essential oils will source their oils from all around the world. For example, France, Bulgaria, and Australia are recognized as producing the finest quality lavender (*lavender officinalis*). This is why the pure, unadulterated essential oils vary in price; some are very expensive (Meyer, 1996). Aromatherapists only use whole essential oils from a single botanical source, which are named according to the genus and species of plant from which they are extracted (Vickers, 1996).

The two most common methods of oil extraction are steam distillation and simple pressing (extraction). Most oils are obtained using the steam distillation process, which isolates the various constituents of the plant.

Essential oils are highly volatile; they dissolve in pure alcohol, fats, and oils but not in water. Therefore they will evaporate readily if left exposed to the air and have a limited lifespan of approximately two years (Lawless, 1992). Because they are also sensitive to heat and light, they are preferably kept in dark glass bottles which should be stored to prevent contamination from other sources (Day & White, 1994; Stevensen, 1995; Tiran, 1996).

Oils are classified by their volatility, being accorded either top, middle, or bass "notes" (Lawless, 1992; Maxwell-Hudson, 1988):

- Top notes evaporate most quickly and are usually uplifting (e.g., lemon, mandarin, basil, tea tree, eucalyptus);
- Middle notes usually have a balancing effect (e.g., geranium, lavender, marjoram, rosewood);
- Base notes are slowest to evaporate and are therefore calming (e.g., patchouli, rose, jasmine, frankincense, and myrrh).

SCIENTIFIC BASIS

An instrument known as a liquid gas chromatograph is used to analyze the chemical components of each essential oil, and internationally accepted levels have been determined. The gas chromatograph can analyze the different chemical properties and compounds in each essential oil, which are thought to give the oil its characteristic therapeutic property. This type of analysis can also demonstrate the proportions of each compound in an oil, and can distinguish between plant varieties, geographical locations and even the life-cycle stage at harvesting (Stevensen, 1995; Vickers, 1996).

The chemical compounds found in essential oils include alcohols, esters, ketones, aldehydes, oxides, coumarins and lactones, phenols and terpenes. Generally speaking, those oils that are high in esters and alcohols are safe for home use and contain healing properties. Esters, for example, are the most common compounds found in essential oils and occur in oils of bergamot, clary sage, lavender, sweet marjoram, and others. They tend to be fruity in aroma and have sedative and fungicidal properties (Lawless, 1992; Price, 1991).

Despite scientific research, the exact therapeutic mechanism of aromatherapy is not completely understood, although there is evidence to suggest that two principal routes are involved: inhalation via the olfactory system, and absorption through the skin.

With olfaction, it is thought that the inhaled essential oil particles are picked up by tiny cilia, each equipped with thousands of receptor cells, located at the roof of the nose. The "smell message" then travels to the brain where it is processed by the limbic system which influences our emotional, hormonal, metabolic and stress responses (Hogan, 1995; Price, 1991; Vickers, 1996).

In the Unitd Kingdom and the United States, the most widely used method of administering essential oils is by adding a few drops to a "carrier" oil or lubricant, which is then applied via massage. It is believed that the tiny essential oil molecules readily permeate the skin through to the capillaries where they are transported around the body (Price 1991; Vickers, 1996).

INTERVENTION

Essential oils can be used in massage (blended with a carrier oil), baths, compresses and inhalations. The oils may also be vaporized in a number of different ways (see below). Ingestion is a contentious issue (Vickers, 1996) and although common in France, is not often seen in the U.K., U.S., or Australia; it is not recommended by the International Federation of Aromatherapists (Meyer, 1996).

General Guidelines

As previously mentioned, there are a number of different ways in which essential oils can be applied. A single favorite oil can be used, or a combination of up to three different oils for the following methods of application:

Massage:	Half the number of essential oil drops to milliliters of massage base oil, e.g., 5 drops essential oil : 10 ml base (carrier) oil.
Inhalation:	4–5 drops essential oil in a bowl of very hot water.
Compress:	3–4 drops essential oil in a bowl of water (temperature depends on condition). Agitate water gently to disperse oil; soak a small cotton or toweling cloth in bowl, ensuring cloth has absorbed oil. Gently squeeze cloth of excess water, and apply to skin.
Baths:	6–8 drops added to bath; agitate surface to disperse molecules. The oils can be mixed with milk before adding to facilitate dispersion. Gently pat the skin dry afterwards to leave a fine layer of oils on the skin for further absorption.
Hand/Footbaths:	2–3 drops essential oil in a bowl of warm water; agitate gently.
Vaporizers:	Candle generated: 8–10 drops essential oil added to water in dish; Electric: 5–6 drops.

Recommended essential oil blends (White & Day, 1994, pp. 13–16) and Meyer (1996) which could be used with one of the above-mentioned methods to promote relaxation and well-being include:

1. Lavender (3 drops), Patchouli (2 drops) and Orange (2 drops)
2. Marjoram (2 drops), Lavender (3 drops) and Sandalwood (2 drops)
3. Geranium (2 drops), Lavender (3 drops) and Cedarwood (2 drops)

USES

Guideline Example: Vaporizing

One method that is practical and effective is vaporizing. Aromatherapists claim that vaporized essential oils can help to eliminate airborne bacteria, therapeutically affect the emotions and mask undesirable odors. Many nurses could undoubtedly find a great need for this in their workplace situation! The beauty of this technique is that patients and staff can all benefit.

It is important to note, however, that as nurses we must always respect the rights and comfort of individual patients. Thus, we need to check the appropriateness of vaporizing in a shared room. Although a particular oil may have certain therapeutic properties, an individual patient may have a negative memory association with a fragrance and find the effect of the oil upsetting or even nauseating (Mackreth, 1995). To vaporize essential oils for a single individual, a few drops of oil can be placed on a tissue, handkerchief, or even a pillow case. Another method is to use a necklace which has a special interchangeable vaporizing disc.

For rooms, light bulb ring burners can be used. These are hollow, circular rings made from either metal or clay which sit over the top of a low-wattage light bulb. Once positioned, a few drops of oil or oils can be placed in the ring, and once the light is turned on, the heat generated helps to permeate the room with aroma.

Vaporizers usually come in three different forms: *aromatizers* which are made of glass and run on electricity, *ceramic electric burners* and *candle-generated* vaporizers of ceramic or metal. The former two are more suitable for hospital usage because the candles present a fire hazard. At home, however, the candle vaporizers help to create a pleasant ambience which adds another therapeutic dimension. A small amount of water (around one to two tablespoons) is placed in the vaporizer bowl, to which approximately 8–10 drops of oil are added (Price 1991). The candle's heat facilitates evaporation and the room soon fills with the chosen scent. The vaporizer bowl should be replenished with water and oil as necessary. In a coronary care unit in Melbourne, Australia, the nurses routinely check the vaporizers once they have checked their drugs of addiction stock at the end of each shift (Hudson, 1996).

Conditions/Populations Suited to Aromatherapy

Although there are a number of ways in which essential oils can be used therapeutically in nursing to treat specific conditions (including nausea, muscular aches and pains, headaches, wound healing, etc.), it is advisable on legal, safety, political and professional grounds to exercise caution. It may be best to leave medical use to the professional aromatherapist.

In the U.K. and Australia, many nurses in professional settings have chosen to use aromatherapy to promote relaxation and to enhance well-being. This path is particularly recommended when venturing into this form of complementary therapies for the first time. Chamomile, lavender, marjoram and ylang ylang are all hypnotics, which induce a calm and restful sleep; for a sedative and calming effect on the nervous system, bergamot, frankincense, sandalwood, rose otto, geranium, orange, or patchouli are just some of the oils that could be used. Different blends of oils can be used to achieve a relaxing environment. *It is strongly advised to consult with a qualified practitioner,* and to also select a simple range of no more than three to four oils to begin with. Any sensitivities or allergies can thus be more readily detected and cost can be held down.

Precautions

Other than what has already been stated, I would like to defer to Caroline Stevensen's "Contraindications for Use" (1995, pp. 55–56):

- If essential oils are administered with massage, then the contraindications for massage apply.
- Essential oils must always be diluted before applying to the skin; the dilution will depend on the particular essential oil used and the age, size, and condition of the patient.
- Sensitive patients or those with allergies should be treated with caution; a simple patch test of the proposed blend of oils should be applied, if in doubt, before proceeding with full massage.
- Oils for inhalation via fragrancers (like vaporizers) should be selected for the individual patient rather than a whole ward.
- Toxicity and contraindications for each oil must be well understood.
- Keep essential oils away from eyes and mucous membranes.
- In pregnancy, many oils are contraindicated due to toxic risk to mother and foetus or risk of spontaneous abortion.
- Many oils are toxic and not recommended for general use.
- Avoid using oils that elicit a negative psychological response from the patient by asking them about their preferences and responses.
- Due to the strong association that smell can have with memory, special care should be taken with patients undergoing chemotherapy or those feeling very unwell or sensitive; the smell of an oil present at an uncomfortable time could, in a subsequent context, induce nausea, vomiting, or negative emotions.

• Aromatherapy is not for dabblers; undergo professional training before treating patients.

RESEARCH QUESTIONS

Andrew Vickers (1996), in his recent publication *Massage and Aromatherapy: A Guide for Health Professionals* has undertaken a thorough and comprehensive review of the literature available on both aromatherapy and massage. In his summary of findings on both the basic and clinical research, he concludes that findings are very disappointing: Although numerous studies have been performed, few are good quality and claims by aromatherapists "remain unevaluated." (p. 169)

He does, however, point out that client group responses have indicated that aromatherapy treatments can be pleasurable and that most people report an improved sense of well-being after an aromatherapy treatment. For health care practitioners who have a keen desire to enhance the quality of patients' lives, the opportunities for research are begging! For example:

1. Does the use of lavender and other relaxing oils reduce aggressive behaviors in elders wiht dementia?
2. What is the length of time to use essential oils to obtain therapeutic results?
3. Does use of stimulating oils have an impact on postoperative patients?

REFERENCES

Davis, P. (1988). *Aromatherapy An A–Z*. Essex, UK: Daniel.

Hudson, S. (1996). Complementary therapies & high tech care. *Australian Nursing Journal, 4*(4), 34–36.

Lawless, J. (1992). *The encyclopedia of essential oils*. Longmead, Shaftsbury, Dorset, UK: Element Books.

Mackreth, P. (1995). Aromatherapy: Nice but not 'essential'. *Complementary Therapies in Nursing & Midwifery, 1*, 4–7.

Maxwell-Hudson, C. (1988). *The complete book of massage*. Brookevale, NSW: Simon & Schuster.

Price, S. (1991). *Aromatherapy for common ailments*. Sydney, Australia: Angus & Robertson.

Stevensen, C. (1995). Aromatherapy. In D. Rankin-Box (Ed.), *The nurses' handbook of complementary therapies.* (pp. 51–58). Edinburgh, UK: Churchill Livingstone.

Tiran, D. (1996). Aromatherapy in midwifery: Benefits and risks. *Complementary Therapies in Nursing & Midwifery, 2,* 88–92.

Tisserand, R. (1994). *The art of aromatherapy* (rev. ed.). Essex, England: Daniel.

Vickers, A. (1996). *Massage and aromatherapy: A guide for health professionals.* London: Chapman Hall.

White, J., & Day, K. (1994). *Aromatherapy for scents & scentuality.* Brighton-Le-Sands, NSW: Nacson.

Worwood, V. (1992). *The fragrant pharmacy.* London: Macmillan.

12

PURPOSEFUL TOUCH

Mariah Snyder and Yoshiko Nojima

Nurses frequently implement touch in patient interactions. Krieger (1975) stated that touch was the imprimatur of nursing (p. 784). Because nurses use touch so frequently, they may not be consciously aware that they are implementing the intervention or how it is affecting the patient. Touch is often a component of many other nursing interventions.

Touch as a nursing intervention is receiving renewed attention throughout the world. The role that touch plays in the healing process has been the focus of numerous articles. The American Holistic Nursing Association and other organizations offer courses in healing touch. Although therapeutic touch is a component of these courses, strategies for implementing purposeful or caring touch are also included.

DEFINITION

Purposeful touch will be described in this chapter. This type of touch has also been termed affective touch (Seaman, 1982), comforting touch (Bottorff, 1993) and empathetic touch (Gadow, 1984). Purposeful touch is the intentional physical contact with the patient by the nurse with the intent of helping. This definition connotes intentionality on the part of the nurse and interpersonal interaction between the nurse and the patient (Schoenhofer, 1989).

Purposeful touch is one of three types of touch identified by Estabrooks (1989). The other two types in Estabrook's paradigm are instrumental and protective. *Instrumental* touch is the touching that is part of assessment and care; taking a patient's pulse is an example of instrumental touch. (Bottorff [1993] used the term *working* touch synonymously.) *Protective* touch is used to protect the patient or others; an example is a nurse restraining a patient's hand or arm so the person is unable to pull out an intravenous line. From an observation study, Bottorff (1993) identified three additional types of touch: connecting, orienting, and social.

Weiss (1979) described six components of purposeful touch: duration, location, action, intensity, frequency, and sensation. *Duration* of touch is the temporal length of the touch from the initiation of the contact to its cessation. *Location* is the area of the body being touched. The most frequent areas touched by nurses are the hands, arms, and shoulders (Pratt & Mason, 1981; Schoenhofer, 1989). Social and cultural norms influence the areas of the body the nurse can acceptably touch. The characteristic of *action* refers to the specific gesture used in touching; examples include holding, touching, patting, rubbing, or squeezing. *Intensity* is the degree of pressure applied. Different situations and areas of the body require different intensities. *Frequency* refers to how often the touching is done. *Sensation* denotes the perceived comfort or discomfort from the touch; past experiences and the integrity of the neurological system affect the sensation experienced. Nurses cannot assume that everyone finds touch to be comforting. Although characteristics of touch identified by Weiss (1979) have been publicized, few studies have examined how the specific characteristics contribute to the outcomes resulting from purposeful touch.

SCIENTIFIC BASIS

The somesthetic system, which includes receptors for touch, vibration, pain, and temperature, is paramount in the efficacy of touch. All or some of these receptors may be involved when touch is used. Stimuli increase the permeability of the receptor cell membrane, generating impulses in the sensory nerves. Depolarization of the sensory nerve fiber follows; this is termed the *generator potential*. The potential varies depending on the strength of the stimulus. Adaptation occurs if the stimulus is applied constantly for a period of time. Impulses from the receptors are transmitted to the brain primarily via the lateral spinothalamic tract and the sensory component of the cranial nerves. The impulses are relayed to the thalamus before terminating in the postcentral gyrus of the parietal lobe. The face, hands, and feet have larger representations in the somatosensory area of the parietal lobe than do other areas of the body.

The process of touching stimulates feelings and thoughts on the part of both the giver and the receiver. According to Schoenhofer (1989), touch brings about changes in the neural, endocrine, muscular, and cognitive systems. It is more than just a physical modality. The feelings and past experiences of the nurse and the patient all have an impact on the outcomes from use of touch.

Touch is also transactional in nature. When a nurse uses purposeful touch, both the nurse and the patient change with the experience. The interaction has an impact on subsequent use and reception of touch. For example, if a patient finds the touch to be comforting, he or she will bring a pleasant memory to the next encounter with touch. Positive responses from patients provide nurses with confidence in using touch in interactions with other patients.

Touch is the most frequent nonverbal type of communication used. Research has shown that holding a patient's hand during stressful situations conveys concern and provides a sense of security (Morales, 1994; Schoenfofer, 1989). According to Kubler-Ross (1969), a gentle pressure on the hand is the most meaningful communication that a nurse can have with a dying patient. Many anecdotal reports substantiate that touch conveys caring and reduces stress.

INTERVENTION

A variety of techniques can be used to implement purposeful touch. These include handholding, stroking or patting a patient's arm, hand, or face; placing one's hand on a patient's shoulder or circling one's arm around the patient's shoulder; and hugging. Tactile stimulation, a form of purposeful touch, is more forceful in nature and is used to achieve arousal in patients with decreased levels of arousal (Helwick, 1994).

Purposeful touch has been equated with caring. Thus, the intent and demeanor of the nurse is an important element of the intervention. Centering oneself prior to implementing purposeful touch focuses the nurse on the patient. Centering is described in Chapter 5.

A number of factors affect the outcomes resulting from purposeful touch. Schoenhofer (1989) examined nurse and patient variables that may have an impact on the outcomes. Nurse variables included the nurse's emotional state and the nurse's level of energy. Patient factors that may influence the impact of touch include the cognitive and emotional status of the patient, past experiences with touch, and the area of the body being touched. Pratt and Mason (1981) noted that the lower arms and the back were the most commonly touched areas for expressing understanding and sympathy. Patients' hands and shoulders were the areas of the body intensive care nurses touched most frequently when using purposeful touch. Cultural practices affect the acceptable areas of the body to use in purposeful touch (Fisher & Joseph, 1989).

Careful assessment of patients is needed before purposeful touch is used. When initially greeting the patient the nurse notes whether the patient extends his or her hand or tends to withdraw. If a handshake is made, is it a strong shake or a floppy one? When touching a patient, what are the facial expressions noted? Past abuses may make some persons reluctant to be touched. Gentle approaches may help to overcome fears. Fisher and Joseph (1989) developed a scale to measure patient attitudes about purposeful touch.

Handholding

In Western cultures, a handshake is often used in establishing a relationship with another person. Extending one's hand to another person is viewed as a sign of friendship or agreement. Extending one's hand for a handshake does not invade another's territory as much as other forms of touch (e.g., an embrace). The person to whom the hand is extended has the opportunity to withdraw or reject the extended hand.

Several techniques can be used for handholding. The nurse can place a hand on top of the patient's hand, grasp the hand as in a handshake, or place one of the patient's hands between two hands. Guidelines for implementing handholding follow. Many variations of this technique can be made depending on the status of the patient and the setting of the interaction.

1. Center self by focusing on the current moment, eliminating distractions, and putting the patient's welfare foremost in your thoughts.
2. Sit next to the patient and talk with the patient for a short period of time. Continue to carry on conversation with the patient throughout the handholding. If the patient is unable to

communicate verbally, talk to the patient. (Entering phase as designated by Estabrooks & Morse, 1992.)
3. Extend your hands slowly toward the patient. (Connecting phase as designated by Estabrooks & Morse, 1992.) Make sure your hands are warm before touching the patient.
4. Put one hand under and one hand on top of one of the patient's hands. Do this in such a manner that the arm of the patient is supported. Hold the hands for several minutes.
5. Gently stroke the hand, if you wish. Your hands may be moved and the pressure lightened or increased depending on the patient's response.
6. During the handholding, observe the patient for reactions and adjust the length of time the hands are held and the pressure used.
7. Remove your top hand slowly and then the bottom hand. Sit for a short period before terminating the interaction. Thank the patient for the time spent. Elicit feedback about the interaction if deemed feasible.

The length of time a hand should be held was not indicated in any of the studies reviewed (Copstead, 1980; Knable, 1981; McCorkle, 1974; Pollack & Goldstein, 1981; Schoenhofer, 1989; Tobiason, 1981). Walleck (1982) stroked the patient's arm or face for 2 minutes in an effort to promote relaxation and reduce intracranial pressure.

Measurement of Effectiveness

The purpose for which purposeful touch is used determines the indexes to be used to measure its effectiveness. Physiological parameters that have been measured include heart rate, intracranial pressure, and blood pressure. Psychological variables that have been examined in touch studies have included comfort level, cognitive ability, and self-appraisal. Obtaining anecdotal information about a patient's response to touch is also useful in planning subsequent uses of the intervention.

USES

Purposeful touch is a widely used nursing intervention with many populations. In a review of nurse-patient touch, Bottorff (1991) reported 12 studies in which touch with children had been explored

TABLE 12.1   Use of Touch

Stress Management
  Decreases in intracranial pressure (Walleck, 1982)
  Lessening of anxiety (Triplett & Arneson, 1979)
  Increase in relaxation (Snyder, Egan, & Burns (1995)
  Reduced arousal (Weiss, 1990)

Communication
  Encouragement (Schoenhofer, 1989)
  Emotional support (Knable, 1981; Schoenhofer, 1989)
  Improved attitude toward task (Lange-Alberts & Shott, 1994)
  Increased feeling of affection (Moore & Gilbert, 1995)
  Positive expectations (Morales, 1994)
  Reawakening of perceptual abilities (Hollinger, 1980)

and 38 studies focusing on touch with adults. The majority of these latter studies were on the use of touch in elders. Table 12.1 lists some of the specific conditions or outcomes for which touch has been used.

Stress Management

The soothing effect that purposeful touch has on persons with high levels of stress has been shown in several studies (American Association of Retired Persons [AARP], 1993; Green, 1994; Richter, Roberto, & Bottenberg, 1995; Weiss, 1990). In an anecdotal report (AARP, 1993), elderly volunteers held the hands of elders undergoing cataract surgery. Outcomes included a feeling of confidence and relaxation and lowered blood pressure. Triplett and Arneson (1979) found use of verbal and tactile stimulation reduced distress in hospitalized children.

Several studies have shown that purposeful touch has contributed to decreases in intracranial pressure. These effects may be due to the impact that touch has on reducing stress. Walleck (1982) used purposeful touching of the face and hands of patients with severe head injuries. Touch resulted in decreases in intracranial pressure; greater decreases were found with touching of the face. Pollack and Goldstein (1981) noted decreases in intracranial pressure in patients with Reyes syndrome following gentle touching.

Communication

Purposeful touch is used extensively to communicate with persons who are confused, have decreased levels of arousal, or who are cognitively impaired. According to Hagland (1995), a great need exists for nurses working with patients in critical care units to expand their repertoire of strategies for communicating with this population. Increased use of purposeful touch is suggested. A gentle touch on the arm or circling an arm around a shoulder communicate to persons who have suffered losses or feel alone that someone else cares.

Use of touch with elders has been emphasized by many nurses. Because of hearing and vision deficits, other means to communicate with elders are needed. Some of the earliest studies on touch explored its use with elders (Barnett, 1972; Copstead, 1980; Tobiason, 1981). In a study by Moore and Gilbert (1995), nursing home residents reported that comforting touch by nurses increased their feelings of affection and immediacy. Smiles and touch were found to be strategies nursing assistants used to communicate with elders who had dementia (Richter et al., 1995). Touch used in conjunction with verbal cuing was found by Lange-Alberts and Shott (1994) to improve the nutritional intake of hospitalized elders.

Precautions

Adequate assessment of patients prior to using touch is essential. Nurses need to be cognizant of cultural differences in relation to touch. Although many times touch is used to establish a relationship with a patient (Schoenhofer, 1989), in some situations touch can only be used effectively after a trusting relationship has been established through other means. Some reluctance has existed in using touch on patients who have cardiac conditions because of the fear that the touching would increase heart rate and blood pressure. Findings from a study by Weiss (1990) indicate that such fears are not founded, and that touch served to reduce arousal.

Patting was noted as being one technique for purposeful touch. Patting, especially of the head, can be interpreted as condescension or being treated like a child (Walters, 1994). Some nurses pat a patient's hand to gain the person's attention. Because of the negative connotations that can be attached to patting, care must be taken in its use.

The intervention of purposeful touch needs to be addressed in nursing curricula. It cannot be assumed that students possess knowledge about assessment or implementation techniques. Observing expert nurses who are role models for use of purposeful touch and discussions about use of touch will help students gain confidence in its use.

FURTHER RESEARCH

As has been noted earlier, considerably more research on use of purposeful touch is needed to provide direction for its use. Weiss (1988), Schoenhofer (1989), and Bottorff (1991) have reviewed studies related to touch and provide multiple suggestions for future research. Specific areas in which research is needed include:

1. Review of the literature to identify whether the investigators have specified the type of touch used. For example, Burgener, Jirovec, Murrell, and Barton (1992) noted that no improvement in behaviors in elders with dementia was found when caregivers touched the elders. However, the type of touch used was not noted. Additional research is needed on reactions to purposeful touch versus procedural and other types of touch.
2. Variations in the impact of the various qualities of touch delineated by Weiss (1988) and others. Knable (1981) reported that in observational study patients reached out and grasped the nurse's hand after the nurse had terminated the handholding. Questions such as, "How long should the nurse hold a patient's hand?" and "When is gentler touch superior to firm touching and vice versa?" need to be explored.
3. The effect of the gender of the nurse on the outcomes achieved from handholding or other types of touch. Both the gender of the nurse and the gender of the patient need to be examined. Snyder, Egan, and Burns (1995) found that the incidence of aggressive behaviors increased in male elders with dementia who received hand massage, in contrast to a decrease in female subjects. Lane (1989) also found differences depending on the gender of the nurse.
4. Patients in critical care units have been identified as one population for whom purposeful touch is important (Estabrooks, 1989; Green, 1994). These patients may benefit not only from purposeful touching by nurses but also by family members. Does touching of the patient by the nurse increase the extent to which family members touch and interact with the patient?

REFERENCES

American Association of Retired Persons. (1993, May–June). Undercover hand holder perks patients. *AARP highlights, 11*(3), 4.

Barnett, K. (1972). A survey of the current utilization of touch by health team personnel with hospitalized patients. *International Journal of Nursing Studies, 9,* 195–209.

Bottorff, J. L. (1993). The use and meaning of touch in caring for patients with cancer. *Oncology Nursing Forum, 20,* 1531– 1538.

Bottorff, J. L. (1991). A methodological review and evaluation of research on nurse-patient touch. In P. L. Chinn (Ed.), *Anthology on caring* (pp. 303–343). New York: National League for Nursing.

Burgener, S. C., Jirovec, M., Murrell, L., & Barton, D. (1992). Caregiver and environmental variables related to difficult behaviors in institutionalized, demented elderly persons. *Journal of Gerontology, Psychological Sciences, 47,* P242–P249.

Copstead, L. (1980). Effects of touch on self-appraisal and interaction appraisal for permanently institutionalized older adults. *Journal of Gerontological Nursing, 6,* 747–752.

Estabrooks, C. A. (1989). Touch: A nursing strategy in intensive care units. *Heart & Lung, 18,* 392–401.

Estabrooks, C. A., & Morse, J. M. (1992). Toward a theory of touch: The touching process and acquiring a touching style. *Journal of Advanced Nursing, 17,* 448–456.

Fisher, L. M., & Joseph, D. H. (1989). A scale to measure attitudes about nonprocedural touch. *The Canadian Journal of Nursing Research, 21*(2), 5–14.

Gadow, S. (1984). Touch and technology: Two paradigms of care. *Journal of Religion and Health, 23,* 63–69.

Green, L. (1994). Touch and visualization to facilitate a therapeutic relationship in an intensive care unit—a personal experience. *Intensive and Critical Care Nursing, 10,* 51–57.

Hagland, M. R. (1995). Nurse-patient communication in intensive care: a low priority? *Intensive and Critical Care Nursing, 11,* 111–115.

Helwick, L. D. (1994). Stimulation programs for coma patients. *Critical Care Nurse, 14*(4), 47–52.

Hollinger, L. (1980). Perception of touch in the elderly. *Journal of Gerontological Nursing, 6,* 741–745.

Knable, J. (1981). Handholding: One means of transcending barriers of communication. *Heart & Lung, 10,* 1106–1110.

Krieger, D. (1975). Therapeutic touch: The imprimatur of nursing. *American Journal of Nursing, 75,* 784–787.

Kubler-Ross, E. (1969). *On death and dying.* New York: Macmillan.

Lane, P. L. (1989). Nurse-client perceptions: The double standard of touch. *Issues in Mental Health Nursing, 10,* 1–13.

Lange-Alberts, M. E., & Shott, S. (1994). Nutritional intake: Use of touch and verbal cuing. *Journal of Gerontological Nursing, 20*(2), 36–40.

McCorkle, R. (1974). Effects of touch on seriously ill patients. *Nursing Research, 23*, 125–132.

Moore, J. R., & Gilbert, D. A. (1995). Elderly residents: Perceptions of nurses' comforting touch. *Journal of Gerontological Nursing, 21*(1), 6–13.

Morales, E. (1994). Meaning of touch to hospitalized Puerto Ricans with cancer. *Cancer Nursing, 17*, 464–469.

Pollack, L., & Goldstein, G. (1981). Lowering of intracranial pressure in Reye's syndrome by sensory stimulation. *Lancet, i*, 732.

Pratt, J., & Mason, R. (1981). *The caring touch.* London: HM & M.

Richter, J. M., Roberto, K. A., & Bottenberg, D. J. (1995). Communicating with persons with Alzheimer's disease: Experiences of family and formal caregivers. *Archives of Psychiatric Nursing, 9*, 279–285.

Schoenhofer, S. O. (1989). Affectional touch in critical care nursing: A descriptive study. *Heart & Lung, 18*, 146–154.

Snyder, M., Egan, E. C., & Burns, K. R. (1995). Efficacy of hand massage in decreasing agitation behaviors associated with care activities in persons with dementia. *Journal of Geriatric Nursing, 16*, 60–63.

Seaman, L. (1982). Affective nursing touch. *Geriatric Nursing, 3*, 162–164.

Tobiason, S. (1981). Touching is for everyone. *American Journal of Nursing, 81*, 728–730.

Triplett, J., & Arneson, S. (1979). The use of verbal and tactile comfort to alleviate distress in young hospitalized children. *Research in Nursing and Health, 2*, 76–80.

Walleck, C. (1982, May). Effect of touch on intracranial pressure. Speech at the American Association of Neurological Nurses, Honolulu, Hawaii.

Walters, A. J. (1994). The comforting role in critical care nursing practice: A phenomenological interpretation. *International Journal of Nursing Studies, 31*, 607–616.

Weiss, S. J. (1979). The language of touch. *Nursing Research, 28*, 76–80.

Weiss, S. J. (1988). Touch. In J. Fitzpatrick, R. Taunton, & J. Benoliel (Eds.). *Annual review of nursing research* (vol.6), (pp. 3–27). New York: Springer.

Weiss, S. J. (1990). Effects of differential touch on nervous system arousal of patients recovering from cardiac disease. *Heart & Lung, 19*, 474–480.

13

PRESENCE

Susan Moch and Carol Schaefer

Presence, as a concept integral to the nurse-patient relationship, has an important place in nursing. Nurses in practice (Cohen & Sarter, 1992; Dossey, 1995; Ferrell, 1993; Marsden, 1990; Smith-Regojo, 1995) and nurse theorists (Gadow, 1980; Paterson & Zderad, 1976; Watson, 1985) discuss presence. Similarities in definition are beginning to emerge, levels of presence have been described (Osterman & Schwartz-Barcott, 1996; McKivergin & Daubenmire, 1994) and research on presence continues (Nelms, 1996; Rogers, 1996). In this chapter, presence is described, current perspectives about presence are presented, and outcome measures for presence are articulated.

DEFINITION

Presence is a process of being available with the whole of oneself and open to the experience of another through a reciprocal interpersonal encounter. This definition is adapted from the definition proposed by Paterson and Zderad (1976). Gardner (1992) defined presence as "the physical 'being there' and the psychological 'being with' a patient for the purpose of meeting the patient's health care needs" (p. 191). True presence, according to Liehr (1989), occurs when one is "genuinely engaging with another" (p. 7). The nurse uses extreme sensitivity to grasp the other's anger, joy, fear, or pain. For true presence to occur, the nurse must bring his or her own humaneness and acceptance of self into the encounter (Liehr, 1989). Dossey (1995) identified presence as being a state of readiness, or "being in the moment," to become available in relationships with client.

Major ideas that stand out in presence definitions are "being with" or being available, engagement, relationship (possibly reciprocal), and bringing more than physical presence. More recently, the spiritual or transcendent nature of presence (Osterman & Schwartz-Barcott, 1996) and the potential of presence "to awaken the client's own healing potential" (Dossey, 1995, p. 69) have been discussed. Earlier, nurse theorists such as Benner and Wrubel (1989), Newman (1986), Paterson and Zderad (1976), and Watson (1985) identified the importance of presence in nursing processes.

SCIENTIFIC BASIS

Theoretical Foundations

Paterson and Zderad (1976) recognized presence as being integral to their theory of humanistic nursing. Presence implies an openness, a receptivity, readiness, or availability on the part of the nurse. Many nursing situations require close proximity to another person, but that in itself does not guarantee presence. In order to experience the lived dialogue of nursing, the nurse responds with an openness to a "person-with-needs" and with an "availability-in-a-helping-way" (Paterson & Zedrad, 1976, p. 28). Reciprocity often emerges through the dialogue.

Vaillot (1966) described the role of a nurse as helping the patient become an authentic person through the illness experience by being present. Another nurse, Ferlic (1968), identified the nurse as a presence to the patient through closeness, perception, awareness, and involvement. According to Anderson (1979), a change happens within the nurse and the patient through presence.

In Newman's (1994) theory of health as expanding consciousness, the nurse is viewed as a partner in pattern recognition; this involves presence. The nurse must be fully aware of self and open to the client's agenda and to being with the client for pattern recognition to occur. According to Newman, "The nurse must be fully present with the client and wait for insight into the meaning of the pattern" (p. 109).

Presence involves the nurse as coparticipant in the caring process (Watson, 1985). Caring is related in part to the nurse's self-knowledge and ability in interpersonal interaction. According to Watson, "A truly caring nurse/artist is able to destroy in the consciousness of the recipient the separation between him or herself and the nurse" (p. 68).

The union or total presencing that happens through the experience leads to healing, discovery, and finding meaning.

Concept Development and Research on Presence

McKivergin and Daubenmire (1994) clarified three levels of presence interactions: physical presence, psychological presence and therapeutic presence. The type of contact identified for physical presence is body to body while psychological presence is mind to mind and therapeutic presence is spirit to spirit. More recently, Osterman and Schwartz-Barcott (1996), building on the definition of presence as being there, described four of presence: presence, partial presence, full presence, and transcendent presence. The nature of the interaction is different within each of the ways of being there. For instance, in presence, the nature of the interaction is very limited and almost self-absorbed, whereas in the description of transcendent presence, a high degree of interrelationship exists, such as human intimacy/love, and there are no boundaries between client and nurse.

Nelms (1996) used Heideggerian hermeneutics to study caring presence in nursing. Her narratives of practice situations illuminate caring presence. The importance of intuition and feeling in the caring presence is noted in her work. One theme in Nelms' research is the "silent call" to take on the presence role with another person. The nurses' stories she recounts depict an inner knowledge of how to authentically relate to the clients.

Rogers (1996) identified presence as a defining attribute of the concept of facilitative affiliation. Using Gardner's (1992) definition of presence, she suggests that psychologically being with a client is necessary for facilitative affiliation. In a study by Cohen, Hauser, & Johnson (1994), patients identified presence as being important. Patients described presence as an attentive attitude which included the nurse's being available and making patients comfortable. Other research (Minick, 1995) has linked presence and caring with early recognition of acute care patient problems.

Presence and Other Ways of Knowing

The concept of presence can be illuminated through examples from and discussion with nurses in practice. Nurses understand presence in their own personal way and often relate examples of being present to clients. For instance, Katie Kraemer, a woman's health care nurse practitioner, describes presence as a way of connecting with clients that is essential in providing client-centered care.

Marcia Manz, (personal communication Nov. 10, 1996) understands presence through a patient encounter:

> Presence. I never really thought about it. So, what! I'm here, tell me what it is you need. I will try to help. The patient, Ms. Jones, didn't appear anxious. I simply asked if she was concerned about surgery. Tears slid down her cheeks.
>
> "It's not the surgery. It's just that I'm so fat. Sometimes fat people don't make it through anesthesia." I listened. She continued with her fear.
>
> Then she told me how the wonderful kids who ride the school bus she drives gave her a card to wish her well. I, too, wished her well and she thanked me for listening.
>
> It seems so simple now. I just invited her to share a piece of herself, which she so openly did. I should be thanking her because today she taught me about presence.

Knowledge of presence may also evolve through personal knowing or practical knowledge. Personal knowing is discovery of self-and-other arrived at through reflection, synthesis of perceptions, and connecting with what is known (Moch, 1990b). Personal knowing emerges through interpersonal processes, life and clinical experiences, and intuition. Knowledge through practice—proposed by Lather (1986) and expanded upon for nursing by Newman (1990), Moch (1990b), and Boyd (1993)—serves to enlarge the body of knowledge on presence. Through this method the researcher engages with the subject in a process of negotiation, reciprocity, and empowerment toward mutual insight of the phenomenon being studied. Knowledge through practice on presence would involve data collection of the experience of the client and the nurse and/or researcher engaged with presence.

Presence as an Outcome Measure

Imagine how health care would be transformed if presence was demanded of at least one member of the team in each client's health care encounter. Consider the following hypothetical statement as a required health care outcome: "Ninety percent of clients served will perceive at least one health care team member as totally present to her or him once during each health care encounter. Health care encounters include such events as office visits, intervention experiences, hospital stays, treatments, or home visits." With the outcome suggested, at least one health care team member would be perceived as "available with the whole of oneself" to the needs of the client seeking assistance in every health care system contact!

A perceived presence outcome could also affect consumer satisfaction and the number of health care encounters needed. Literature suggests that clients in the current high technology environment have high touch needs which may be met through presence interventions by health care team members. According to Marsden (1990), presence "can be an antidote for the dehumanizing effects of technology" (p. 541).

INTERVENTION

Preparation for Presence

Presence entails conscious attention in getting ready to engage in the process. To be available with the wholeness of oneself and to be open to the experience of another, the nurse must focus on self as the instrument. Thus, the nurse consciously attends to the moment by centering self so that being available to the other is possible. This process may involve a period of quiet attention to self before a planned encounter, for example, simply taking a deep breath and closing one's eyes in order to center self and detach from other distractions.

The centering process promotes openness and readiness for caring, which are essential to interpersonal presence. The attitude of openness and readiness may be the most important criterion for presence to occur. Possession of compassion, sympathy, and empathy, also facilitates presence (Schaefer, 1990). Without a willingness on the part of the nurse to be open and to take a risk, presence cannot occur. The risk involves a choice on the part of the nurse. A student nurse aptly reflected in a journal of her practical experience: "I think the only way to be present is to choose to allow the real you to be there for someone at a given time" (T. Kelcher, personal communication, March 9, 1990).

The skills needed for engaging in presence are centering, listening, seeing (observing), and feeling (Schaefer, 1990). Listening is an active process of searching for meaning. It also requires the ability to be silent and to be open to the other person. Through silence, acceptance and caring can be portrayed.

Excellent observational, or seeing, skills are important for presence. Observation skills reveal subtleties in expression and communication that are cues for being with clients. Feeling skills are brought to bear on observation when the nurse listens to really hear or to really see what the patient is saying. Often the nurse feels what the patient is saying through his or her unspoken words.

Technique

The techniques of presence involve openness, unknowing, attention, and connectedness. If the nurse is open, he or she can be available with the whole self. *Openness* can be likened to Travelbee's (1966) use of the term *transcendence* for "the ability to get beyond and outside of self in order to perceive and respond to the human being in the patient" (p. 47).

Unknowing is approaching another with a question (Sarosi, 1986), a desire to know more coupled with the confidence that the other person will be the teacher, a position of knowing that there is much more for the nurse to know about the situation. Unknowing involves vulnerability—the nurse becomes the learner rather than the traditionally, knowing teacher.

Presence requires the attention of the nurse. *Attention* is focused completely on the other person. Focus points include the sensations, emotions, cognitions, and spiritual elements in the client's experience and the sensations, emotions, and spiritual elements of the nurse that arise through the interactions with the client (Sarosi, 1986).

Through presence, a connectedness with the patient emerges. Both the nurse and the client experience a sense of union or joining for a moment in time. In describing one such connection experience a nursing student identified how her knowing from experience immediately connected her with a client. The client described a wish to ask his deceased parents some questions, which was a wish the student had because her parents, too, had died. She said, "I was truly touched because I really understood" (J. Vorwald, personal communication, 1990).

Measurement of Effectiveness

Measuring outcomes of presence interventions will involve both the client and the nurse because of the reciprocal interaction in presence. The client could complete an assessment of whether or not certain key areas of presence were experienced. Some ideas for such an assessment have been suggested by Katie Kraemer (personal communication, 1996), women's health care nurse practitioner. They are:

I felt understood.
I decided what to talk about on at least one occasion.
I felt cared about.
At least one health care team member took time for me and my real needs.

Another way to measure presence would be to determine whether the client felt the nurse practiced the elements of the technique of presence. For instance, did the nurse demonstrate centering, openness, unknowing, attention and connectedness? Language clearly describing the elements would be needed to help clients readily understand the elements being assessed.

Assessment of presence on the part of the nurse could include whether or not key elements of presence for the nurse were experienced. Through presence with clients, Moch (1988) experienced knowing of another, awe and respect for the other, and awareness of self. Measuring whether these aspects or other identified nurse outcomes of presence occurred in nurse-client encounters could facilitate evaluation.

USES

Presence can be used in any nursing situation. Persons struggling with an illness are especially in need of moments of presence. A psychosocial intervention involving presence has also been identified as important to the nursing care of women diagnosed with breast cancer (Moch, 1990a, 1995). Presence is especially indicated with patients experiencing a high level of anxiety (Marsden, 1990) and with persons coping with loss (Smith-Regojo, 1995).

Precautions

The major precaution is the necessity for taking the cue from the patient and not forcing a presence encounter. A true presence encounter considers the wants and the needs of the patient. If the nurse is "available with the whole of oneself and open to the experience" of the client, as the definition states, the nurse will be following the patient and will thus act in accordance with his or her wishes.

RESEARCH QUESTIONS

The need for presence interventions within the nursing discipline is evident through nursing clinical, theoretical, and scientific literature. The time has come for considering outcome measures for presence and measuring whether presence occurs in nurse-client encounters. Further research should address the questions of:

1. What are effective measures to determine whether or not presence occurs?
2. How can we measure the outcomes of presence?
3. How can we assess a client's need for presence?
4. How can we better assure compatibility between nursing's theoretical world and the practice arena?

ACKNOWLEDGMENTS

The first author gratefully acknowledges Melissa Avery, JoAnn Butrin, Ann Kelly, Marilyn Loen, and Margot Nelson for earlier development of presence ideas.

REFERENCES

Anderson, N.D. (1979). Human interaction for nurses. *Supervisor Nurse, 10,* 44–50.

Benner, P., & Wrubel, J. (1989). *The primacy of caring: Stress and coping in health and illness.* Menlo Park: Addison-Wesley.

Boyd, C. O. (1993). Toward a nursing practice research method. *Advances in Nursing Science, 16*(2), 9–25.

Cohen, M. Z., & Sarter, B. (1992). Love and work: Oncology nurses' view of the meaning of their work. *Oncology Nursing Forum, 19,* 1481–1486.

Cohen, M. Z., Hausner, J., & Johnson, M. (1994). Knowledge and presence: Accountability as described by nurses and surgical patients. *Journal of Professional Nursing, 10,* 177–185.

Dossey, B. M. (1995). Nurse as healer. In B. M. Dossey, L. Keegan, C. E. Guzzetta, & L. G. Kolkmeier, *Holistic nursing: A handbook for practice* (2nd ed.), (pp. 61–82). Gaithersburg, MD: Aspen.

Ferlic, A. (1968). Existential approach in nursing. *Nursing Outlook, 16,* 30–33.

Ferrell, B. R. (1993). To know suffering. *Oncology Nursing Forum, 20*(10), 1471–1477.

Gadow, S. (1980). Existential advocacy: Philosophical foundation of nursing. In S. Spiker and S. Gadow (Eds.). *Nursing images and ideals* (pp. 79–101). New York: Springer.

Gardner, D. L. (1992). Presence. In G. M. Bulechek & J. C. McCloskey (Eds.), *Nursing interventions: Essential nursing treatments* (2nd ed., pp. 191–200). Philadelphia: Saunders.

Lather, P. (1986). Research as praxis. *Harvard Educational Review 56*(3), 257–277.

Liehr, P. R. (1989). The core of true presence: A loving center. *Nursing Science Quarterly 2*(1), 7–8.

Marsden, C (1990). Ethical issues in critical care. *Heart & Lung, 19,* 540–541.

McKivergin, M., & Daubenmire, J. (1994). The essence of therapeutic presence. *Journal of Holistic Nursing, 12*(1), 65–81.

Minick, P. (1995). The power of human caring: Early recognition of patient problems. *Scholarly Inquiry for Nursing Practice: An International Journal, 9*(4), 303–317.

Moch, S. D. (1988). *Health in illness: Experiences with breast cancer.* Unpublished doctoral dissertation, University of Minnesota, Minneapolis, MN.

Moch, S. D. (1990a). Health within the experience of breast cancer. *Journal of Advanced Nursing, 15,* 119–123.

Moch, S. D. (1990b). Personal knowing: Evolving research and practice. *Scholarly Inquiry for Nursing Practice: An International Journal 4,* 155–165.

Moch, S. D. (1995) *Breast cancer: Twenty women's stories.* New York: National League of Nursing.

Nelms, T. P. (1996). Living a caring presence in nursing: A Heideggerian hermeneutical analysis. *Journal of Advanced Nursing, 24,* 368–374.

Newman, M. A. (1986). *Health as expanding consciousness.* St. Louis: Mosby.

Newman, M. A. (1990). Newman's theory of health as praxis. *Nursing Science Quarterly, 3*(1), 37–41.

Newman, M. A. (1994). *Health as expanding consciousness* (2nd ed.) New York: National League for Nursing.

Osterman, P., & Schwartz-Barcott, D. (1996). Presence: Four ways of being there. *Nursing Forum, 31*(2), 23–30.

Paterson, J. G., & Zderad, L. T. (1976). *Humanistic nursing.* New York: Wiley.

Rogers, S. (1996). Facilitative affiliation: Nurse-client interactions that enhance healing. *Issues in Mental Health Nursing, 17,* 171–184.

Sarosi, G. M. (1986). *An experiment in understanding: The nurse is the laboratory.* Unpublished paper, University of Minnesota, Minneapolis, MN.

Schaefer, C. C. (1990). *Concept clarification of presence.* Unpublished masters thesis, University of Wisconsin-Eau Claire, Eau Claire, WI.

Smith-Regojo, P. (1995). "Being with" a patient who is dying. *Holistic Nursing Practice, 9*(3), 1–3.

Travelbee, J. (1966). *Interpersonal aspects of nursing.* Philadelphia: Davis.

Vaillot, M. C. (1966). Existentialism: A philosophy of commitment. *American Journal of Nursing 66,* 500–502.

Watson, J. (1985). *Nursing: Human science and human care, a theory of nursing.* Norwalk, CT: Appleton-Century-Crofts.

14

Active Listening

Muriel B. Ryden

The therapeutic use of self has long been a primary independent nursing intervention. The ability of the nurse to use her personality consciously and in full awareness in an attempt to establish related-ness was described by Travelbee (1966) as a disciplined intellectual approach, not mere kindly feelings. The potential for nurses to be a healing force was emphasized by Ujhely (1968). Both in the presence or the absence of high technology, the instrument "self" is available to the nurse and helpful to the client. Listening represents one of the essential components in the use of the self as an intervention to bring about desired outcomes for clients. Listening, according to Fromm-Reichmann, is "a basic psychotherapeutic instrument" (1950, p. 7).

A listener does not require verbal communication by the sender in order to respond, since all behavior is a form of communication. The nonverbal component of social meaning is estimated by Birdwhistell (1970) to be 65% of the communication. The interpretation of emotion from facial expression and body movement across cultures has been studied extensively by Ekman and Friesen (1969, 1971). Six basic human emotions (happiness, sadness, anger, fear, surprise, and disgust) have been found to be associated with a quite limited range of facial muscle movements that were judged correctly from pictures by subjects from various cross-cultural groups (Ekman, 1972). When words contradicted silent messages, Mehrabian (1971) found that communicators relied on nonverbal cues; facial expression and tone of voice were more important than words in determining the impact of a total message. Nonverbal behavior can confirm what is said by the degree of congruence with verbal statements, or it can "leak" messages (Ekman & Friesen, 1969), since it is not as easily subject to control as are verbal messages.

DEFINITION

The dictionary definition of *listen* is "to make a conscious effort to hear; to attend closely, so as to hear" (*Webster's New Twentieth Century Dictionary*, 1983, p. 1055). Because the word has a passive connotation, the term *active listening* has come to be used to refer to a disciplined, skilled interpersonal communication style. Active listening is the skill of understanding what another is saying and feeling. The active listener will also paraphrase the message back to the speaker (Gerrard, Boniface, & Love, 1980). In discussing holistic listening, Rowan (1986) describes many levels of listening, from obvious acknowledgement of what the other says to the deepest level of entering into an intuitive relationship with the other person.

Listening is a part of the classic communication model, which consists of a sender who encodes a message and transmits it through some medium to a receiver, who must listen and hear to decode the message (Arnold & Boggs, 1989). The independent intervention of listening essentially involves the helper remaining in the role of the receiver, assisting the sender/client to more clearly understand his or her own message. In the words of Davis, "Listening is receiving with nothing to prove" (1984, p. 4). An active listener, like a sounding board, does not employ interpersonal strategies that send new messages. Therefore, changing the frame of reference, using self-disclosure, and providing information—all of which may be useful actions in some situations—would not be part of active listening.

Active listening also is called "empathic listening." The literal meaning of empathy is "feeling into," or "emotional knowing" (Greenson, 1960). The definition of empathy by Truax and Carkhuff approximates that of active listening: "Accurate empathy involves both the therapist's sensitivity to current feelings and his [sic] verbal facility to communicate this in a language attuned to the client's feelings" (1967, p. 46). Empathy, warmth, and genuineness are three qualities necessary and sufficient for therapeutic change to occur in the other, according to Rogers (1957); they are the essence of his "client-centered approach." What is involved is profound listening, harkening to the other in order to truly hear, know, and understand (Jackson, 1992).

Empathy is viewed by Gerrard and colleagues (1980), as having three components. The affective component is sensitivity to feelings; the cognitive component observes and processes messages; and the communicative component restates in response what the receiver has sensed. These authors assert that active listening is the cognitive and communicative component of empathy.

SCIENTIFIC BASIS

In the nursing literature, listening tends to be addressed in an anecdotal and an exhortatory mode more frequently than in a scientific mode. For example, Magnan and Benner (1989) assert that listening allows nurses to become catalysts for recovery and healing; in the process, the authors assert, nurses are also taught by their clients. Listening is identified by Burnard (1987) as the first and most important aspect of counseling persons in spiritual distress. Texts describing interpersonal communication skills in nursing consistently include listening as an essential skill, but tend not to document the scientific basis for its use. In the field of counseling, Rogers (1975) asserts that research points strongly to the conclusion that a high degree of empathy in a relationship is possibly the most potent, and certainly one of the most potent factors in bringing about change and learning in clients (Cartwright & Lerner, 1966; Mullen & Abeles,1971; Rogers, Gendlin, Kiesler, & Traux, 1967).

The research in nursing that relates to listening has been done primarily from an educational perspective, not from a clinical outcomes perspective. Researchers have studied the effectiveness of methodologies designed to increase empathic listening skills in students and practicing nurses (Daniels, Denny, & Andrews, 1988; Hardin & Halaris; 1983; Norris, 1986; Olson & Iwasiw, 1987). Some studies have suggested that nurses as a group possess low levels of empathy (Friedrich, Livcely, & Sachacht, 1985; Lamonica, Carew, Winder, Haase, & Blanchard, 1976). However, in a comparison of the helping styles of psychotherapists, crisis interveners, and trained individuals with those of undergraduate junior nursing students completing a course in interpersonal relationships, the nursing students were found to be similar to trained psychotherapists in their use of statements reflecting affect and content—in other words, empathic listening (Ryden, McCarthy, Lewis, & Sherman, 1991). This discrepancy in research findings is puzzling. Does the pressure of practicing nursing in short-staffed, high-tech environments result in the loss of listening skills, or were these skills never learned or only minimally valued by many nurses?

A study of the relationship between the quality of interpersonal skills used by practitioners and the level of satisfaction with care of 38 clients of a community mental health center in England revealed that those who perceived the practitioner to be using skills of empathy, listening, openness, and genuineness tended to more satisfied (Sheppard, 1993). The author suggests that, in an era of cost-conscious managed care, the contribution of interpersonal skills to clients' perceptions of the quality of care should be given high priority.

In contrast to the positive findings in Sheppard's study, results of a study of the relationship between distress in cancer patients and primary nurses' empathy skills (Reid-Ponte, 1992) did not support the effectiveness of empathy in reducing distress. Cancer patients rated nurses, for the most part, below the 50th percentile on the La Monica Empathy Profile. The investigator found that nurses with more education were rated lower in perceiving, feeling, and listening than nurses with less education; older and more experienced nurses were rated as responding less empathically than younger, more inexperienced nurses. The distress scores of patients, whose mean level of pain and distress was low, were negatively associated with perceiving, feeling and listening ratings of their primary nurses. This study points to the complexities of disentangling relationships between interpersonal skills and patient outcomes.

INTERVENTION

Active listening requires the receiver to be exquisitely tuned to the sender—to vibrate on the same frequency. The metalanguage communicated through the nuances of tone, fleeting facial expressions, hesitancies over words, silences, and telling body language may escape the casual listener. "Listening with the third ear," is the term used by Reik (1951) to describe the capacity to catch the unstated message. To really *hear* the content of the spoken message takes concentration and an ability to differentiate between what is actually said and what one wants or expects to hear. Listening with an attitude of "cultivated naivet," is advocated by Schlesinger (1994); he urges abandoning assumptions that might lead one to hear what he or she thinks the patient ought to say. The active listener is wholly focused on trying to determine what the client is really saying, recognizing themes and patterns, and hearing what is left unsaid. Active listening can be hard work. After listening to some clients, you may feel as exhausted as you do when traveling abroad, where you try to make sense of communications in a language that is foreign to you. In other situations, the challenge may be not so much the difficulty of interpreting unclear messages as a problem in really hearing the messages of clients you find difficult to relate to (Egan, 1986). Also, it is difficult to listen to what you don't want to hear (Kelly, 1984). Since the brain is capable of processing information much more rapidly than the rate at which the average persons talks (which approximates 150 words per minute) the listener is left with free brain time (Davis, 1984). Often this allows the receiver to become distracted, or to focus attention on what to say in response, rather than concentrating totally on the other person in an attempt to fully understand the messages and the metamessages being communicated.

Technique

Active listening requires at least three different skills: (a) skill in interpreting the verbal and nonverbal messages from the client; (b) skill in assisting the client to communicate a message more clearly; and (c) skill in communicating to a client your understanding of his or her verbal and nonverbal messages. Being able to really *hear* (observe and listen) and to *read* (interpret the meaning of what you hear) a client message is essential to understanding. Frequently the jumbled turmoil of thoughts experienced by persons under stress is expressed in communication that lacks clarity. The receiver's difficulty in decoding such a message may reflect the sender's own lack of self-understanding. Therefore, the external feedback from a skilled active listener which helps a client to communicate more clearly to others also can be a direct means of helping clarify the client's own thinking. This "sounding board" effect can be achieved by reflecting the essence of what you have understood the client to say, by asking for elaboration, by encouraging specificity and concreteness in place of vague global statements, and by pointing out discrepancies in communication.

Interpreting the meaning of what is heard is dependent not only on the quality of listening, but also on the critical thinking skills of the listener, such as analysis, inference, and evaluation (Facione, 1990). Some of the critical thinking dispositions identified as part of the 1990 American Philosophical Association Delphi Study (Facione, 1990) seem to be foundational to active listening: they include the disposition to truthseeking, openmindedness, and cognitive maturity.

The adeptness and sensitivity of the listener in communicating to the patient what is understood is also an important aspect of effective active listening. Make your response as accurate a reflection of the overt or covert message as possible. Attempt to match the intensity of the feeling that has been communicated, rather than overstate or minimize. Phrase your interpretation in a tentative way rather than as a dogmatic assertion. Allow the patient's response to determine the direction of the subsequent interaction.

Examples of Active Listening

Active listening may be demonstrated in the following ways:

1. The receiver attempts to clarify a message that was unclear.
   Client: Well, I came to the clinic because it seemed like the thing to do. I would really rather not, but you know how it is.
   Nurse: I am not sure I understand what you are saying about your reason for coming here. Can you explain further what you mean?
2. The receiver paraphrases the content and/or feeling that the sender has overtly communicated.
   Client: I am so tired of trying one thing after another and having absolutely no success! I have spent thousands of dollars and I am no better than I was when I started!
   Nurse: It is discouraging and frustrating to invest a lot of time, energy, and money and not get the results you hoped for.
3. The receiver responds by putting into words content and/or feelings that the sender has only covertly communicated.
   Client: I am so tired of trying one thing after another and having absolutely no success! I have spent thousands of dollars and I am no better than I was when I started!
   Nurse: I wonder if what you are saying is that you feel very hopeless about ever getting better.
4. The receiver responds to a client who is verbally noncommunicative:
   Nurse: It seems that talking about this is not something you are comfortable with doing right now.
   [Or, to a comatose client:] I wish you could tell me how you are feeling; you look uncomfortable in that position. I am going to rub your back and turn you to the other side, and prop you with some pillows to try to make you more comfortable.

Measurement of Effectiveness

Outcomes of listening as a nursing intervention are not easily measured. Instruments that have been designed to measure the psychosocial constructs of trust, rapport, self-understanding, self-efficacy, and client satisfaction are possible outcome indicators of effective listening. Physiologically based indicators of healing and traditional health care indexes such as length of stay are other variables whose sensitivity of response to a listening intervention warrant testing. However, there are methodological challenges in isolating active listening as an independent variable.

USES

The purpose of active listening is for the client to better understand self and to experience being understood by another caring person. This experience is likely to lead to a number of positive consequences.

First, energy, which previously was channeled into abortive attempts to be understood, may be released for healing, problem solving, and other priorities of the client. Orlando, in her classic text on the nurse-patient relationship (1961, p. 23), points out that patients frequently are unable to communicate their needs clearly. The responsibility of nurses to prevent depletion of energy resources by eliminating not only physiological but also psychological energy wasters is described by Miller (1983).

Second, trust is enhanced as the client perceives the nurse as someone who cares enough to try to genuinely hear and understand. Bok has said, "*Whatever* matters to human beings, trust is the atmosphere in which it thrives" (1978, p. 31). The experience of being truly heard is nourishing for the client. Being understood can enable the other to open a private world and allow the nurse to enter, to discover "whatever matters," and be present as a resource.

A third possible consequence is increased self-understanding, which may empower a client to greater autonomy and independence in health care concerns (Greenberg & Kahn, 1979). The goal of nursing is not to create a continuing need for nursing care by the client, nor to paternalistically make decisions in this client's best interest. Through active listening a client may come to understand self and the present situation more clearly, even though the nurse may only partially comprehend. Such self-knowledge may contribute to self-efficacy (Bandura, 1982), and enable the client to act more independently and authentically to achieve goals. For a physically dependent person, it may become possible to be self-determining by directing others to take action on his or her behalf.

A fourth consequence of listening is a clearer grasp by the nurse of the client's perception of the situation. This provides the nurse with valid data to use in determining what health-related goals should have priority and what subsequent interventions might offer the greatest probability of helping the client achieve those goals. This understanding by the nurse can allow for collaborative efforts with the client who can then be an agent for his or her own health.

Finally, listening has a healing quality: ". . . . the good listener is the best physician for those who are ill in thought and feeling" (Johnson, 1956, p. 20). The healing value of listening as a therapeutic intervention with those in grief is poignantly described by Gibbons (1993). She suggests that the tendency of nurses to be action oriented may lead them to minimize and underestimate the significance and the power of just listening.

At a time when cost-conscious managed health care systems pressure primary care providers to spend limited time with each client, we need to ensure that listening does not become a lost intervention. "The healer learns about the sufferer in direct proportion to the quantity *and* quality of his listening" (Jackson, 1992, p. 1631.) Therefore, clinical outcomes of care are likely to be related to the quality of listening. A sense of being heard also influences client satisfaction with care (Johnson, 1981).

Precautions

There is a need for a willingness to acknowledge one's limitations. Being a good listener is not equivalent to having the advanced practical knowledge and skills that are requisite for the role of psychotherapist. Knowing when to seek help or refer a client to other health care professionals is essential.

In studies by Ford (1981) and Larson (1984), nurses identified listening as the behavior most representative of their caring for clients. However, rankings of nurses' caring behavior that were made by persons with cancer in Larson's study (1984) showed that clients ranked competency behaviors higher than listening behaviors as indicative of caring. While listening can at times be the best choice for independent nursing intervention, more often it has its value as the medium through which direct, hands-on nursing care is given. Listening cannot be a substitute for expertise in other aspects of nursing, but, as Benner (1984) describes, it is an integral part of the professional's development from novice to expert.

RESEARCH QUESTIONS

Within nursing there appears to be such a strong belief in the intrinsic merit of listening that attempts to carry out a controlled study in which a group of clients was deliberately *not* listened to probably would be considered unethical. However, studies of the outcomes of an "enriched" intervention of listening might provide answers to the following questions:

1. What is the effect of listening on psychological variables such as anxiety, depression, trust, self-efficacy, and self-esteem?
2. What is the effect of listening on physiological variables such as client's healing time and physiological indicators of stress?
3. What is the effect of listening on cognitive variables such as self-understanding, and learning?
4. How do the variables of the time, frequency, and duration of a listening intervention influence client outcomes?
5. How does the effectiveness of listening as a nursing intervention differ for client groups with specific characteristics?
6. To what extent is client satisfaction with health care affected when listening is used as a nursing intervention?

REFERENCES

Arnold, E., & Boggs, K. (1989). *Interpersonal relationships: Professional communication skills for nurses*. Philadelphia: Saunders.

Bandura, A. (1982). Self-efficacy mechanisms in human agency. *American Psychologist, 37,* 122–147.

Benner, P. (1984). *From novice to expert: Excellence and power in clinical nursing practice*. Menlo Park, CA: Addison-Wesley.

Birdwhistell, R. (1970). *Kinesics and context*. Philadelphia: University of Pennsylvania Press.

Bok, S. (1978). *Lying*. New York: Pantheon.

Burnard, P. (1987). Spiritual distress and the nursing response. Theoretical considerations and counselling skills. *Journal of Advanced Nursing, 12*(3), 377–382.

Cartwright, R.D., & Lerner, B. (1966). Empathy, need to change, and improvement in psychotherapy. In G. E. Stollak, B. G. Guerney, Jr., & M. Rothberg (Eds.), *Psychotherapy research: Selected readings* (pp. 537–545). Chicago: Rand McNally.

Daniels, T. G., Denny, A., & Andrews, D. (1988). Using microcounseling to teach RN nursing student skills of therapeutic communication. *Journal of Nursing Education, 27*(6), 246–252.

Davis, A. J. (1984). *Listening and responding.* St. Louis: Mosby.

Egan, G. (1986). *The skilled helper* (3rd ed.). Monterey, CA: Brooks/Cole.

Ekman, P. (1972). Universal and cultural differences in facial expression of emotion. In J. K. Cole (Ed.), *Nebraska symposium on motivation.* Lincoln: University of Nebraska Press.

Ekman, P., & Freisen, W. V. (1969). The repertoire of nonverbal behavior: Categories, origin, usage and coding. *Semiotica, 1,* 49–98.

Ekman, P., & Freisen, W. V. (1971). Constants across cultures in the face and emotion. *Journal of Personality and Social Psychology, 17*(2), 124–129.

Facione, P. A. (1990). *The Delphi Report and critical thinking: A statement of expert consensus for purposes of educational assessment and instruction.* (ERIC Document Number: ED 315 423)

Ford, M. (1981). Nurse professionals and the caring process. *Dissertation Abstracts International, 43,* 967B–968B. (University Microfilms No. 81–19278)

Friedrich, R. M., Livcely, S. I. & Sachacht, E. (1985). Teaching communication skills in an integrated curriculum. *Journal of Nursing Education, 24*(4), 164–166.

Fromm-Reichmann, F. (1950). *Principles of intensive psychotherapy.* Chicago: University of Chicago Press.

Gibbons, M. B. (1993). Listening to the lived experience of loss. *Pediatric Nursing, 19*(6), 597–599.

Gerrard, B. A., Boniface, W. J., & Love, B. H. (1980). *Interpersonal skills for health professionals.* Reston, VA: Reston.

Greenberg, L. S., & Kahn, S. E. (1979). The stimulation phase in counseling. *Counselor Education and Supervision, 19,* 137–145.

Greenson, R. R. (1960). Empathy and its vicissitudes. *International Journal of Psychoanalysis, 41,* 418–424.

Hardin, S. B., & Halaris, A. L. (1983). Nonverbal communication of patients and high and low empathy nurses. *Journal of Psychosocial Nursing and Mental Health Services, 21*(1), 14–20.

Jackson, S. W. (1992). The listening healer in the history of psychological healing. *American Journal of Psychiatry, 149,* 1623–1632.

Johnson, B. L. (1981). *Empathy in nursing: Its effect on patient satisfaction and adherence.* Unpublished doctoral dissertation. Yale University, New Haven, CT.

Johnson, W. (1956). *Your most enchanted listener.* New York: Harper.

Kelly, C. H. (1984). Listen to what you don't want to hear. *Geriatric Nursing, 5*(2), 83.

Lamonica, E. L., Carew, D. K., Winder, A. E., Haase, A. M. B., & Blanchard, K. (1976). Empathy training as the major thrust of a staff development program. *Nursing Research, 25*(6), 447–450.

Larson, P. J. (1984). Important nurse caring behaviors perceived by patients with cancer. *Oncology Nursing Forum, 1*(6), 46–50.

Magnan, M. A., & Benner, P. (1989). Listening with care. *American Journal of Nursing, 89*(2), 219–221.

Mehrabian, A. (1971). *Silent messages.* Belmont, CA: Wadsworth.

Miller, J. F. (1983). *Coping with chronic illness: Overcoming powerlessness.* Philadelphia: Davis.

Mullen, J., & Abeles, N. (1971). Relationship of liking, empathy and therapist's experience to outcome of therapy. *Journal of Counseling Psychology, 18*(1), 39–43.

Norris, J. (1986). Teaching communication skills: Effects of two methods of instruction and selected learner characteristics. *Journal of Nursing Education, 25*(3), 102–106.

Olson, J. K., & Iwasiw, C. L. (1987). Effects of a training model on active listening skills of post-RN students. *Journal of Nursing Education, 26*(3), 104–107.

Orlando, I. J. (1961). *The dynamic nurse-patient relationship.* New York: Putnam.

Rogers, C. R. (1957). The necessary and sufficient conditions of therapeutic personality change. *Journal of Consulting Psychology, 21,* 95–103.

Rogers, C. R. (1975). Empathic: An unappreciated way of being. *Counseling Psychologist, 5,* 2–10.

Rogers, C. R., Gendlin, E. T., Kiesler, J. J., & Truax, C. B. (Eds). (1967). *The therapeutic relationship and its impact. A study of psychotherapy with schizophrenics.* Madison: University of Wisconsin Press.

Reid-Ponte, P. (1992). Distress in cancer patients and primary nurses' empathy skills. *Cancer Nursing, 15*(4), 283–292.

Reik, T. (1951). *Listening with the third ear: The inner experience of a psychoanalyst.* Garden City, NY: Garden City Books.

Rowan, J. (1986). Holistic listening. *Journal of Humanistic Psychology, 26*(1), 83–102.

Ryden, M. B., McCarthy, P. R., Lewis, M. L., & Sherman, C. (1991). A behavioral comparison of the helping styles of nursing students, psychotherapists, crisis interveners, and untrained individuals. *Annals of Psychiatric Nursing, 5*(3), 1–4.

Schlesinger, H. J. (1994). How the analyst listens: The pre-stages of interpretation. *International Journal of Psycho-Analysis, 75,* 31–37.

Sheppard, M. (1993). Client satisfaction, extended intervention, and interpersonal skills in community mental health. *Journal of Advanced Nursing, 18,* 246–259.

Travelbee, J. (1966). *Interpersonal aspects of nursing.* Philadelphia: Davis.

Truax, C. B., & Carkhuff, R. R. (1967). *Toward effective counseling and psychotherapy.* Chicago: Aldine.

Ujhely, G. (1968). *Determinants of the nurse-patient relationship.* New York: Springer.

Webster's New Twentieth Century Dictionary. (1983). (2nd unabridged ed.) New York: Prentice Hall.

15

Positioning

Mary Fran Tracy

Positioning is an intervention frequently used by nurses in many settings. Positioning is one of the interventions most often used by nurses in critical care units (Doering, 1993; Fontaine & McQuillan, 1989; Gawlinski, 1993; Kinney, 1984). However, Fontaine and McQuillan cited evidence that 63% of nurses working in critical care units who were surveyed stated no awareness about the use of therapeutic positioning techniques in providing nursing care.

Positioning is used to promote comfort, to prevent complications such as decubitus ulcers, and to facilitate the performance of diagnostic or therapeutic procedures. When a nurse walks into a patient's room and sees that the patient has slid toward the foot of the bed, it is almost automatic to reposition the patient to promote comfort. Nurses assist in positioning patients for diagnostic and therapeutic procedures, such as spinal taps and chest drainage. Repositioning critically ill and bedridden patients every 2 hours is a practice with a long history in nursing. Teaching patients positions that will promote better ventilation in conditions such as chronic obstructive pulmonary disease and providing information about positions that will reduce pain for persons with chronic back problems are other examples of how nurses use the intervention of positioning. Thus, strong evidence exists to support positioning as an independent nursing intervention.

Another aspect of positioning is how the nurse is positioned when interacting with patients. Sitting down to talk with patients who are in bed or in wheelchairs, maintaining a distance so as to respect the patient's space, and understanding how one's body language affects a patient are important components of patient-nurse interactions. Although these aspects of positioning are critical to nursing, they will not be included in this chapter.

DEFINITION

Titler and colleagues (1991) from the Iowa Classification of Nursing Interventions team defined positioning as movement of a patient or part of a patient to promote comfort, skin integrity and healing, and to reduce skin breakdown. In addition, positioning may be used to faciliate the implementation of therapeutic and diagnostic procedures (Tyler, 1984). During positioning for procedures, the nurse must still be cognizant of comfort and try to decrease the amount of discomfort experienced. Prevention of complications other than skin breakdown is another important purpose for the use of certain positions and the changing of positions.

SCIENTIFIC BASIS

The scientific basis for the use of positioning varies depending on the purpose for which it is being used. Proper positioning not only increases patient comfort, but it has major implications for the functioning of body systems such as the circulatory and respiratory systems. Correct positioning avoids pressure on certain areas, thus providing for adequate circulation to all body areas. Correct positioning promotes ventilation and oxygenation of the lungs. The scientific basis for positioning to promote skin integrity, to facilitate gas exchange, to promote cerebral perfusion, and to promote comfort will be presented.

Skin Care

Positioning in relation to skin care has received considerable attention in nursing (Copeland-Fields & Hoshiko, 1989; Ebersole & Hess, 1990; Steffel, Schenk, & Walker, 1980). Turning schedules, use of assistive devices, and proper positioning are critical in the care of persons who have decreased mobility and sensation. Forces on an area of the body that are of sufficient strength and for a long enough period of time so as to obstruct blood flow will result in tissue necrosis. If the pressure forces exceed normal capillary pressure (14 mm

Hg for venous flow and 35 mm Hg for arterial flow) damage may occur. Pressure forces and related tissue damage are dependent on many factors, such as length of time of excessive pressure, the surface the patient is positioned on, the patient's body structure, the patient's nutritional status, and the patient's hemoglobin. In persons with normal sensation and mobility, automatic position changes are made. However, persons with decreased mobility, sensation, or alertness require assistance in changing positions, and they need to be taught strategies that they can use to decrease constant pressure.

Ventilation

Hurn (1988) noted that the use of specific body positions would maximize oxygenation and ventilation even in the presence of lung pathology. In healthy persons, ventilation-perfusion ratios are increased in the dependent lung bases when the person is upright (Fontaine & McQuillan, 1989). The volume of ventilation is greater at the base of the lungs, but the perfusion ratio is greater at the apex of the lungs. The effects of various positions on ventilation have been examined. Piehl and Brown (1976) reported that patients in respiratory failure had improved PaO_2 (a measure that reflects the amount of oxygen dissolved in the blood) after being placed in a prone position; in most instances this positioning was achieved through the use of a Circ-O-Lectric bed. In a study by Langer, Mascheroni, Marcolin, and Gattinoni (1988), it was found that eight of thirteen patients with moderate to severe adult respiratory distress syndrome (ARDS) responded with at least a 10 mm Hg increase in PaO_2 after 30 minutes in the prone position. Recommendations included placing ARDS patients in the prone position at least as a brief test to identify those patients that would show an improvement in oxygenation. A number of researchers have shown that oxygenation is increased in patients with unilateral lung problems when the patient is positioned so that the lung with no pathology is dependent (Banasik, Bruya, Steadman, & Demand, 1987; Rivara, Artucio, Arcos, & Hiriart, 1984). It is thought that this position promotes optimal ventilation-perfusion matching.

Cerebral Perfusion

Adequate cerebral tissue perfusion in patients with head injuries is an objective of many therapies used in the care of this population. Maintaining normal intracranial pressures or reducing increased pressures aids in cerebral tissue perfusion. Positioning plays a key role in the attainment of this objective. Elevating the head of the bed 30 degrees assists in decreasing intracranial pressure (Parsons & Wilson, 1984; Shalit & Umansky, 1977). However, elevating the head of the bed to a 90–degree position may increase pressure, as it results in sharp flexion of the hips (Fontaine & McQuillan, 1989). Keeping the head and neck in alignment reduces interference with venous return (Mitchell & Mauss, 1978; Mitchell, Ozuna, & Lipe, 1981). Use of proper positioning techniques decreases cerebral tissue compromise in persons prone to increases in intracranial pressure.

Comfort

Appropriate positioning of a patient to promote comfort is a skill most nurse possess, yet it is often overlooked as a simple method to prevent or relieve pain. Positioning is especially helpful for those patients who are inactive and unable to correctly position themselves. Proper positioning of the joints places them into an anatomically relaxed position called the "loose packed" position (McCaffery & Wolff, 1992). This positioning ensures the joint receives the least stress from the skin, muscle, and tendon anatomy. Proper alignment prevents pull on body structures. For example, unless a paralyzed arm is supported, tremendous pull on the shoulder socket and muscles occurs.

INTERVENTION

Techniques

Numerous techniques for positioning exist. Fundamentals of nursing texts contain many pages on positioning techniques to promote skin integrity, to prevent contractures, and to achieve adequate ventilation. Content in these texts addresses the various positions that are used for respiratory therapy, diagnostic tests, such as lumbar punctures or barium enemas, and positions to be used postoperatively for various surgical procedures. Correct use of these and other techniques does much to promote positive patient outcomes.

Positioning should be considered a dynamic, not static, process (McCaffery & Wolff, 1992). Even an anatomically correct position should not be maintained for long periods of time. The patient should be considered a partner in the process and positioning techniques used only as guidelines, especially when using positioning to promote comfort. Altering a patient's position should promote a reduction, not an increase, in pain and anxiety. Basic tools such as pillows, small towels, and foam wedges are often needed to maintain the preferred position.

To illustrate the use of positioning as a nursing intervention, the research base of positioning patients with increased intracranial pressure (ICP) is presented. Findings from research studies will be used as the basis to describe techniques.

An Example of Technique: Positioning in Increased Intracranial Pressure

Although much research is still required in the area of positioning of persons with increased intracranial pressure (ICP), or the potential for it, the studies that have been completed provide a basis for the positioning of patients to promote cerebral perfusion (Mitchell, 1986). Elevation of the head of the bed, flexion and extension of body parts, and turning schedules have been examined.

Durward, Amacher, DelMaestro, & Sibbard (1983) found that elevating the head of the bed 15 to 30 degrees resulted in the lowest intracranial pressure readings, and the cerebral perfusion and cardiac output remained stable when subjects were in this position. Elevating the head of the bed in excess of a 45–degree angle often results in increases in ICP (Mitchell et al., 1981). Although horizontal or head down positions are often listed as contraindications for persons with increased ICP, Lee (1989) reported that 20% of the patients in his study demonstrated reduction in ICP in this position. Based on findings from studies, it can be recommended that patients with ICP or potential for increased ICP be placed in a position with the head of their bed elevated 15 to 30 degrees.

Positioning the patient to avoid sharp flexion of the hips will assist in maintaining the ICP within normal range. Turning the patient may result in increases in ICP, but these changes are often transient in nature (Parsons & Wilson, 1984). Maintaining the head and neck in alignment with the trunk of the body has been demonstrated to be a critical factor in preventing increases in ICP when turning and positioning patients (Mitchell et al., 1981). Williams and Coyne (1993) found that putting the head and neck in the left, right, or flexed positions significantly increased a patient's ICP when compared to either an extension or a neutral position. Using two or three persons to turn the patient and placing rolls or small pillows to keep the head and neck in alignment are needed.

USES

Conditions/Populations

The preceding content described the scientific foundation for positioning of patients as well as a research-based technique for positioning patients with increased ICP. It is encouraging to see the body of research that is developing regarding the use of this independent nursing intervention (Fontaine & McQuillan, 1989; Mitchell, 1986; Noll & Fountain, 1990; Quaglietti, Stotts, & Lovejoy, 1988). The use of this intervention in patients who have cardiovascular diseases and for patients who are prone to spasticity because of neurological problems will be examined.

Cardiovascular Disease.   Effects of positioning on the physiological status of postmyocardial infarction patients has been studied. Quaglietti and colleagues (1988) studied the effects that several types of position changes had on the rate pressure product (RPP) of persons who were recovering from an uncomplicated myocardial infarction. Findings reveal that assumption of a supine, semi-Fowler's position at 70 degrees or sitting in a chair did not significantly alter the RPP of the subjects. The investigators state that these findings are congruent with those of others who have examined positioning in persons with myocardial infarction.

Noll and Fountain (1990) examined the effect that a backrest position had on the mixed oxygen saturation in patients who had had coronary artery bypass surgery. The effects of three positions—head elevated 20 degrees, head elevated 40 degrees, and head flat—were studied. No significant differences were found among the oxygen saturation measurements taken for each position. The investigators concluded that that head of the bed could be elevated to a 40–degree angle to promote patient comfort. The sample used in the study included 30 subjects who were hemodynamically stable and under 70 years of age. Thus, additional studies are needed before these findings can be generalized.

Several research studies have measured changes in mixed venous oxygenation with lateral position changes in coronary artery bypass surgery patients (Pena, 1989; Shively, 1988; Tidwell, Ryan, Osguthorpe, Paull, & Smith, 1990). While oxygen saturations in these patients did significantly decrease immediately after lateral position changes, the majority of patients' saturations returned to baseline readings within 5 minutes of turning. Though most patients will have a transient and clinically insignificant decrease in mixed venous oxygen saturation with turning, it is recommended that nurses be alert for those patients who may exhibit a more extended and severe decrease after turning.

Spasticity in Patients with Neurological Conditions. Proper positioning plays a key role in preventing contractures in persons who have neurological pathology (Ferido & Habel, 1986). Use of side-lying, semiprone, and high Fowler's positions help to inhibit abnormal posturing in persons who have suffered head trauma. The prone and semiprone positions are effective, since they alter the effects of the tonic labyrinth and tonic reflexes (Palmer & Wyness, 1988). In persons with conditions in which spasticity may occur, rapid change in positions often results in increased muscle tone (Palmer & Wyness, 1988). Thus, slow, gentle changing of positioning is needed.

Precautions in Use

Incorrect positioning of patients can have serious deleterious effects. Knowledge from research studies will guide nurses in choosing the correct positions to use for a patient with a particular pathology. Keeping a patient with a head injury in a flat position may precipitate increases in intracranial pressure. Patients with alterations in autonomic function, such as diabetes and the elderly, may have limited ability to respond to changes in position which result in changes in blood volume distribution. Patients on prolonged bedrest may also have difficulty compensating for hemodynamic changes that occur with position changes. Turning critically ill patients can initiate negative responses such as cardiac dysrhythmias, hypotension, and decreased cardiac output. Therefore, nurses should be cognizant of how the patient's underlying pathology and condition may affect their ability to tolerate position changes.

Nurses also should be aware of environmental safety issues when repositioning patients. Positioning patients away from the edge of the bed, using side rails as appropriate, and ensuring that patients with impaired sensation are not positioned against hard or sharp objects is important.

Positioning for diagnostic procedures, such as x-rays, may be paramount to getting accurate diagnostic results. However, patients left in untherapeutic positions for protracted periods of time may develop complications such as injury or prolonged discomfort. Precautions must be taken to closely monitor the patient during these situations.

FURTHER RESEARCH

Nurses have begun to examine the outcomes resulting from the use of various positions for patients having specific conditions. In some instances, myths have been dispelled. Other findings have pointed to the need for increased caution in turning and positioning patients. In almost all studies on positioning, the sample sizes have been very small, preventing the generalization of findings. The following are some of the areas in which further research is necessary so as to provide a more scientific basis for the use of positioning in nursing therapeutics:

1. What are the effective mechanisms for maintaining the head and neck in alignment in persons who have suffered a head injury and who have decreased levels of responsiveness? In many instances these persons are restless and move from the position in which they were placed. This often results in flexion of the neck, which interferes with venous return and leads to an increase in intracranial pressure.
2. Validation of the positioning protocols that have been developed for patients with various conditions, such as the one for trauma patients that has been proposed by Norton and Conforti (1985), is needed. Many protocols are presented in the literature, but few have been subjected to clinical trials.
3. What are assessments nurses should make to determine if the patient is in a comfortable position? Students and novices need to become more attuned to these observations.
4. Is repositioning of patients every 2 hours postoperatively optimal? While that has been the long standing practice in nursing, research suppporting the optimal time interval for repositioning is needed.

REFERENCES

Banasik, J. L., Bruya, M. A., Steadman, R. E., & Demand, J. K. (1987). Effect of position on arterial oxygenation in postoperative coronary revascularization. *Heart & Lung, 16,* 652–657.

Copeland-Fields, L. D., & Hoshiko, B. R. (1989). Clinical validation of Braden and Bergstrom's conceptual schema of pressure sore risk factors. *Rehabilitation Nursing, 14,* 257–260.

Doering, L. V. (1993). The effect of positioning on hemodynamics and gas exchange in the critically ill: A review. *American Journal of Critical Care, 2*(3), 208–216.

Durward, Q. J., Amacher, A. L., DelMaestro, R. F., & Sibbard, W. (1983). Cerebral and cardiovascular responses in head elevation in patients with intracranial hypertension. *Journal of Neurosurgery, 59,* 938–944.

Ebersole, P., & Hess, P. (1990). *Toward healthy aging.* St. Louis: Mosby.

Ferido, T., & Habel, M. (1986). Spasticity in head trauma and CVA patients: Etiology and management. *Journal of Neuroscience Nursing, 20,* 17–22.

Fontaine, D. K., & McQuillan, K. (1989). Positioning as a nursing therapy in trauma care. *Critical Care Nursing Clinics of North America, 1,* 105–112.

Gawlinski, A. (1993). Effect of postioning on mixed venous oxygen saturation. *Journal of Cardiovascular Nursing, 7*(4), 71–81.

Hurn, P. D. (1988). Thoracic injuries. In V. Cardona, P. Hurn, R. Mason, A. M. Scanlon-Schlipp, & S. W. Veise-Berry (Eds.), *Trauma nursing from resuscitation through rehabilitation* (pp. 449–490). Philadelphia: Saunders.

Kinney, M. R. (1984). The scientific basis for critical care nursing practice: 1972 to 1982. *Heart & Lung, 13,* 116–123.

Langer, M., Mascheroni, D., Marcolin, R., & Gattinoni, L. (1988). The prone position in ARDS patients: A clinical study. *Chest, 94,* 103–107.

Lee, S. (1989). Intracranial pressure changes during positioning of patients with severe head injury. *Heart & Lung, 18,* 411–414.

McCaffery, M. & Wolff, M. (1992). Pain relief using cutaneous modalities, positioning, and movement. *Hospice Journal—Physical, Psychosocial, & Pastoral Care of the Dying, 8*(1/2), 121–153.

Mitchell, P. H. (1986). Intracranial hypertension: Influence of nursing care activities. *Nursing Clinics of North America, 21,* 563–576.

Mitchell, P. H., & Mauss, N. K. (1978). Relationship of patient-nurse activities to intracranial variations: A pilot study. *Nursing Research, 27,* 4–10.

Mitchell, P. H., Ozuna, J., & Lipe, H. P. (1981). Moving the patient in bed: Effects of turning and range of motion on intracranial pressure. *Nursing Research, 30,* 212–218.

Noll, M. L., & Fountain, R. L. (1990). Effects of backrest position on mixed venous oxygen saturation in patients with mechanical ventilation after coronary artery bypass surgery. *Heart & Lung, 19,* 243–251.

Norton, L. C., & Conforti, C. G. (1985). The effects of body position on oxygenation. *Heart & Lung, 14,* 45–51.

Palmer, M., & Wyness, M. A. (1988). Positioning and handling: Important considerations in the care of the severley head-injured patient. *Journal of Neuroscience Nursing, 20,* 42–49.

Parsons, L. C., & Wilson, M. M. (1984). Cerebrovascular status of severe closed head injured patients following passive position changes. *Nursing Research, 33,* 68–75.

Pena, M. A. (1989). The effect of position change on mixed venous oxygen saturation measurements in open heart surgery patients during the immediate postoperative period. *Heart & Lung, 18,* 305.

Piehl, M. A., & Brown, R. S. (1976). Use of extreme position changes in acute respiratory failure. *Critical Care Medicine, 4,* 13–14.

Quaglietti, S. E., Stotts, N. A., & Lovejoy, N. C. (1988). The effect of selected positions on rate pressure product of the postmyocardial infarction patient. *Journal of Cardiovascular Nursing, 2*(4), 77–85.

Rivara, D., Artucio, H., Arcos, J., & Hiriart, C. (1984). Positional hypoxemia during artificial ventilation. *Critical Care Medicine, 12,* 436–438.

Shalit, M. N., & Umansky, F. (1977). Effect of routine bedside procedures on intracranial pressure. *Israel Journal of Medical Science, 13,* 881–886.

Shively, M. (1988). Effect of position change on mixed venous oxygen saturation in coronary artery bypass surgery patients. *Heart & Lung, 17,* 51–59.

Steffel, P., Schenk, E., & Walker, S. (1980). Reducing devices for pressure sores with respect to nursing care procedures. *Nursing Research, 29,* 228–230.

Tidwell, S. L., Ryan, W. J., Osguthorpe, S. G., Paull, D. L., & Smith, T. L. (1990). Effects of position changes on mixed venous oxygen saturation in patients after coronary revascularization. *Heart & Lung, 19*(5), S574–S577.

Titler, M. G., Pettit, D., Bulechek, G. M., McCloskey, J. C., Craft, M. J., Cohen, M. Z., Crossley, J. D., Denehy, J. A., Glick, O. J., Kruckeberg, T. W., Maas, M. L., Prophet, C. M., & Tripp-Reimer, T. (1991). Classification of nursing interventions for care of the integument. *Nursing Diagnosis, 2*(2), 45–56.

Tyler, M. (1984). The respiratory effects of body positioning and immobilization. *Respiratory Care, 29,* 472.

Williams, A., & Coyne, S. M. (1993). Effects of neck position on intracranial pressures. *American Journal of Critical Care, 2*(1), 68–71.

16

Sensation Information*

Jo Ann B. Ruiz-Bueno

"If you knew how unreasonably sick people suffer from reasonable causes of distress, you would take more pains about these things" (Nightingale, 1869/1969, p. 104). Traditionally, an accepted responsibility for nurses has been to assess and intervene when patients demonstrate distress associated with encounters with illness and with the health care system. Sensation information is a preparatory intervention provided to the patient prior to a test or procedure. Sensation information, has received continuing support from research. The simplicity of this intervention makes it an important element of nursing's armamentarium. Unfortunately, sensation information is not consistently used in clinical practice (Garvin, Huston, & Baker, 1992).

DEFINITION

Sensation information (also known as sensory information or concrete objective information) gives an objective description of what a person will see, hear, smell, taste, and feel in a specific situation. The information concerns the neurological sensory data received by an individual as a result of direct stimulation of the sense organs (e.g., sour taste or cold skin). The information does not concern generalized reactions or affective states (e.g., feeling uncomfortable or experiencing fear). This is a very important distinction to make. Unfortunately, the terms *feeling* and *sensation* have been used to de-

---

*Material in this chapter is based on content by A. Marilyn Sime and Mariah Snyder in previous editions.

scribe experiences varying from sense organ stimulation to vague generalized states of being. In this chapter, sensation refers specifically to sense organ stimulation, and sensation information to the description of that stimulation.

SCIENTIFIC BASIS

In 1962, Schachter and Singer reported the effects of sensation information on psychological responses to stressful situations. In their study, subjects who were told what bodily sensations they would experience from an epinephrine injection responded with less emotion than subjects who did not receive sensation information. Subsequently, this knowledge was incorporated into nursing by Jean Johnson through her systematic program of research, spanning over a decade. She has been largely responsible for contributing to our understanding of the effect of sensation information as a preparation for stressful or threatening situations and for influencing a cadre of nurse researchers to further expand the knowledge base in this area.

Johnson began her research in the laboratory (Johnson, 1973; Johnson & Rice, 1974) using the inflation of a blood pressure cuff to produce ischemic pain. The series of experiments that followed compared the effects of sensation information to procedural information. Her findings led to the following initial conclusions:

1. Descriptions of typical sensations reduced the amount of distress experienced but not the intensity of pain sensations.
2. Attending to the sensations per se did not reduce distress.
3. Sensation information did not reduce the perceived danger of the threatening event or its expected intensity.
4. All typical sensations did not need to be described for distress reduction.
5. Atypical sensations resulted in elevated distress.

Johnson theorized that a cognitive process involving expectations about sensations was the factor implicated in distress reduction. Specifically, emotional responses during threatening encounters were reduced when there was congruency between expected and experienced sensations.

As Johnson applied this theory to clinical research, she reached somewhat different conclusions about the cognitive processes involved in the use of sensation information. In a series of studies which included endoscopy (Johnson & Leventhal, 1974), orthopedic cast removal (Johnson, Kirchhoff, & Endress, 1975), pelvic examination (Fuller, Endress, & Johnson, 1978), and abdominal surgery (Johnson, Fuller, Endress, & Rice, 1978; Johnson, Rice, & Endress, 1978), Johnson and her colleagues found the following:

1. Sensation information reduced negative emotional responses in endoscopy, pelvic examination and cast removal; it also reduced restlessness, tranquilizers needed, heart rate acceleration, and gagging in the endoscopy studies.
2. In cholecystectomy, sensation information reduced negative postoperative moods only for those who were relatively fearful before surgery. It also reduced length of hospital stay and shortened the length of time before venturing from home.
3. There was no effect in herniorrhaphy subjects.

In this series of studies, sensation information had a greater effect on coping behaviors than on emotional responses. Accordingly, Johnson, Fuller, et al. (1978) concluded that knowing the sensations commonly experienced during the event provides a reality-oriented cognitive image (schema) that give the person a sense of control over the situation and enhances the person's ability to use available coping strategies, rather that merely providing congruence. Leventhal and colleagues (Leventhal, Brown, Schacham, & Engquist, 1979) further demonstrated that congruence or accuracy of the sensation information per se is not the critical factor in distress reduction. When a pain warning was added to sensation information, distress reduction was blocked. They interpreted this finding to mean that information on the potential strength of a stimulus elicits an emotional interpretation of the stimulus, rather than an objective encoding of the information. Arousal information, or descriptions of generalized states (such as apprehension, tension, excitement), was demonstrated to have little impact on distress during the encounter with the stressor. According to Leventhal, such information does not seem to assist persons to construct a schema of the features of the stimulus. If the schema is accurate, the person is assured that the experience is typical and he/she will be more likely to cope effectively with the situation and not experience undue emotional distress. Thus, an effective sensation information message should not contain information about generalized reactions or affective states.

INTERVENTION

Technique

Sensation information provided to a patient about to undergo a threatening procedure or test is believed to stimulate cognitive processes that assist the patient in developing a mental image or schema of the upcoming event. This schema provides a framework within which the patient can interpret and understand the experience, thereby reducing emotional response and promoting effective coping. To accomplish this objective, the information in the sensation information script must contain a specific and accurate description of the typical experience for the particular event and must be administered prior to the event.

Development of Intervention. Sometimes sensation information scripts are available by request from authors of previous research studies. The script should contain descriptions of both the subjective features and the objective features of the event that will assist the person to develop a schema of the upcoming test or procedure. Sometimes published reports provide sensory descriptions to assist in developing a script.

When a script or sensory description are not available, one must be developed. To develop a script, sensation information that is common to a particular diagnostic procedure or test that is thought to be stressful must be identified. Specific instructions are included in the following six steps for developing a sensation information intervention.

Step 1. Using a literature review or a preliminary study, identify procedures/events that are perceived as being stressful. It is important to verify that the event identified by health care professionals as stressful is also perceived as stressful by the client. If it is not, then sensation information is not necessary. Conversely, events that health care professionals do not consider stressful may indeed produce distress in clients who will be having the test or procedure (Ruiz-Bueno & Clement, 1996). Men and women who are undergoing the event or procedure may respond differently (Davis, Maguire, Haraphongse, & Schaumberger, 1994). Therefore, when determining the stressfulness of an event, gender differences need to be assessed.

Step 2. After determining that an event produces stress, observe clients during the event to obtain concrete information about stages, temporal aspects, and spatial features connected with the procedure.

The numbers needed to obtain these data will vary. Ruiz-Bueno (1987) secured sufficient information about genetic amniocentesis to develop an effective script after observing four subjects.

Step 3. Common sensations experienced during the test or procedure are identified by interviewing patients. This is best done after the test or procedure in order to obtain the subjective and objective features patients experienced during the event. Subjective features are the sensations the person directly experienced and are verifiable only by that person. Objective features are aspects of the situation verifiable by the experiencing person as well as anyone observing the event; objective features include temporal ordering of activities and spatial features of the environment. Approximately 10 to 15 interviews are needed to yield sufficient information about short procedures or tests (Cason & Landis, 1995; Sime & Libera, 1985). Lengthy procedures can be divided into stages with information obtained on each stage; such division increases the accuracy of recall. When the procedure is common to both men and women, both are included in the sample so as to avoid gender differences in descriptors (Cason & Landis, 1995). Open-ended questions are used to elicit information about what clients saw, heard, tasted, or felt. When terms such as "had pain" are used, follow-up questions are necessary to determine the sensations associated with pain. Behaviors or responses such as "couldn't swallow" or "jumped" also need to be clarified through additional questions to determine the associated sensations. To obtain a complete description of the sensations experienced throughout the procedure, clients may need to be asked about aspects of the procedure not initially described. Information obtained in step 2 can serve as the basis for questions to ask. It is important to ascertain the temporal order of the sensations the patient is reporting so that these sensations can be anchored with the specific objective features of the event. When saturation is reached (no new sensations being reported in interviews), the interviewing process can cease. Leventhal and Johnson suggested that sensations considered typical for the procedure are those reported by 50% of the respondents (1983).

Step 4. Typical sensations identified by patients in the first sample are validated in a second sample of 10 to 15 patients (Sime & Libera, 1985). One hundred percent verification about a sensation is needed for inclusion of the sensation in the script.

Step 5. In this final step, a script including the validated sensations is developed. The developer needs to decide whether the sensation information will be administered to subjects by audiotape, audiotape and photographs, or videotape. Conveyance of the sensation information script in a pamphlet is discouraged because clients may misread or only partially read the content. Davis, Maguire, Haraphongse, and Schaumberger (1994) found that administration of sensation and procedural information by means of a booklet increased anxiety before cardiac catheterization. As opposed to in-person delivery, these modalities are efficient and effective and ensure standard, complete delivery of information. It is important that the information be accurate, clear, logically organized, anchored to objective events, and objectively presented. Information about impressions, interpretations, or evaluations are not included. To insure completeness of the content, a written script is developed which includes both the subjective and the objective features of the event that were identified and validated by patients undergoing the event. For example, the following is a portion of the script developed for clients having genetic amniocentesis:

> For the ultrasound, the nurse will squirt a generous amount of a gel on your abdomen. The gel may feel warm as it is applied, then cools off. The light will be dimmed to make it easier for the doctor to see the images on the screen. (Ruiz-Bueno, 1987, p. 185)

Note that no evaluative statements were included.

Step 6. The final script is produced for administration by audiotape or videotape. The person selected to read the script for media production should have a clear, pleasant voice that is accent free. The script should be read without emotional inflection that might influence interpretation.

Administering the Intervention.   When a test or procedure is of a fairly short duration, the script is provided to the patient immediately before the procedure. For surgical procedures, sensation information can be provided the evening before surgery (Johnson, Rice, & Endress, 1978b). However, with the advent of same-day surgery, administration of the sensation information script may be done when pre-admission testing is scheduled. Administration should not be done so long in advance that the person forgets the information. Table 16.1 gives an example of the administration protocol developed for women undergoing genetic amniocentesis (Ruiz-Bueno, 1987).

TABLE 16.1   Sensation Information Protocol for Genetic Amniocentesis

1. Sensation information is described to clients scheduled for genetic amniocentesis.
2. Immediately or up to 30 minutes before the procedure (during "waiting room" time), the sensation information script is administered using an audiotape and earphones (administration time 4.75 minutes).
3. After listening to the audiotape, the client continues the normal routine of the office for the procedure.

Measurement of Effectiveness

The effectiveness of sensation information is thought to be the result of stimulation of cognitive processes which, in turn, help to reduce emotional responses to stressors and improve coping responses. Therefore, measuring the client's emotional state and coping processes during and after the event is considered to be appropriate. Self-reported moods and observations of the patient's behaviors during and after the event have been employed to reveal information on emotional states (Johnson, Morrissey, & Leventhal, 1973; Johnson, et al., 1975; Sime & Libera, 1985). Other investigators have interviewed patients following a procedure to determine the specific coping strategies used (King & Parrinello, 1988). Outcomes specific to surgery may also be examined. Johnson and colleagues (Johnson, Fuller, et al., 1978, Johnson, Rice, & Endress, 1978) looked at longer term effects, such as length of hospital stay and postdischarge convalescence period. Time before venture from home and resumption of normal activities have been measured for patients having abdominal surgery (Johnson, Fuller, 1978) or cataract surgery (Hill, 1982).

USES

The judgment of whether or not to use sensation information as an intervention is based on the nature of the diagnostic test or procedure, whether it is perceived as stressful by the patient, characteristics of the patient, and desired outcomes. Table 16.2 lists procedures and tests in which research has demonstrated the effectiveness of sensation information. Persons planning to use sensation information with similar populations may wish to contact the investigator for a copy of the developed script; however, frequent changes in techniques for

TABLE 16.2   Procedures/tests for which Sensation Information has been Used

Procedure/test	Author(s)
Amniocentesis	Ruiz-Bueno (1987)
Barium enema	Hartfield, Cason, & Cason (1981)
Cardiac catheterization	Davis et al. (1994)
Cast removal	Johnson et al. (1975)
Dental surgery	Sime & Libera (1985)
Femoral arteriography	Clark & Gregor (1988)
Endoscopy	Johnson et al. (1973)
Pelvic examination	Fuller et al. (1978)
Surgery	Hill (1982); Johnson, Fuller, et al. (1978a)

procedures and surgery may require updating the script. Although most research investigating the effectiveness of sensation information has involved adult subjects, it has also been shown to be effective with children (Johnson et al., 1975). Individual client characteristics (e.g., pre-event anxiety, desire for control, preferences for involvement) must also be considered when selecting sensation information as an intervention employed to reduce anxiety. Individual client characteristics have received limited attention in research studies.

Sensation information has not always been effective for all populations for whom it has been utilized. Flam and colleagues (Flam, Spice-Cherry, & Amsel, 1989) found no anxiety reduction in persons having a myelogram. Likewise, Wells (1992) found no effect in first-trimester abortion. However, neither of these studies included pre-event anxiety in the analysis of intervention outcome.

Precautions

One precaution in the use of sensation information relates to the script content. A common problem in some scripts has been the inclusion of generalized reactions or affective states rather than objective sensation information. Evaluations of sensations can increase distress (Leventhal et al., 1979; Padilla et al., 1981). Also, the inclusion of atypical sensations has resulted in elevated distress (Johnson, 1973; Johnson & Rice, 1974).

A second precaution concerns selection of candidates for the intervention. Before administering the script, patients must be adequately assessed. Then administer sensory information only to clients who have shown some degree of anticipatory concern or anxiety. Sime and Libera (1985) found that periodontal surgery patients with low pre-event anxiety who received sensation information reported less positive self-statements; sensation information may interfere with established coping responses in patients with low anxiety. Also, Padilla and colleagues (1981) found that sensation information given to some clients who were having a nasogastric tube inserted caused an increase in anxiety for patients who had expressed no desire for control over their experience.

Finally, sensation information will not be effective unless it is given at the right time.

FURTHER RESEARCH

Although the effectiveness of sensation information in reducing anxiety in a number of populations has been investigated, many theoretical and research questions still remain unanswered. To provide explanations, some research projects are suggested below.

1. A meta-analysis of previous nursing research would provide information about the overall efficacy of sensation information on coping with stressful health care encounters, updating the Suls and Wan (1989) meta-analysis of early nursing and nonnursing research on interventions using sensation information.
2. When studying the effects of sensation information, scrutinize scripts to ascertain that only pure sensation information is included. Other cognitive interventions, such as behavioral instruction or cognitive coping instruction, may achieve outcomes similar to sensation information; however the processes underlying these interventions are not clearly understood and further study is required to develop theoretical formulations that explain these differential effects. In some situations, combining cognitive/behavioral strategies may produce optimal outcomes. Therefore, careful study of the interactive effects of these interventions is mandatory.
3. Although a few studies have examined characteristics of subjects (Padilla et al., 1981; Ruiz-Bueno, 1987; Sime & Libera, 1985), considerably more information is needed to provide direction for nurses who are selecting candidates for the intervention. Emotional arousal, coping dispositions and preferences, and other

personal characteristics which interact with sensation information, must be investigated. Gender and life span differences in the perception of threat, and in response to intervention are also important areas for future investigation.

REFERENCES

Cason, C. L., & Landis, M. (1995). Women's sensory experiences during cardiac catheterization. *Cardiovascular Nursing, 31*, 33–36.

Clark, C. R., & Gregor, F. M. (1988). Developing a sensation information message for femoral arteriography. *Journal of Advanced Nursing, 13*, 237–244.

Davis, T. M. A., Maguire, T. O., Haraphongse, M., & Schaumberger, M. R. (1994). Preparing adult patients for cardiac catheterization: Informational treatment and coping style interactions. *Heart & Lung: Journal of Critical Care, 23*, 130–139.

Flam, B., Spice-Cherry, P., & Amsel, R. (1989). Effects of preparatory information of a myelogram on patients' expectations and anxiety levels. *Patient Education and Counseling, 14*, 115–126.

Fuller, S. S., Endress, M. P., & Johnson, J. E. (1978). The effects of cognitive and behavioral control on coping with an aversive health examination. *Journal of Human Stress, 4*, 18–25.

Garvin, B. J., Huston, G. P., & Baker, C. F. (1992). Information used by nurses to prepare patients for a stressful event. *Applied Nursing Research, 5*, 158–163.

Hartfield, M. T., Cason, C. L., & Cason, G. J. (1981). Effects of information about a threatening procedure on patients' expectations and emotional distress. *Nursing Research, 31*, 202–206.

Hill, B. J. (1982). Sensory information, behavioral instructions and coping with sensory alteration surgery. *Nursing Research, 31*, 17–21.

Johnson, J. E. (1973). Effects of accurate expectations about sensations on the sensory and distress component of pain. *Journal of Personality and Social Psychology, 27*, 261–275.

Johnson, J. E., Fuller, S. S., Endress, M. P., & Rice, V. H. (1978). Altering patients' responses to surgery: An extension and replication. *Research in Nursing and Health, 1*, 111–121.

Johnson, J. E., Kirchhoff, K. T., & Endress, M. P. (1975). Altering children's distress behavior during orthopedic cast removal. *Nursing Research, 24*, 404–410.

Johnson, J. E., & Leventhal, H. (1974). Effects of accurate expectations and behavioral instructions on reactions during a noxious medical examination. *Journal of Personality and Social Psychology, 29*, 710–718.

Johnson, J. E., Morrissey, J. F., & Leventhal, H. (1973). Psychological preparation for an endoscopic examination. *Gastrointestinal Endoscopy*, *19*, 180–182.

Johnson, J. E., & Rice, V. H. (1974). Sensory and distress components of pain: Implications for the study of clinical pain. *Nursing Research, 23*, 203–209.

Johnson, J. E., Rice, V. H., & Endress, M. P. (1978). Sensory information, instruction in a coping strategy, and recovery from surgery. *Research in Nursing and Health, 1*, 4–17.

King, B. K., & Parrinello, K. A. (1988). Patients perceptions of recovery from coronary artery bypass grafting after discharge from the hospital. *Heart & Lung, 17*, 708–715.

Leventhal, H., Brown, D., Schacham, S., & Engquist, G. (1979). Effects of preparatory information about sensation, threat of pain, and attention on cold pressor distress. *Journal of Personality and Social Psychology, 37*, 688–714.

Leventhal, H., & Johnson, J. E. (1983). Laboratory and field experimentation: Development of a theory of self-regulation. In P. J. Wooldridge, M. H. Schmitt, J. K. Skipper, Jr., & R. C. Leonard (Eds.), *Behavioral science and nursing theory*, (pp. 189–262). St. Louis: Mosby.

Nightingale, F. (1969). *Notes on nursing: What it is and what it is not.* NY: Dover. (Original work published 1869)

Padilla, G. V., Grant, M. M., Raines, B. L., Hansen, B. C., Bergstrom, N., Wong., H. L., Hanson, R., & Kubo,. W. (1981). Distress reduction and the effects of preparatory teaching films and patient control. *Research in Nursing and Health, 4*, 375–387.

Ruiz-Bueno, J. B. (1987). *Preferences for health care, pre-event anxiety, informational interventions and coping during genetic amniocentesis.* Unpublished doctoral dissertation, University of Minnesota, Minneapolis, MN.

Ruiz-Bueno, J. B., & Clement, E. (1996). *Experience of third trimester nonstress testing.* Unpublished manuscript.

Schachter, S., & Singer, J. E. (1962). Cognitive, social, and physiological determinants of emotional state. *Psychological Review, 69*, 379–399.

Sime, A. M., & Libera, M. B. (1985). Sensation information, self-instruction and responses to dental surgery. *Research in Nursing and Health, 8*, 41–47.

Suls, J., & Wan, C. K. (1989). Effects of sensory and procedural information on coping with stressful medical procedures and pain: A meta-analysis. *Journal of Consulting and Clinical Psychology, 57*, 372–379.

Wells, N. (1992). Reducing distress during abortion: A test of sensory information. *Journal of Advanced Nursing, 17*, 1050–1056.

17

Journal Writing

Mariah Snyder

Journals have been used extensively throughout history. Libraries abound with volumes of personal journals while countless other journals are stashed away in desks and attics. Journals provide a unique perspective on history and on personal struggles and growth.

Although much anecdotal evidence exists about the beneficial effects resulting from journaling, there is little documentation about the use of journals as a nursing intervention. The majority of nursing literature that exists focuses on the use of journals as a teaching strategy. Mayo (1996) proposed that "journaling is a new paradigm teaching technique" (p. 27) that provides students with an opportunity to reflect on and analyze their experiences. Her contention is congruent with Progoff (1975), a psychologist, who asserted that journaling enables persons to reflect and grow. Journal writing is a creative intervention that requires active involvement by the client. Despite the lack of empirical data to support its use as a nursing intervention, this author proposes that nurses explore the use of journal writing with patients.

DEFINITION

The terms *journal* and *diary* are often used interchangeably. However, major differences exist. According to Baldwin (1977), a diary is a more formal pattern of entries in which observations and experiences are recorded. Diaries are more superficial than journals, which are tools for recording the process of one's life (Baldwin, 1977). Events and experiences are noted in journals, but the emphasis is placed on the person's reflections about these events. In journal writing, an interplay between the conscious and unconscious often occurs.

Baldwin (1977) enumerated three assumptions she believed were implicit in journaling:

1. A person is capable of having a relationship with one's own mind.
2. The mind is seeking that which is waiting for attention in the unconscious.
3. This activity is valid and assists in promoting a person's well-being.

SCIENTIFIC BASIS

Making journal entries integrates memory, musculoskeletal system, and sensory systems, promoting harmony in a person. Because writing is slower than talking, it allows for more reflection on its content (Surbeck, Han, & Moyer, 1991).

Progoff (1975), a Jungian psychologist, has developed a systematized method for journaling, the "intensive journal." He views this transpsychological approach as, "providing active techniques that enable the individual to draw upon his inherent resources for becoming a whole person" (p. 9). Progoff noted

> The *intensive journal* process and its procedures for the person's work provide an instrument and a method by which we can develop interior capacities strong enough to be relied upon in meeting trials of our life. It gives us a means for private and personal discipline with which to develop our inner muscles. When we rely on these, we are indeed self-reliant because these inner capacities are ourselves. (p. 15)

Through journal recordings, persons are able to connect themselves with the continuity of their lives and thus enhance wholeness. Awareness of this continuity occurs as the person reflects on specific events, records them, and then carries on a dialogue linking the past and present.

INTERVENTION

Many techniques for journaling exist. However, some general guidelines or rules apply to all techniques. Journals are private; persons may volunteer to share entries they have made, but this should never be an expectation when instructing a patient about journal writing. Entries are made in a special notebook; this may be a fancy journal book or an inexpensive spiral notebook. Since pencil recordings fade over time, a pen should be used as it is helpful to re-read past entries. Establishing a specific time of day to make entries is helpful. Cameron (1992) suggested making entries in the early morning as it is easier to access the unconscious upon awakening. Many recommend making entries on a daily basis. However, Simons (1978) noted that journal writing needs to be the servant and not the master.

Techniques

Free Flow Journaling.   Free flow writing is the most common type of journaling. Cameron (1992) describes free flow journaling as "the act of moving the hand across the page and writing down whatever comes to mind. Nothing is too petty, too silly, too stupid, or too weird to be included" (p. 10). No attention is given to grammar, punctuation, or spelling. The main goal is to put one's thoughts on paper. Writing three pages a day has been suggested by Cameron (1992).

Occasionally persons are supplied with a stimulus that serves as a basis for their recordings. For example, fresh cinnamon rolls may be brought to a group journaling session. The smell and sight serve as stimuli on which a person can reflect and write. For some, recalling their mother's baking while for others, thinking about visits with a friend over a cup of coffee and a cinnamon roll will stimulate the flow. Even when a particular stimulus is used, persons write freely with no attention given to the structure of what is written. No constraints are imposed.

Intensive Journal.   Progoff (1975) developed the *Intensive Journal* method, a systematic way of making entries and conducting dialogue with and between topics. The process proposed by Progoff is aimed at enabling persons to reflect upon their lives and to grow. Directions are provided to assist persons to explore specific areas of their lives. An entry relating to one area often evokes thoughts in another area; thus, persons move between and among various areas.

Table 17.1 presents the 19 topics or sections of an *Intensive Journal*. These topics fit into three dimensions: life/time, dialogue, and depth. Each has a specific role in helping persons to explore their lives and

TABLE 17.1   Sections in the *Intensive Journal*

Life/Time Dimension
  Life history log
  Steppingstones
  Intersections
  Roads taken and not taken
  Now: the open moment

Dialogue Dimension
  Dialogue with persons
  Dialogue with work
  Dialogue with society
  Dialogue with events
  Dialogue with the body

Depth Dimension
  Dream log
  Dream enlargements
  Twilight imagery log
  Imagery extensions
  Inner wisdom dialogue
Period Log
Daily Log

Note. Adapted from *At a Journal workshop,* by I. Progoff, 1975, NY: Dialogue House Library.

become more self-reliant. In addition, a period log and a daily log are used.

The first dimension, "Life/Time," focuses on aspects of the person's life. It is central to the rest of the process in that all experiences occur within a time frame. All phenomena that relate to the progression of experiences and cumulatively form one's life history are included. According to Progoff (1975)

> Working in our life history is progressive. Its cumulative effect is to draw our life into focus so that we have a basis for making decisions that are pressing at the moment, and also to give us a perspective of the pattern and context of our life as a whole (p. 98).

In the "Steppingstones" section, the person records the significant points of movement from life's beginning to the present time. The area of "Intersections" explores moments of choice and why certain decisions are made. Unlived possibilities can be explored in "Roads Taken and Not Taken." "Now: The Open Moment" provides the person with an opportunity to decide on the way to proceed.

The "Dialogue" dimension helps persons to examine various life areas and their interrelations. Relationships with the various areas are explored as the person writes down the active conversations that occurs between self and work, society, events, and body.

In the "Depth Dimension" sections persons move from more tangible areas of life to deeper, unconscious areas. Considerable attention is given to dreams as these often reflect the tensions and anxieties of life. The twilight imagery and imagery sections are similar to meditation. A greater awareness of one's inner wisdom is sought.

The "Daily Log" section provides writers with opportunities to record events and their reactions to these events as they happen. Progoff (1975) noted that the focus should be on the essence of the experience. Accompanying mental images and emotions should be recorded. Writing thoughts and feelings may be therapeutic in and of itself.

Although Progoff saw the *Intensive Journal* as being a complete process, sections of the *Intensive Journal* can be used separately. For example, "Dialogue with Body" could be used by persons diagnosed with a chronic illness or a condition. Journaling may help them become more accepting of the illness and moving forward. "Roads Taken and Not Taken" can be used when persons are faced with decisions about their future. Persons review past choices and explore what might have occurred if a different choice had actually been made. These reflections may provide insights about the current decision to be made.

Measurement of Effectiveness

Many of the outcomes of journal writing may be not discernable immediately. Some of the possible areas to measure are improvement in self-esteem, reduction in anxiety, and acceptance of a chronic condition. Because journaling is very personal, it may be difficult for the nurse to evaluate the specific outcome, but the patient could report changes that have resulted from use of journal writing.

USES

Journals can be used to achieve outcomes such as increasing self-esteem and confidence, gaining personal knowledge, and improving overall well-being. As has been noted throughout this chapter, no research on the use of journals in nursing has been found.

Recording one's perspectives in a journal may help persons to increase knowledge about themselves and to uncover hidden resources or strengths. Cameron (1992) urged persons to provide positive affirmations to themselves. Writing positive statements and then reading these may help persons to gain confidence in their abilities. According to Simon (1978), keeping a journal provides a person with a clearer sense of self. Baldwin (1977) noted that persons often have an intuitive feeling that something is wrong but are unable to identify the precise problem. Journaling may help in uncovering the underlying concerns. Journals have been used as a teaching strategy to increase students' sense of social responsibility (Mayo, 1996). Johnson and Kelly (1990) described using journaling with cancer patients to help them in gaining insights about their lives.

Anecdotal evidence suggests that journaling helps to improve well-being. Runions (1984) instructed the mother of a seriously ill adolescent to keep a journal. The mother found journaling assisted her in coping with the stressful situation. Responses of high school students who used journaling suggested that journaling assisted them to accept their potentialities and develop techniques for managing conflict (Hall, 1990).

Precautions

Fear that others will find and read journal entries is a common concern. This fear prevents some persons from being completely open in expressing their perspectives. The heightened anxiety about the journal being found may prevent unconscious thoughts from entering consciousness and thus decrease the efficacy of the intervention. Caution is needed in using journaling with persons who are extremely introspective. However, Simons (1978) noted that journal writing may be useful in helping persons heal memories and become less introspective. Discussions or interactions with the person will assist the health professional in assessing if journal writing is helpful.

FURTHER RESEARCH

Research on the efficacy of journals is truly in its infancy. Studies are needed to determine the acceptance and efficacy of specific journaling techniques. Likewise, studies are needed to identify conditions and persons for whom journal writing would be helpful. McKinney

(1982) reported that 43% of the students in his study were enthusiastic about keeping a journal. Although journaling may appear to have a more feminine appeal, history abounds with examples of males who have kept journals. Information about characteristics of persons who enjoy journaling is needed so as to guide nurses in suggesting the interventions for patients.

REFERENCES

Baldwin, C. (1977). *One to one.* New York: Evans.

Cameron, J. (1992). *The artist's way.* New York: Putnam.

Hall, E. G. (1990). Strategies for using journal writing in counseling gifted students. *The Gifted Child Today, 13*(4), 2–6.

Johnson, J. B., & Kelly, A. W. (1990). A multifaceted rehabilitation program for women with cancer. *Oncology Nursing Forum, 17,* 691–695.

Mayo, K. (1996). Social responsibility in nursing education. *Journal of Holistic Nursing, 14,* 24–43.

McKinney, F. (1982). Free writing as therapy. In E. Nickerson & K. O'Laughlin (Eds.), *Helping through action: Action-oriented therapies* (pp. 60–65). Amherst, MA: Human Resources Development Press.

Progoff, I. (1975). *At a journal workshop.* New York: Dialogue House Library.

Runions, J. (1984). The diary: a self-directed approach to coping with stress. *Canadian Nurse, 80*(5), 24–28.

Simons, G. (1978). *Keeping your personal journal.* New York: Paulist Press.

Surbeck, E., Han, E. P., & Moyer, J. E. (1991). Assessing reflective responses in journals. *Educational Leadership, 48*(6), 25–27.

18

REMINISCENCE

Mariah Snyder

"Mrs. Johnson is living in the past. That's all she talks about." Comments similar to these are frequently made by nurses caring for elders. Often, elders' reflections about their past have been viewed negatively (Coleman, 1986). Reminiscing about the past, however, can have positive outcomes such as helping elders make adaptations necessary for meaningful living or contributing to their self-esteem. Reminiscence has been largely used as a planned intervention with elders. Since persons begin to reminiscence at about age 10 (Havighurst & Glaser, 1972), use of the intervention with younger populations needs further exploration (Chubon, 1980; Jones, 1995; Nugent, 1995). Reminiscence can be a part of the intervention armamentarium of nurses.

DEFINITION

In reading the literature on reminiscence, the intervention of "life review" is frequently cited interchangeably with reminiscence. Reflection on one's past life through memory and recall is common in the two interventions. Many authors fail to distinguish between life review and reminiscence. However, differences exist. Intermingling of reminiscence and life review has contributed to difficulties in interpreting the results of research studies. However, differences exist.

Butler (1963) defined life review as:

A naturally occurring, universal mental process characterized by the progressive return to consciousness of past experiences, and particular-

211

ly, the resurgence of unresolved conflicts; simultaneously, and normally, these reviewed experiences and conflicts can be surveyed and integrated. (p. 6)

Life review, according to Haight and Burnside (1993) is a critical analysis of one's past. The goal of life review is to facilitate the achievement of integrity.

Reminiscence has been defined in numerous ways. King (1982) defined reminiscence as "memory that has been filtered through time and altered by the person's other life experiences" (p. 22). In King's definition, reminiscent memories do not necessarily have to match life facts. Reminiscence, according to Kovach (1991) is "a cognitive process of recalling events from the past that are personally significant and perceived as reality based" (p. 14). Although persons reminisce spontaneously, reminiscence as a nursing intervention is a planned strategy in which persons are helped to recall past events, interactions, experiences, and feelings.

Kovach (1991) identified two types of reminiscence: validating and lamenting. In validating reminiscence the memories confirm or validate that the person's life has been fruitful and enriching. Lamenting reminiscences, in contrast, focus on negative elements of events or experiences and include difficulties in the person's past. Merriman (1989) presents a different paradigm: recreational and therapeutic reminiscence. Recreational reminiscence is what occurs when persons sit around and recall "the good old days." Therapeutic reminiscence is done to achieve a specific goal and may be difficult or painful.

SCIENTIFIC BASIS

Erikson's developmental stages (1950) have been used by some as the basis for the efficacy of reminiscence. Ego integrity vies with despair in Erikson's final developmental stage. Ryden (1981) viewed reminiscence as an adaptive strategy that helps elders to compensate for the many losses they have had and are experiencing. Reminiscence is a part of letting go, a realization that the past is past and that what happened during that part of life was alright. Ebersole (1976) contended that until persons have dealt with feelings about the past they are unable to deal with the present. Reminiscence provides persons with opportunities to resolve conflicts and to rid oneself of guilt. Studies provide support for using reminiscence to gain pride in accomplishments (Matteson & Munsat, 1982), increase interest in personal hygiene (Hala, 1975), and maintain self-esteem (Newbern, 1992).

The continuity theory has been proposed by Parker (1995) as a theoretical perspective that accounts for the therapeutic effects of reminiscence. In continuity theory, change is associated with one's past life and there is continuity in one's inner psychological functioning. Reminiscence provides persons with a sustaining sense of self and a mechanism for connecting the many developmental stages through which they have progressed. Recalling the past helps persons to adapt to life's changes and thus provide a sense of continuity. Parker contends that individuals reminisce more during times of personal transitions than during more stable periods. Within the continuity perspective, reminiscence would be an appropriate intervention to use with persons of any age group who are experiencing a transition in their lives. While the continuity theory appears to provide a logical basis for the efficacy of reminiscence, research is needed to validate this relationship.

INTERVENTION

Technique

Many different techniques have been used for assisting persons to reminisce. Group versus individual (Burnside & Haight, 1994) and structured versus unstructured (Haight & Burnside, 1993) are two of the different approaches that have been used. Each of these strategies will be discussed.

Individual and Unstructured. After discussing the intervention with the patient and obtaining patient's approval, the nurse assures the patient's comfort. In unstructured reminiscing, the patient is invited to talk about past experiences or feelings; no specific topic upon which to reflect is suggested. Good listening skills on the part of the nurse are essential. The nurse extends the reminiscence by providing comments that are supportive of the ideas or feelings being expressed. When a patient repeats an idea or returns to it, the nurse may suggest that this topic seems to be important to the person and encourage the person to talk about the associated memories or feelings. Expression of both positive and negative feelings are accepted. If a nurse does not feel competent in dealing with strong negative feelings, a referral to a psychiatric clinical nurse specialist can be offered to the patient as an option.

The patient may wish to audiotape the memories recalled. A tape can serve as a legacy to the family. Some patients may wish to record their memories in a journal. However, confidentiality regarding recorded or written memories is necessary and sharing should only be done with the patient's permission.

The number of reminiscence sessions used with a patient will vary and many times these cannot be predicted when initiating the intervention. Sessions may be held several times a week or on a weekly basis. No specific length of time for sessions has been established; the frailty of the patient and the nature of the reminiscing are factors to consider in determining the length of sessions.

Individual reminiscence sessions have a number of advantages. One-to-one sessions facilitate establishing a good relationship between the patient and the nurse. Unstructured individual sessions require less preplanning and less coordinating than do group sessions. One-on-one sessions tend to be best for persons who have moderate to severe cognitive deficits or who are shy. However, individual reminiscence sessions are time consuming and may not be feasible in busy nursing homes or senior centers.

Group Structured Sessions.   Because of time constraints, group structured reminiscence is used more frequently than is individual reminiscence. Various group sizes have been proposed. McMordie and Blom (1979) proposed groups of four to eight participants. If elders who are confused or cognitively impaired are group participants, the size of the group should be smaller. Whether the group will be open (i.e., anyone can join at any session) or closed (only those present at the first session will attend subsequent sessions) needs to be discussed and a group consensus achieved. The specific focus for the sessions may contribute to the decision about groups being open or closed.

Conducting a reminiscence group requires that the nurse be skillful in group techniques. It is important that everyone in the group has an opportunity to share reminiscences; however, no one should feel pressured to do so. Some group participants may need encouragement to share their memories. Several meetings of the group may be needed before all of the members feel comfortable in sharing their memories with others. The leader needs to be aware that despite the presumed pleasantness of the suggested topic, such as a holiday, some participants may have sad or negative memories associated with the topic.

For a structured reminiscence group, a special topic or theme is chosen. Props are often used to provide an atmosphere that helps the group recall memories related to the theme. For example, if the theme is holidays, decorations and foods for a particular holiday will help members "get in the mood." Flags, band music, and watermelon to eat could be used when the Fourth of July is the theme.

Table 18.1 provides guidelines for using structured reminiscence with a group.

TABLE 18.1 Technique for Group Structured Reminiscence

1. Contact potential participants.
   Decide on size of group (4–8).
   Determine length (45–60 minutes), date, and time of session.
   Establish whether it will be an open or closed group.
   Select number of sessions to hold (6–10) on a weekly basis.
2. Select as meeting place a quiet space, pleasant environment. Arrange the room with comfortable chairs.
3. Remind participants about session and arrange for participants to attend.
4. At first session, introduce self and have participants introduce themselves.
   Take time for persons to get to know each other.
   Describe the purpose of reminiscence and format of sessions.
   Have group establish ground rules, such as occasions for all participants to share their reminiscences.
5. Introduce the theme for the session. (Grade school, for example, would be a good topic if the group is beginning in September because it is relatively unthreatening.)
   Use pictures (e.g., schools) schools and other props.
   Ask participants to share memories (e.g., of their first day of school or early school days).
   Allow sufficient time for persons to respond and others to ask questions and contribute their memories; if the group is hesitant, the leader can share her or his own memories; ask probing questions to elicit other memories.
   If conversation drifts from chosen topic, a decision must be made whether to bring the discussion back to the topic.
6. When about 10 minutes remain, scan the group and see if all members have had an opportunity to share their memories; provide them with an opportunity to share.
7. The leader frequently scans the group to determine members' reactions, such as smiles, alertness, withdrawal, etc.; if any untoward reactions are noted, individual discussion with the member should occur at the conclusion of the session.
8. Summarize the general memories that have been shared; thank the members for their contributions; provide members with a schedule of the next meetings and the topics.

Measurement of Effectiveness

A variety of psychological variables have been examined to determine the efficacy of reminiscence. Since most of the studies have been with elders, one questions whether the tests used have been developed for use with elders. Few studies have included measures that would capture any untoward reactions to the use of reminiscence. In addition to the measurement of psychological factors, anecdotal recordings by the nurse about the personal reactions, both immediate and longer term, would provide a more extensive picture about the impact that reminiscence has on participants.

USES

Elders

Reminiscence has been used extensively with elders. The majority of the outcomes explored relate to improved mood state. Some of the specific outcomes tested include improvement of self-esteem (Nugent, 1995), lessening of depression (Ha, 1993; Youssef, 1990), improving life satisfaction (Ha, 1993; Sherman, 1987), and decreasing stress/anxiety (Beadleson-Baird & Lara, 1988; Rybarczyk & Auerbach, 1990). Because of the multiplicity of techniques used, including segments of life review, it is difficult to determine which technique or techniques would be most beneficial to use. However, the overall evidence is that reminiscence does produce beneficial effects when implemented with elders.

Other Populations

Suggestions in the literature about the use of reminiscence with other populations is becoming more common. It appears that in most instances reminiscence has been used with persons who have terminal conditions or are critically ill. Chubon (1980) used reminiscence for patients who had end-stage renal disease. Results showed that reminiscence/life review helped the patients gain a better sense of their self-worth. Use of reminiscence in critical care units has been suggested by Jones (1995). Outcomes from the use were to encourage communication between the nurse and the patient, to provide a relief from stressful situations, and to promote interaction between the family and the patient. Nugent (1995) provided case studies to illustrate the use of reminiscence with patients who had cancer. Nurses should consider use of reminiscence with patients and families who may be experiencing high levels of stress, especially stress associated with transitions (Parker, 1995).

Precautions

Assessment of individuals prior to initiating reminiscence will help to avoid its use with individuals for whom it may produce negative effects. According to Ryden (1981), elders who are functioning in Erikson's generativity developmental stage may be adversely affected if attention is focused on recalling past events and experiences. Conversely, some persons may use reminiscence as an escape from the present situation.

Reminiscence may result in the recall of painful memories. Lashley (1993) noted that nurses need to be alert to unresolved grief or guilt that may result from reminiscence sessions. Difficulty in sleeping, eating, and concentrating are several of the symptoms that may indicate a person has unresolved life conflicts that reminiscence has brought to consciousness. Recalling past memories may make some persons feel more lonely and isolated. Awareness that outcomes of reminiscence may not always be pleasant and positive will help nurses to detect symptoms suggesting persons who may require professional assistance in resolving conflicts from earlier years.

FURTHER RESEARCH

A number of authors (Burnside, 1990; Kovach, 1990; Merriman, 1989) have done critical reviews of the research on reminiscence. A major problem has been the lack of specificity in describing the technique used and the mixing of components of reminiscence and life review. Merriman (1989) noted that the lack of consistency in findings may be the result of using various techniques. The following are a few of the areas in which further research is needed:

1. Groups are frequently used for reminiscence. However, studies have not examined whether the results are due to the use of reminiscence or to being part of a group. Similarly, few data exist to guide practitioners on which persons would benefit most from reminiscence on a one-to-one basis.

2. Clear differentiations have been made between life review and reminiscence (Burnside & Haight, 1994). However, studies are needed to determine conditions/populations for which each intervention would be the intervention of choice.
3. Explorations on the outcomes resulting from the use of reminiscence with younger populations are needed. The majority of findings on its use with younger populations have been anecdotal.

REFERENCES

Beadleson-Baird, M., & Lara, L. L. (1988). Reminiscing: Nursing actions for acutely ill geriatric patients. *Issues in Mental Health Nursing, 9,* 83–94.

Burnside, I. (1990). Reminiscence: An independent nursing intervention for the elderly. *Issues in Mental health Nursing, 11,* 33–48.

Burnside, I., & Haight, B. (1994). Reminiscence and life review: Therapeutic interventions for older people. *Nurse Practitioner, 19,* 55–61.

Butler, R. (1963). The life review: An interpretation of reminiscence in the aged. *Psychiatry, 26,* 65–76.

Chubon, S. (1980). A novel approach to the process of life review. *Journal of Gerontological Nursing, 6,* 543–546.

Coleman, P. (1986). Issues in the therapeutic use of reminiscence with elderly people. In I. Hanley & M. Gilhooly (Eds.), *Psychological therapies for the elderly* (pp. 41–64). New York: New York University Press.

Ebersole, P. (1976). Problems of group reminiscing with institutionalized aged. *Journal of Gerontological Nursing, 2,* 23–27.

Erikson, E. (1950). *Childhood and society.* New York: Norton.

Ha, Y. S. (1993). The effect of group reminiscence on the psychological well-being of the elderly. *The Seoul Journal of Nursing, 7*(1), 35–60.

Haight, B., & Burnside, I. (1993). Reminiscence and life review: explaining the differences. *Archives of Psychiatric Nursing, 7*(2), 91–98.

Hala, M. (1975). Reminiscing group therapy project. *Journal of Gerontology, 27,* 245–253.

Havighurst, R., & Glaser, R. (1972). An exploratory study of reminiscence. *Journal of Gerontology, 27,* 245–253.

Jones, C. (1995). 'Take me away from all of this' . . . can reminiscence be therapeutic in an intensive care unit? *Intensive and Critical Care Nursing, 1,* 341–343.

King, K. (1982). Reminiscing psychotherapy with aging people. *JPN and Mental Health Services, 20*(2), 20–25.

Kovach, C. R. (1990). Promise and problems in reminiscence research. *Journal of Gerontological Nursing, 16*(4), 10–14.

Kovach, C. (1991). Reminiscence: Exploring the origins, processes, and consequences. *Nursing Forum, 26*(3), 14–20.

Lashley, M. E. (1993). The painful side of reminiscence. *Geriatric Nursing, 14,* 138–141.

Matteson, M. & Munsat, E. (1982). Group reminiscing therapy with elderly clients. *Issues in Mental Health Nursing, 4,* 177–189.

McMordie, R., & Blom, S. (1979). Life review therapy: Psychotherapy for the elderly. *Perspectives in Psychiatric Care, 27,* 162–166.

Merriman, S. B. (1989). The structure of simple reminiscence. *The Gerontologist, 29,* 761–767.

Newbern, V. B. (1992). Sharing the memories: The value of reminiscence as a research tool. *Journal of Gerontological Nursing, 18*(5), 13–18.

Nugent, E. (1995). Try to remember . . . reminiscence as a nursing intervention. *Journal of Psychosocial Nursing, 33*(11), 7–11.

Parker, R. G. (1995). Reminiscence: A continuity theory framework. *The Gerontologist, 35,* 515–525.

Rybarczyk, B. D., & Auerbach, S. M. (1990). Reminiscence interviews as stress management interventions for older patients undergoing surgery. *The Gerontologist, 30,* 522–528.

Ryden, M. B. (1981). Nursing intervention in support reminiscence. *Journal of Gerontological Nursing, 7,* 461–463.

Sherman, E. (1987). Reminiscence groups for community elderly. *The Gerontologist, 27,* 569–572.

Youssef, F. A. (1990). The impact of group reminiscence counseling on a depressed elderly population. *Nurse Practitioner, 15*(4), 32–37.

19

Storytelling

Paula Dicke

Storytelling is as old as history itself. Throughout time, humans have used stories to entertain, to instruct, and to share a part of themselves with others. Storytelling is a natural and very common part of every-day conversation. Stories are constructed to tell a tale, to convey our understanding and view of an experience, and to increase listeners' comprehension of ideas.

Philosophers and physicians, even Hippocrates, taught through story-telling prose, sharing their wisdom with stories about illness (Borkan, Miller, & Reis, 1992). Storytelling has long been used as a teaching tool and as a therapeutic intervention by nurses, but its use has been poorly documented. One explanation might be that nurses do not always recognize these therapeutic stories because storytelling is used so frequently in everyday conversation. Another explanation for this dearth of reports, especially qualitative studies on the effectiveness of the intervention, may reflect the difficulty nurses experience research-ing the benefits of storytelling. Nurses frequently combine storytell-ing with other interventions, making it difficult to distinguish which benefits come from intervention.

Therapeutic storytelling can take many forms. The story can be told in a group or shared by the nurse and an individual patient. The story can be constructed and shared by the nurse or the patient, or it can be created together. Stories may flow from normal activities, as a patient telling their health history (Bornstein, 1988), or be a purpose-ful part of a therapeutic intervention (Wenckus, 1994). Stories found in literature can also be told.

Storytelling is an effective therapeutic intervention for all ages. Very young children and elders can derive pleasure and therapeutic benefit from stories. Those that are most vulnerable because of limited cognition, language skills, emotional distress, or social isolation benefit from the story as well as the interaction itself (Cohen, 1987; Gotterer, 1989; Wenckus,1994; Wynne, 1987).

Storytelling has many goals:

- to promote the release of tension and emotions
- to gain insight into feelings and behavior
- to develop or change attitudes and values
- to learn effective ways of solving problems and making decisions
- to increase the sense of shared experiences and decrease the sense of isolation

DEFINITION

Storytelling is the oral narration of fact or fiction (Gustafson, 1988). For storytelling to be therapeutic, the patient needs to feel involved in the story and identify with the experience shared in the story. The story benefits the patient when there is insight and catharsis.

Metaphors are extensively used in storytelling. Kopp (1971) defined metaphor as a way of speaking in which one thing or situation is expressed in terms of another. This bringing together of the two ideas casts light on the nature of what is being described.

SCIENTIFIC BASIS

Gotterer (1989), identified three functions of therapeutic storytelling: (a) to change time and place, (b) to stimulate strong emotions, and (c) to encourage communication. The story helps patients make a transition from day-to-day routines to other times and places, where therapeutic benefits can be realized. Active imaging is often triggered, allowing a release of emotional energy that may assist the person in resolving conflicts and gaining a new awareness of their feelings and needs.

According to Barker (1985), for psychotherapeutic interventions to bring about rapid change, the right hemisphere of the brain must be involved. Metaphors or stories are classified as right brain interventions. The following example depicts this.

Todd was a 12-year-old undergoing a bone marrow transplant requiring multiple blood draws and biopsies. Todd was very stressed and anxious about these procedures. At that time, *Star Wars* was a popular movie. A nurse recounted the story to Todd and he was able to quickly identify with one of the characters, Han Solo. By imaging himself as Han Solo, Todd was able to share with staff the adventures he created for Han and his space ship. He was able to escape pain, fear and anxiety by flying off into the stars having new and empowering adventures. Todd used his imaging and storytelling ability whenever a threatening procedure was occurring. He would end the story when the procedure was complete, feeling empowered and not victimized.

Wallis (1985) noted that stories work because persons bring the story into the framework of their own experience. Persons attempt to make sense of the story in relation to their lives. Wallis stated

> Although the content of the story is a metaphor which evokes but does not literally reproduce the actual circumstances of clients' lives, they can accept what the story seems to imply about their problems and consider new solutions within the framework of their own lives. (p. 5)

Smith and Hoppe (1991) stated that every patient has a story that reflects the interaction of the biological, psychological, and social components of his or her life. These stories are rich with information needed for diagnosis of health problems as well as treatment of the problems.

Because stories can also deal indirectly with a patient's problems and their meanings are veiled, they may be less threatening than dealing with the problems directly (Barker, 1985). The various meanings that are presented are interpreted and used on the unconscious level. Stories may provide ideas for the resolution of a problem.

Based on the principle used in group hypnotherapy sessions, it can be assumed that the patient attends only to the message that make sense to him or her and will disregard other messages (Krietemeyer & Heiney, 1992). A story rich in metaphor can be shared with a group or separately with many individuals and still meet the very personal individual needs of the listener. Messages that are not of value to the listener will do no harm.

INTERVENTION

A variety of storytelling techniques are used by nurses. Sometimes literature provides the story; at other times, creating a story for a specific purpose is part of the process.

Technique

Creating an atmosphere for storytelling is important, whether on an individual or group basis. You and your patient need to be comfortable. Encourage a receptive mood by helping the patient relax. Be familiar with the story you will tell or read.

Selecting the story to use is critical to the success of the intervention. The nurse can draw on a wide variety of stories from literature. Bettelheim (1976), Bornstein (1988), and Levine (1980) describe the great value of fairy tales in psychotherapy. The lesson of the tale is safely learned with little defensiveness because it is not a specific representation of the patient's life experiences. A nurse can share a fairy tale with a patient because of this distancing without fear of loosing control of the situation. An example for using a story from literature follows:

Elaine was 43 years old and receiving intensive therapy for her cancer. She had experienced many setbacks that had kept her hospitalized for weeks in protective isolation. Her family visited when they could but school and work kept them occupied and away from Elaine for days at a time. Elaine had expressed initial pleasure that her family could function without her and her children seemed to settle in well to home, school, and social activities. As the days in the hospital grew longer and her isolation became unending, Elaine stopped initiating conversation with staff and visitors, seemed uninterested in her appearance, and complained about the television shows, the noise in the hall, the cleaning staff, the food and so on.

During a visit with Elaine, the nurse therapist shared a picture book, "The Story of a Mouse Trapped in a Book," (Felix, 1980). Elaine studied the book over and over, keeping it at her bedside for days. Her behavior began to change, she talked more freely of her feelings of being trapped and of losing the opportunity to share the wonderfully normal life her family was living. Elaine had gained insight from the story of the mouse, had understood that the life experiences and feelings of the mouse were mirrors of her own sense of powerlessness. She learned from the mouse that there are actions she could take to gain some measure of control over her life. All of this was from a book without words but full of metaphors.

Appendix A lists sources for stories that may be used in storytelling. Gotterer (1989) selected short stories when working with a group of elderly women patients. Native American stories, Hasidic tales, Chinese folklore, and stories by contemporary authors were used during a once-a-week, 90-minute sessions for 10 weeks. The overall goal was to provide elders a consistent opportunity to share their thoughts and feelings by talking, listening and writing. Stories were shared to stimulate discussion at the beginning of the session and another was shared to knit together the day's session and provide closure.

The structure of the group and the stories used are defined by the purpose. Alcoholics Anonymous is a support group that is run in large part by members telling their own stories as they relate to alcoholism. Other groups, encouraging socialization and understanding of a shared experience, might create a group story. The leader starts the story and provides a bridge for a group member to continue the story. The story moves around the group, everyone having an opportunity to help create the story (Krietemeyer & Heiney, 1992).

When sharing a story during a stressful procedure, the nurse should be close enough to the patient to be seen and become the patient's center of attention without shouting or invading the patient's personal space. The story should be short enough to complete in one sitting and needs to be rich in detail to catch the interest of the listener. It helps to know the patient's interests and issues. The story should encourage some interaction from the patient, especially if distraction is a goal. The following example illustrates this:

A young adolescent girl waiting for a liver transplant had to go through many procedures. One of her nurses had a 3-year-old son, Shawn, who had very typical 3-year-old adventures. The patient loved to be told tales of this toddler because she and Shawn were struggling with similar issues, mastering the world they lived in. The nurse added humor to the tales to further release the tension.

McQuellon and Hurt (1993), introduce popular literature on the theme of illness and health as a therapeutic tool for increasing a patient's understanding of the illness experience. Sharing a story written by someone with similar experiences to the patient's is a powerful tool that can decrease the sense of isolation and fear and provide knowledge for managing what is to come.

It is important to provide time for the patient to digest the story and to respond to it. Many persons need time to think about the story before being ready to express themselves and talk about the relation the story has to his or her life. The storyteller must be attentive to the cues, both verbal and nonverbal, being displayed. Emphasizing that stories are rich in meaning and that individuals have very different interpretations may assist persons in responding to the story.

Measurement of Effectiveness

Depending on the purpose for which storytelling is being used, various parameters can be used to measure the effectiveness of the intervention. Instruments that measure decreases in anxiety or depression could be used when improvement in mood is desired. Comparisons of patterns of communication and social isolation before and after storytelling would be appropriate for determining the effectiveness of storytelling in achieving improved social interaction. Most important, subjective reports of improved functioning are beneficial in determining effectiveness of storytelling as an intervention.

USES

Storytelling has been used with a number of patient populations to achieve a variety of goals. Bornstein noted that nurses could use stories in explaining procedures, in evoking hope for a successful outcome of a diagnostic procedure, in obtaining information about the patient, and in helping resolve conflicts.

Coles (1989) detailed the use of literature in teaching medical students and working with patients. Storytelling is one of the teaching strategies included in the *Teacher's Desk Reference* (Gustafson, 1988). This author has found that novels and autobiographies assist nursing students to gain an appreciation of the impact that a chronic condition has on a person's life.

McQuellon and Hurt (1993) reviewed six powerful cancer stories and found the stories, though different in form and style, gave the reader useful insights into life-threatening illness and the common themes shared by patients and their families. These stories can affect the practice of nursing and can provide a framework for patients to see themselves and adapt to life changes.

Stories and metaphors have been used extensively in psychotherapy. Milton Erickson, the father of modern hypnosis, employed metaphorical stories to assist persons in resolving their conflicts. Using the basic premise that therapy first models the patient's world and then role-models the patient's world, Erickson was able to weave metaphors into personalized stories and indirectly deliver therapeutic suggestions (Heiney, 1995).

A classic example of Erickson's style is seen in the metaphor he created for a retired florist experiencing severe cancer pain. Erickson used the metaphor of a garden and of planting a tomato seed. He inserted comfort phrases about the seed resting, sleeping comfortably, at peace. After the session the patient was able to return home and lived pain free for several more months (Heiney,1995).

Precautions

Many fear that because they are not trained psychotherapists, they are not ready to use metaphors and stories as therapeutic interventions. Stories may elicit powerful responses and nurses must be prepared for these feelings and behaviors. Some patients will ignore the story and the storyteller, others might argue the theme of the story, and others might show anger, fear or sadness when listening to the story. All of these are appropriate responses. To extend the story's therapeutic benefit the nurse needs to accept the response and explore other healthy views and options coming from the story.

However, for the patient exhibiting psychological problems, a nurse should only use stories rich with metaphors under the guidance of a trained therapist.

FURTHER RESEARCH

Nurses have used stories and metaphors for many years, but they have not fully documented their effectiveness in achieving patient outcomes. A variety of techniques relating to storytelling have been used. Techniques being used must be fully described so that comparisons can be made across studies and among various techniques. Protocols that can be easily implemented need to be designed. The following are several of the many areas in which research on storytelling is needed:

1. What are the conditions/situations for which the various story-telling techniques would be most appropriate?
2. Which techniques for storytelling are most effective with specific patient populations?
3. What conditions/situations require psychotherapeutic skills when using storytelling?
4. What methodologies would be most appropriate for studying the effectiveness of persons telling their own story?
5. What are the stories/metaphors that practicing nurses use?

APPENDIX A: SOURCES FOR STORIES TO USE IN STORYTELLING

Chase, R. (1943). *The jack tales.* Boston: Houghton Mifflin.
Clarkson, A., & Cross, G. B. (1980). *World folktales: A Scribner collection.* Chicago: Scribner.
Dorson, R. M. (Ed.). (1975). *Folktales told around the world.* Chicago: University of Chicago Press.
Glassie, H. (Ed.). (1985). *Irish folktales.* New York: Pantheon Books.
Lankton, C. H., & Lankton, S. R. (1989). *Goal-oriented metaphors for adults and children in therapy.* New York: Brunner/Mazel.
Lobel, A. (1980). *Fables.* New York: Harper & Row.
Wallis, L. (1985). *Stories for the third ear.* New York: Norton & Co.

REFERENCES

Barker, P. (1985). *Using metaphors in psychotherapy.* New York: Brunner/Mazel.
Bettelheim, B. (1976). *The uses of enchantment: The meaning and importance of fairy tales.* New York: Knopf.
Borkan, J. M., Miller, W. L., & Reis, S. (1992). Medicine as storytelling. *Family Practice, 9*(2), 127–129.
Bornstein, E. M. (1988). Therapeutic storytelling. In R. Zahourek (Ed.), *Relaxation and imagery. Tools for therapeutic communication and intervention* (pp. 101–118). Philadelphia: Saunders.

Cohen, L. J. (1987). Bibliotherapy: Using literature to help children deal with difficult problems. *Journal of Psychosocial Nursing, 25*(10), 20–24.

Coles, R. (1989). *The call of the stories.* Boston: Houghton Mifflin.

Felix, M. (1980). *The story of a mouse trapped in a book.* La Jolla, CA: Green Tiger.

Gotterer, S.M. (1989). Storytelling: A valuable supplement to poetry writing with the elderly. *The Arts in Psychotherapy, 16,* 127–131.

Gustafson, M. (1988). *Teacher's desk reference: Vol. 2.* Unpublished manuscript, School of Nursing, University of Minnesota, Minneapolis.

Heiney, S.P. (1995). The healing power of story. *Oncology Nursing Forum, 22*(6), 889–904.

Kopp, S. (1971). *Guru: Metaphors from a psychotherapist.* Palo Alto, CA: Science and Behavior.

Krietemeyer, B. C., & Heiney, S. P. (1992). Storytelling as a therapeutic technique in a group for school-aged oncology patients. *Children's Health Care, 21*(1), 14–20.

Levine, E. S. (1980). Indirect suggestions through personalized fairy tales for treatment of childhood insomnia. *The American Journal of Clinical Hypnosis, 23*(1), 57–63.

McQuellon, R. P., & Hurt, G. (1993). The healing power of cancer stories. *Journal of Psychosocial Oncology, 11*(4), 95–108.

Smith, R. C., & Hoppe, R. B. (1991). The patient's story: Integrating the patient- and physician-centered approaches to interviewing. *Annals of Internal Medicine, 115,* 470–477.

Wallis, L. (1985). *Stories for the third ear.* New York: Norton.

Wenckus, E. M. (1994). Storytelling: Using an ancient art to work with groups. *Journal of Psychosocial Nursing, 32*(7), 30–32.

Wynne, E. (1987). Storytelling: In therapy and counseling. *Children Today, 16*(2), 11–15.

20

Validation Therapy

Lois B. Taft

Validation is a therapeutic approach for interacting with disoriented elderly individuals. The goals of validation are to relieve anxiety, maintain dignity, and prevent further deterioration and withdrawal. The validation worker focuses on accepting a person's emotional reality and validating feelings rather than insisting on the accuracy of facts and orientation to the present.

Validation was originated by Naomi Feil based on her experience working with confused older adults. Feil grew up in the Montefiore Home for the Aged in Cleveland, Ohio where her father, a psychologist, and her mother, a social worker, pioneered services for the elderly in the 1940s (N. Feil, 1985). Feil returned to the Montefiore Home in 1963 as a social worker and applied *reality orientation*—an intervention designed to reorient confused elderly individuals. Feil became disillusioned with this strategy and explored other forms of group therapy (N. Feil, 1967). She refocused therapeutic interactions on validating and supporting the residents' feelings in whatever time or location was real to them. The treatment she developed was initially known as validation/fantasy therapy; but currently it is generally referred to simply as *validation.*

Feil is now the executive director of the Validation Training Institute in Cleveland, Ohio. She has published books on applying validation techniques (N. Feil, 1982, 1993), written film scripts which demonstrate validation in individual and group settings (E. Feil, 1972, 1978, 1980), and conducted numerous validation workshops throughout the United States and Canada. Validation books and films have been translated into Dutch, German, Finnish, Swedish, Danish, and

French (Kohn, 1993), and validation techniques are used by practitioners in Europe, North America, and Australia.

DEFINITION

Validation therapy is

> a method of therapeutic communication with disoriented clients which focuses on the emotional rather than the factual content of their speech. It assumes that the behavior and speech of the disoriented person has an underlying meaning, and that disoriented people return to the past in an attempt to resolve unfinished conflicts. (Cumulative Index to Nursing & Allied Health Literature, 1996, p. 328)

As a communication technique, validation is not new. Therapeutic communication skills require the recognition of both feeling and content components in a transaction. Clarifying and reflecting feelings are strategies that are integral to therapeutic communication and the establishment of a therapeutic relationship. Validation is a strategy employed in the therapeutic use of self. According to Naomi Feil (1985), "Validation is a combination of empathy, touch, eye contact, mirroring body movements, matching voice and rhythms, picking up cues about feelings and putting them into words, accepting without judging, and genuine total listening" (pp. 91–92).

At a validation workshop in 1987, Feil used the following example to illustrate the application of validation techniques. A woman in her late fifties arrived at a nursing home to visit her 85-year-old mother. The old woman looked up from her chair, smiled at her daughter, and said "Mama." The younger woman was exasperated by her mother's confusion and responded by saying, " I'm not your mother. I'm your daughter. Your mother died a long time ago." This response produced pain and frustration. According to validation, there is wisdom in the old woman's behavior. She has retreated to the world of love, security, and dependence that she experienced as a child. Her eyesight isn't good. The daughter reminds her of her mother. Both are people she loves. Instead of insisting on "reality," the daughter could respond to her mother's emotional reality with affection. Further communication could be facilitated by encouraging reminiscence. The daughter could respond, "What do you remember about your mother?" Validating responses build trust and communicate empathy.

SCIENTIFIC BASIS

Theoretical Support

Feil proposed that her work extends Erikson's theory of developmental stages (Erikson, 1963). Erikson identified eight stages of development throughout the life span and described a psychological conflict at each stage. The developmental crisis of old age focuses on ego integrity versus despair. According to Feil, older adults who are unable to achieve integrity may retreat to the past to express feelings and resolve old conflicts. Feil identified this last life stage as resolution versus vegetation (Feil, 1985). Validation promotes resolution, allows unresolved feelings to be expressed, and restores dignity and self-worth through acceptance.

Assumptions underlying validation therapy are that (a) all behavior has meaning, (b) early learned emotional memories replace rational thinking in the disoriented old-old, and (c) retreat to the past is purposeful (Feil, 1982). The last assumption has been questioned (Miller, 1995), because individuals with dementia may lack the necessary cognitive abilities to think abstractly, analyze, and initiate purposeful behavior. Validation theoy counters that the process occurs on a subconscious level.

Humanistic principles of client-centered therapy as developed by Rogers (1951) support validation therapy (Babins, 1986, 1988). Client-centered therapy focuses on the internal world of the client and emphasizes the dignity of each individual and his or her right to be unique. The role of the therapist is to be accessible to the client and to convey an attitude of genuineness, empathy, and unconditional positive regard. In validation, empathy is used to tune in to the world of the disoriented old person. Validation requires a nonjudgmental attitude that recognizes each person as unique and conveys respect and acceptance.

Research

Feil reported positive outcomes using validation therapy, but she has not substantiated clinical impressions with research. Although a few research studies have been conducted on the effectiveness of validation therapy, there is still a lack of research-based support because of serious methodological pitfalls. Several attempts have been made to test the effectiveness of validation groups with disoriented elderly residents in institutional settings (Babins, 1985; Morton & Bleathman, 1991; Peoples, 1982; Robb, Stegman & Wolanin, 1986; Scanland & Emershaw, 1993). In each of these studies, however, there were serious methodological problems including very small sample sizes, attrition of participants, between-group differences, lack of control groups, and questions about the sensitivity, reliability, and validity of the research instruments.

In response to validation, Babins (1985) reported improvements in verbal and nonverbal communication skills and a slowing of mental deterioration. Additional researchers noted improvements in communications skills of residents participating in validation groups (Morton & Bleathman, 1991; Peoples, 1982). Other research failed to document significant improvements in mental status, morale, social behavior, depression, or functional status (Robb et al., 1986; Scanland & Emershaw, 1993).

Conceptual generality is explained as the accumulation of similar findings in different studies with different subjects, situational factors, and other variations in study procedures. Such aggregate results lead to greater confidence in conclusions regarding the merit of clinical interventions. Robb, Stegman, & Wolanin (1986) proposed that "conceptual generality represents a potential solution to the problem of obtaining valid results from studies that lack methodological rigor because they focus on human behavior in complex health care environments" (p. 113).

In a recent study, Fine & Rouse-Bane (1995) examined the application of validation techniques in one-to-one interactions rather than group settings. This study was conducted on a dementia unit in a retirement community, and results supported the use of validation techniques to respond effectively to agitated behavior. This study documented successful psychotropic dose reductions in 25% of the sample, and a reduction in incident reports related to behavior problems. These results are encouraging, but they cannot be generalized because of methodological concerns, such as the lack of a control group.

Qualitative methodologies provide a mechanism for evaluating the impact of validation therapy. Zachow (1984) reported a case study in which she used validation as an intervention to establish rapport with an extremely withdrawn, disruptive nursing home resident. The staff documented changes in the resident's behavior including a decrease in verbal agitation and an increase in alertness. The resident was able to feed herself more frequently and was more coherent in verbal communication. Nighttime sleep patterns improved, and the use of prn Thorazine decreased by 50%. Such observations support validation as a promising intervention for interacting with disoriented, elderly individuals.

Bleathman and Morton (1992) used a single-case study design on a validation group consisting of 5 residents. The most striking finding in their study was "the contrast between the minimal social interaction observed outside the group and the greatly improved social function in the group setting" (Bleathman & Morton, 1991, p. 20). Based on their research and their clinical experience in England, they concluded that validation therapy is a beneficial psychological treatment worthy of further investigation.

INTERVENTION

Techniques

Validation can be used on an individual basis or as a focus for group work with disoriented elderly residents. Validation strategies are designed according to the stage of disorientation.

Stage One. This stage is labeled *mild confusion* (van Amelsvoort Jones, 1985), or *malorientation* (Feil, 1982). Individuals in stage one are oriented to person, place, and time, and they are verbal and generally ambulatory. Their coping strategies include denial and blaming. Disorientation in this group revolves around old conflicts. These conflicts may be expressed in forms that are labeled as symptoms of confusion. As caregivers, we rarely know with what unresolved conflicts individuals are struggling. But, using validation techniques, it is possible to accept the reality of their feelings, to actively listen, and to empathize.

At this stage, feelings of loss are validated by listening and exploring the individual's experience. The use of key words or rephrasing confirms active listening and allows the older person to lead the conversation. Recognizing and using the preferred sense (auditory, visual, or kinesthetic) is another technique to tune into the older person's language and confirm an understanding of their experience. Nonthreatening, exploring questions begin with *who, what, when, where,* and *how,* but avoid *why.* Other types of questions that can be used include: polarity questions (When is it the worst?), life review questions (What happened before . . . ?), and questions that invite the resident to imagine an opposite situation (What would it be like if. . .?).

Touch is used only if the person is ready. Persons in this stage often retreat from intimate relationships and are threatened by the expression of feelings.

Stage Two.   When physical and social losses accumulate and an individual gives up trying to hold on to reality, they enter stage two, time confusion. In this stage, individuals lose track of present time and retreat inward. They lose communication skills and often create unique word forms from past memories and use pronouns without specific references. They use symbols to represent people and events remembered from the past. Therapeutic responses include the use of vague pronouns (such as *he, she, it, someone,* or *something*) to explore the person's experience and maintain the flow of conversation. Questions similar to those used in Stage 1 are used to explore the person's experience in Stage 2.

The person in Stage 2 expresses feelings in words, through symbols, with movements, and through behavior. The validation worker reflects the feelings, links behavior with universal human needs and feelings, and expresses them out loud. In this way the emotional reality experienced by the individual is validated. At this stage, the person is generally responsive to the use of touch, direct eye contact, and a clear, low nurturing voice.

Stage Three.   Many of the characteristics of individuals in Stage 2 and 3 are similar, but greater withdrawal is apparent in the individual in Stage 3, the repetitive motion stage (Feil, 1993). Communication skills and speech may be lost. Repetitive sounds and repetitive movements may be used to stimulate, reassure, and help resolve feelings. These individuals generally have profound sensory losses and use what Feil refers to as kinesthetic memory or motion to trigger emotions, give pleasure, and control anxiety.

Individuals in Stage 3 are more difficult to reach. They do not respond unless stimulated through a combination of nurturing touch, voice-tone, and direct eye contact; in addition, they respond well to music and rhythms. It may be possible to reach an individual in this stage by mirroring their body movements. Another technique is attempting to link behavior with the feelings that person is experiencing. It is generally necessary to use trial and error. If you hit the right feelings, the person may respond with a nod, with eye contact, or with words. It may be possible to restore some speech, some rational thinking, and some social interaction through a genuine validating relationship.

Stage Four. This stage is labeled *vegetation* and occurs when the individual completely shuts out the outside world and gives up the struggle to live. Feil (1982) reports minimal evidence of response to validation techniques once an individual reaches this level of disorientation.

Table 20.1 summarizes validation techniques that are used in interaction with disoriented older adults. The first five techniques are used with persons in the first stage of disorientation, and the remaining strategies are added when communicating with persons in Stages 2 and 3.

Validation Therapy Groups

Validation techniques may be used in group work in addition to interpersonal communication. Those in the second stage of disorientation are most responsive to group work. Individuals in Stage 1 may assist in a leadership role, but they generally feel threatened if they are included as a group member.

Validation groups with five to ten members generally meet for 20 minutes to an hour once or twice a week. In validation groups, social roles are assigned to each member. Examples of such roles

TABLE 20.1 Validation Techniques

1. Listen with empathy. Do not correct or contradict.
2. Rephrase. Repeat key words.
3. Reminisce. Review the past.
4. Recognize and use words from the person's preferred sense.
   * Visual: look, picture, watch
   * Auditory: listen, hear
   * Kinesthetic: feel, touch
5. Ask nonthreatening questions.
   * Use *who, what, when, where,* and *how* questions, avoid *why*
   * Use polarity: ask the extreme (*worst, best, how bad, how often*)
   * Imagine the opposite (*What would happen if . . .*)
   * Use ambiguity: use vague pronouns such as *he, she, it, somebody*
6. Link behavior to needs (love, safety, activity, usefulness).
7. Reinforce social roles.
8. Sing and interact using music.
9. Use supportive touch (gentle touch to cheek, shoulder, arm, or hand).
10. Maintain eye contact.
11. Observe and mirror body movements.
12. Match and express emotions (love, anger, fear, grief).

include a welcomer to greet each member, a hostess to pass out refreshments, a song leader, or a chair arranger. Universal feelings such as anger, separation, or loss provide the focus of discussion. The goal in validation groups is not to reorient, but simply to help the group members feel better. Music and rhythm are important parts of the group session and refreshments are served to conclude the meeting. "Groups trigger memories of family roles, of former social group roles, of social controls. People begin to listen. Speech improves. They care about others as they model the nurturing validation worker . . . and they validate each other" (Feil, 1982, p. 62).

Guidelines for Validation with Agenda Behavior

Rader, Doan, and Schwab (1985) coined the term *agenda behavior,* to describe "verbal and nonverbal planning and actions that cognitively impaired persons use in an effort to fulfill their felt social, emotional, and physical needs" (p. 196). Wandering is a form of agenda behavior which may threaten the safety of the disoriented elderly person. The proposed approach in response to agenda behavior is an adaptation of validation therapy. The following steps are recommended:

1. Face the resident and make direct eye contact if this does not appear to be threatening.
2. Gently touch the resident's arm, shoulder, back, or waist if he or she does not move away.
3. Listen to what the resident is communicating verbally and nonverbally. Link this to the resident's feelings.
4. Identify the agenda, the resident's plan of action, and the emotional needs the agenda is expressing.
5. Repeat specific words or phrases from the agenda ("fix supper," "your children") or state the need or emotion ("You need to go home?," "You're worried that you family won't be fed?") (Rader, Doan, & Schwab, 1985, p. 198).

If these five steps are followed consistently throughout the day, agenda behavior can be diminished or eliminated. These validation techniques may be successful because residents feel safe and understood and no longer need to fantasize or actually seek a past environment to feel connected with others and secure.

Measurement of Outcomes

Patterns of ambulating, eating, and speaking can be documented to determine the impact of validation techniques on functional abilities. Mental status scales measure cognitive responses to validation. However, it is important to maintain realistic expectations. If the goal of validation is to reduce anxiety and maintain dignity, emotional and behavioral responses may be the most significant variables to measure. Scales that measure depression, morale, and anxiety as well as measures of affect such as smiling or crying are some indicators that can be used for measuring progress. Sleep patterns may also reflect emotional comfort. Behavioral outcomes include social behavior such as alertness, responsiveness, and the number of social interactions. Problematic behaviors such as verbal agitation and aggressive behavior can also be monitored.

USES

In their classic text on confusion, Wolanin and Phillips (1981) state that confusion can be a decompensating reaction resulting from disruption of pattern and meaning. The stressors of old age including losses, powerlessness, and rejection can result in disorientation. According to Wolanin and Phillips, the nurse can best intervene by providing support and by providing opportunities for meaningful social interaction. Validation can be effectively used to treat individuals whose confusion results from disruption of pattern and meaning.

Feil (1985) advocates the use of validation for disoriented old people who have retreated to the past to resolve old conflicts or escape painful feelings. She points out that individuals with a dementia such as Alzheimer's disease do not choose to withdraw, and they may not respond to validation. However, validation techniques have been effectively used as an intervention for clients with dementia (Bleathman & Morton, 1992; Gold, 1994; Olds, 1995; Rader, 1995).

Precautions

Although validation provides a promising therapeutic approach for working with confused, elderly individuals, it is not an appropriate intervention in all cases of confusion. Validation is not appropriate when confusion is due to acute, reversible causes. The abrupt onset or sudden change in the severity of confusion should prompt the nurse to suspect physiological causes. Physical assessment and prompt medical treatment are required.

FURTHER RESEARCH

Long-term care of the cognitively impaired elderly is often custodial rather than therapeutic. The use of validation offers the caregiver an opportunity to intervene therapeutically. Validation techniques may be useful in relieving anxiety and maintaining dignity despite the ravages of old age. The following are areas in which research investigations would provide data on the application and merit of validation therapy.

1. What assessment strategies can determine the stage of disorientation?
2. What are the characteristics of persons who benefit from validation?
3. What are the characteristics of persons who benefit most from one-to-one validation versus group sessions?
4. What are the behavioral, emotional, and functional patient outcomes associated with validation therapy?
5. What are the longitudinal effects of validation therapy?
6. Can validation provide an alternative to the use of physical and chemical restraints?
7. How can validation techniques be effectively implemented by nonprofessional staff and/or family members?
8. What is the impact of a validation therapy program on staff morale and on the stress of family caregiving?

REFERENCES

Babins, L. (1985). *Group approaches with the disoriented elderly: Reality orientation and validation therapies.* Unpublished Master's thesis, McGill University, Montreal.

Babins, L. (1986). A humanistic approach to old-old people: a general model. *Activities, Adaptation, and Aging, 3–4*(8), 57–63.

Babins, L. (1988). Conceptual analysis of validation therapy. *International Journal of Aging and Human Development, 26*(3), 161–168.

Bleathman, C., & Morton, I. (1991). Validation therapy with the demented elderly. *Nursing Standard, 5*(45), 20.

Bleathman, C., & Morton, I. (1992). Validation therapy: extracts from 20 groups with dementia sufferers. *Journal of Advanced Nursing, 17,* 658–666.

Cumulative Index to Nursing & Allied Health Literature 1996 subject heading list (Vol. 41). (1996). Glendale, CA: Cinahl Information Systems.

Erikson, E. *Childhood and society* (2nd ed.). (1963). New York: Norton.

Feil, E. (Producer). (1972) *The Tuesday group* [Film]. Cleveland. OH: Edward Feil Productions.

Feil, E. (Producer). (1978). *Looking for yesterday* [Film]. Cleveland, OH: Edward Feil Productions.

Feil, E. (Producer). (1980). *The more we get together* [Film]. Cleveland, OH: Edward Feil Productions.

Feil, N. (1967). Group therapy in a home for the aged. *Gerontologist, 7*(3), 192–195.

Feil, N. (1982). *Validation: the Feil method.* Cleveland, Ohio: Edward Feil Productions.

Feil, N. (1985). Resolution: The final life task. *Journal of Humanistic Psychology, 25*(2), 91–105.

Feil, N. (1993). *The Validation breakthrough: Simple techniques for communicating with people with Alzheimer's-type dementia.* Baltimore: Health Professions.

Fine, J. I., & Rouse-Bane, S. (1995). Using validation techniques to improve communication with cognitively impaired older adults. *Journal of Gerontological Nursing, 21*(6), 39–45.

Gold, M. (1994). Bringing focus to the mind of dementia. *Provider, 20*(5), 43–46, 122.

Kohn, L. S. (1993). Validating current validation therapy (letter). *Journal of Gerontological Nursing, 19*(11), 6.

Miller, L. (1995). Validation therapy: The human face of elderly care? *Complementary Therapies in Nursing & Midwifery, 1*(4), 103–105.

Morton, I. & Bleathman, C. (1991). The effectiveness of validation therapy in dementia—A pilot study. *International Journal of Geriatric Psychiatry, 6,* 327–330.

Olds, J. (1995). Strategies of care for patients with dementia. *Professional Nurse, 10*(9), 585–587.

Peoples, M. (1982). *Validation therapy versus reality orientation as treatment for disoriented institutionalized elderly.* Unpublished Master's thesis, University of Akron, Akron, Ohio.

Rader, J. (1995). *Individualized dementia care.* New York: Springer.

Rader, J., Doan, J., & Schwab, M. (1985). How to decrease wandering, a form of agenda behavior. *Geriatric Nursing, 6,* 196–199.

Robb, S. S., Stegman, C. E., & Wolanin, M. O. (1986). No research versus research with compromised results: A study of validation therapy. *Nursing Research, 35*(2), 113–118.

Rogers, C. R. (1951). *Client-centered therapy: It's current practice, implications, and theory.* Boston: Houghton Mifflin.

Scanland, S. G., & Emershaw, L. E. (1993). Reality orientation and validation therapy: Dementia, depression, and functional status. *Journal of Gerontological Nursing, 19*(6), 7–11.

van Amelsvoort Jones, G. (1985). Validation therapy: A companion to reality orientation. *The Canadian Nurse, 81*(3), 20–23.

Wolanin, M. O., & Phillips, L.(1981). *Confusion: Prevention and care.* St. Louis: Mosby.

Zachow, K. M. (1984). Helen, can you hear me? *Journal of Gerontological Nursing, 10*(8), 18–22.

21

Music Therapy

Linda Chlan

Music has been used since ancient times as a treatment modality. Over 4,000 years ago the Egyptians noted that incantation affected the fertility of women. The Bible details how David used the harp to cure King Saul's depression. Plato and Aristotle have been designated by Alvin (1975) as the fathers of music therapy; they prescribed music for treating numerous diseases. According to Plato, health of mind and body could be obtained through music. Aristotle provided hyperactive children with musical rattles for the purpose of calming the youngsters. Since the time of Aesculapius, music has been used to treat the mentally ill. Cicero and Seneca studied the effects that music had on behavior. Nightingale recognized the healing power of music in her care of the sick (1860/1969).

Music therapy evolved as a distinct profession in the late 1940s. Although music therapists are found in many larger health care facilities and would be chiefly responsible for planning and instituting the therapeutic use of music, many occasions and situations exist in which nurses are in a prime position to implement music as an intervention. Nurse can integrate music into the patient's care plan and effectively utilize music in professional practice with patients (Cook, 1986; Herth, 1978). Although the majority of the early literature on the use of music in nursing was primarily anecdotal, the number of experimental design studies on the use of music as an intervention is increasing.

DEFINITION

Webster's dictionary defined music as "the science or art of ordering tones or sounds in succession, in combination, and in temporal relationships to produce a composition having unity and continuity" (Woolf, 1979, p. 752).

Music used for therapeutic purposes has been termed music therapy. Munro and Mount (1978) defined music therapy as the controlled use of music and its influence on the human being to aid in physiologic, psychologic, and emotional integration during treatment of an illness or disability. From a nursing perspective, music used for therapeutic purposes includes promotion of patient/client health and well-being.

Alvin (1975) delineated five elements of music: (a) frequency (pitch), (b) intensity, (c) tone color (timbre), (d) interval (creates melody and harmony), and (e) duration (creates rhythm and tempo). The character of the music and its effects depend on the qualities of these elements and their relationships to each other. Rhythm has particularly strong influence.

Pitch is produced by the number of vibrations per second of a sound. Rapid vibrations (high-pitched sounds) tend to act as a stimulant, whereas slow vibrations bring about relaxation.

Intensity refers to the volume of the sound. It is related to the amplitude of the vibrations. A person's like or dislike of a musical piece often depends on the intensity of the music. Intensity can be used to produce effects such as intimacy (soft music), protection (loud music), and power. Emotions are affected by the intensity of the music.

Tone color (or *timbre*) is a nonrhythmical, purely sensuous property and results from the harmony present or the characteristics of a voice or instrument. Psychological significance results from the tone color of a piece because the person associates it with past events or feelings. A musical piece sung by two different artists can produce very different effects on an individual because of the tone color (Alvin, 1975).

The interval is the distance between two notes and is related to pitch. The sequence of intervals results in the melody and harmony of a piece. Cultural norms determine what is deemed enjoyable and pleasant. Musical compositions may contain dissonances, but the expectation in Western culture is that these will be relieved and that the ending of the piece will be a pleasant cadence. The harmonic progression in a musical piece holds the person's attention until the conclusion.

Duration and *rhythm* are similar. Duration refers to the length of sounds, and rhythm is a time pattern fitted into a certain speed. Rhythm is the most dynamic aspect of music and is a key factor for selecting particular pieces to use in specific situations. Rhythms (respiration, heart beat, speech, gait) are an integral part of human life, and music can play an instrumental role in harmonizing these internal rhythms. In some pieces, the rhythm conveys peace and security. Repetitive rhythms can elicit feelings of depression. Continuous sounds that are repeated at a slow pace and become gradually slower produce decreased levels of responsiveness. Strong rhythms can awaken feelings of power and control. Of all the five elements to consider in selecting music for a patient population, rhythm requires the closest scrutiny.

SCIENTIFIC BASIS

Because music is complex and affects all aspects (physiological, psychological, spiritual) of human beings, it is difficult to differentiate the precise effects because of the constant interplay between and among them. Over the centuries philosophers, musicians, and psychologists have debated whether the physiological or psychological system is affected first. Guzzetta (1995) stated that music first affects the mind, then influences the body. Alvin (1975) stated that responses to music are influenced by one's physical receptivity to sound, the innate or acquired sensitivity to music, and state of mind. Responses to music are also influenced by one's preferences, environment, education and other nonmusical factors that cannot be ignored.

Entrainment is a process whereby two objects vibrating at similar frequencies will tend to cause mutual sympathetic resonance (Moranto, 1993). Musical tempos may be used to synchronize or entrain the physiological state; changes in body rhythms (e.g., heart rate) are caused by musical variations (Bonny, 1986). Music has the potential to entrain heart rate via its pulse, or to entrain breathing through its rhythm (Moranto, 1993). Bonny (1986) noted that entrainment can utilize not only the tempo of a musical selection, but also the mood of the music to effect changes in mood state and body rhythms.

In addition to entrainment of body rhythms, music also affects the limbic system, which is integrally involved in emotions and feelings. In particular, the pitch and rhythm of music affect the limbic system (Guzzetta, 1995). Psychophysiologic responses occur because of the impact the musical selection has on the limbic system. Guzzetta (1995) notes that musical vibrations in harmony with a person's fundamental vibratory pattern may produce healing and restore regulatory functions.

INTERVENTION

Adequate assessment is needed before using music as an intervention. Determination of a person's likes or dislikes regarding musical selections is essential. This assessment will provide information on how frequently music is listened to, musical preferences and the purpose for which the person listens to music. For some, the purpose for listening to music may be relaxation and restfulness while others may listen to music for stimulation and invigoration. It is only after sufficient data have been gathered that decisions can be made regarding the type of selections and the technique that would be most feasible to use.

Type of Music

Careful attention to the selection of the music contributes to the therapeutic effects obtained. For example, music to induce relaxation has a regular rhythm, no extremes of pitch or dynamics, and a melodic sound that is smooth and flowing (Bonny, 1986). Because past experiences influence one's response to music, careful assessment of the patient precedes initiation of the therapy. Specific selections may be associated with happy or sad past experiences. Mason (1978) recommends having available recordings of old-time songs and dances; theme music from plays; television and radio programs, and movies; national and folk songs; Viennese waltzes, polkas, and marches; and popular classics for use with the elderly. Many elderly persons prefer patriotic and popular songs, and hymns with slower tempos played with familiar instruments (Moore, Staum, & Brotons, 1992).

Religious music may be welcomed by many. Hymns are not readily available on the radio, and providing tapes will fill a void for many who are unable to attend church or synagogue services. Playing these at the time of the scheduled service may help to make the person feel less isolated.

Classical music is thought to evoke greater enjoyment and interest with repeated listening, while popular music declines in effectiveness with repetition (Bonny, 1986). Bonny feels that patients in a weakened state respond less to popular music and are more receptive to meaningful stimuli of classics that have lived through time. Providing a choice and consideration of individual musical preferences are key (Bonny, 1986).

New-age or nontraditional music has become very popular. New-age music lacks traditional music's characteristic tension and release (Guzzetta, 1995). According to Guzzetta, new-age music is thought to be a vibrational language that helps the bodymind attune itself, and is frequently used for promoting relaxation. However, varying opinions exist as to the appropriateness of new-age music for relaxation (Bonny, 1986; Hanser, 1988); further investigation is needed.

Techniques

Use of music can take many forms, from listening to a tape to singing or to playing an instrument. The nurse must keep a number of factors in mind when considering the use of music as an intervention: (a) type of music and personal preferences, (b) active versus passive involvement, (c) use in a group or on an individual basis, (d) length of time to use music, and (e) the desired outcomes.

Listening. Providing means for patients to listen to musical selections is the technique most frequently employed activity. Cassette tapes and compact disks make it easy to provide music for patients in all types of settings. Tapes have many advantages. The machines are relatively inexpensive; they are small and can be used in even the most crowded confines, such as critical care units. Auto-reverse capabilities on tape players allow the patient to listen to music for any length of time without having to be interrupted to turn the tape over. Compact disks (CDs), although more expensive than tapes, have superior sound clarity, and track-seeking that allows immediate selection of a desired piece. Comfortable headphones allow patients private music listening that does not disturb others, whether with a tape or CD player.

For a very modest outlay of money, a nursing unit can establish a tape library containing a sufficiently wide variety of selections to meet various musical preferences. It is also easy to individualize tapes to meet the preferences of each patient. Attention to copyright laws is needed in reproducing tapes. Permission from the production company is needed. A number of commercial companies, such as Halpern's Inner Peace Music, produce long-playing tapes that are appropriate for hospital use.*

---

*Halpern's Inner Peace Music, 524 San Anselmo Ave., Suite 700, San Anselmo, CA 94960-2614.

A variety of types of music is readily available on the radio. However, commercial messages and talk are deterrents to music therapy intervention. Also, one cannot control the quality of the radio signal reception nor the specific selection of music.

Active Involvement.   The purpose for which music is being used dictates the types of patient involvement. Active involvement is often used to elicit responses from withdrawn patients. Hoskyns (1982) had a group of patients with Huntington's chorea play instruments as a means of stimulation and to increase involvement with others. Mason (1978) used tambourines, triangles, castanets, sleigh bells, chime bars, cymbals, and drums with an elderly population as a means for increasing social interaction. Active participation requires more planning and time involvement on the part of the nurse than does the use of taped selections for individual listening.

Individual Versus Group.   Music has been used widely for groups of patients. Alvin viewed music as a powerful integrating force in a group of people. Music creates interrelationships among the members, and between the listener and the music. Music has been used as a modality for fostering group social interaction with the elderly and with persons who have psychiatric disorders. A group of Canadian nurses on a chronic care unit have used karaoke to enhance the patients quality of life by connecting with others on the unit and with memories of people from the past (Mavely & Mitchell, 1994). Unless an appropriate research design is used, it is difficult to determine if the effects obtained from the use of music are due to the music or to the interaction and support provided from being part of a group.

Diversity in the preferences of individuals in a group or the lack of an appropriate site for a group session may necessitate implementing music on an individual basis. Assessment findings provide data from which the nurse makes the decision about which method is the preferred one for a specific patient.

Guidelines for Music as Relaxation

Individuals in stressful situations, such as hospitalization, respond to music in a positive manner which can be used to promote relaxation (Hanser, 1988). Music as a relaxation technique utilizes music as a pleasant stimulus to block out sensations of anxiety, fear, and tension, and to divert attention from unpleasant thoughts (Thaut, 1990). A minimum of 20

TABLE 21.1 Guidelines for Music Intervention for Relaxation

1. Ascertain patient has adequate hearing.
2. Ascertain patient's like/dislike for music.
3. Assess music preferences and previous experience with music for relaxation; assist with tape selection as needed.
4. Determine mutually agreed upon goals for music intervention with patient.
5. Complete all nursing cares prior to intervention; allow at least 20 minutes of uninterrupted listening time.
6. Gather equipment (cassette tape player, cassette, headphones, batteries) and ensure it is in good working order. Provide the patient a choice of soothing selections for relaxation.
7. Assist patient to a comfortable position, as needed; ensure call-light is within easy reach.
8. Assist patient with equipment as needed.
9. Enhance environment to suit patient (draw blinds, close door, turn off overhead lights, etc.).
10. Post a "Do not disturb" sign to minimize unnecessary interruptions.
11. Encourage and provide patient with opportunities to practice relaxation with music.

minutes are probably necessary to induce relaxation with some form of relaxation exercise, like deep breathing, before initiating the music intervention (Guzzetta, 1995). Guzzetta postulated four necessary elements for promoting relaxation: a quiet environment; a comfortable position, a passive attitude, and focused concentration on the music.

While the definition of relaxing music may be unique to the individual, factors affecting the response to music also include musical preferences and familiarity. Selections with slow tempos, lengthy phrases, and soft dynamics (Hanser, 1988), and with a tempo of 70–80 beats per minute (Cook, 1981) are considered relaxing. One of the most widely used classical music selections for relaxation is the Pachebel *Canon in D,* which is frequently included in commercially available relaxation tapes. As with any relaxation intervention, practice enhances effectiveness. Table 21.1 outlines the basic steps for utilizing music intervention to promote relaxation.

Measurement of Outcomes

The outcome indexes selected for evaluating the effectiveness of music vary depending on the purpose for which music was implemented.

TABLE 21.2 Uses of Music

Orientation/Minimizing Disruptive Behaviors
  Elderly (Gerdner & Swanson, 1993; Janelli et al., 1995; Sambandham &
    Schirm, 1995)
  Psychiatric Patients (Courtright et al., 1990)

Decreasing Anxiety
  Pediatrics (Klein & Winkelstein, 1996; Pfaff, Smith, & Gowan, 1989)
  Surgical (Augustin & Hains, 1996; Kaempf & Amodei, 1989; Moss, 1988;
    Steelman, 1990; Stevens, 1990)
  Coronary Care Unit (Bolwerk, 1990; White, 1992)

Pain Management
  Acute Pain (Good, 1995)
  Chronic Pain (Schorr, 1993)
  Childbirth (Durham & Collins, 1986)
  Cancer-related Pain (Beck, 1991)

Stress Reduction and Relaxation
  NICU (Burke, et al., 1995; Collins & Kuck, 1991)
  Ventilator-dependent ICU Patients (Chlan, 1995)
  Adult ICU Patients (Updike, 1990)
  Coronary Care Patients (Guzzetta, 1989)

Stimulation
  Elderly Depression (Hanser & Thompson, 1994)
  Elderly Sleep Disturbances (Mornhinweg & Voignier, 1995)
  Head-injury (Jones et al., 1994)

Music-Thanatology
  Dying Patients (Schroeder-Sheker, 1994)

Outcomes may be physiological and/or psychological alterations and include a decrease in anxiety, an increase or decrease in arousal, an increase in social interaction, promotion of relaxation, and an increase in overall well-being. Table 21.2 provides the reader with measurement indexes that have been used with specific populations. In addition to those listed in the table, salivary cortisol (Miluk-Kolasa, Obminski, Stupnicki, & Golec, 1994) and serum immune measures (Bartlett, Kaufman, & Smeltekop, 1993) have also been examined in response to music; results are mixed and require further investigation.

USES

Conditions/Populations in Which Music Therapy has been Used

Music has been tested as a therapeutic intervention with many different patient populations; a majority of the nursing literature focuses on individualized music intervention. Table 21.2 lists those common populations for which music has been used as an intervention. General uses of music include orienting, minimizing disruptive behaviors, decreasing anxiety, pain management, stress reduction, relaxation, and stimulation.

Orienting and Minimizing Disruptive Behaviors. Music stimulates free association of ideas, helping persons recall past experiences, events, and feelings, and integrate these into the present. Playing familiar songs prompted reminiscence, created and facilitated communication, and increased socialization in a group of elderly residents with Alzheimer's disease (AD) (Sambandham & Schirm, 1995). Music has also been found to mask noise and provide for a more relaxing environment at meal-time with institutionalized psychiatric patients (Courtright, Johnson, Baumgartner, & Webster, 1990).

Individualized music intervention for confused AD residents has been used successfully for agitation management (Gerdner & Swanson, 1993). Elderly medical/surgical patients who were restrained demonstrated more positive behaviors while listening to music, which was thought to be a familiar stimulus (Janelli, Kanski, Jones, & Kennedy, 1995).

Decreasing Anxiety. One of the strongest effects of music is anxiety reduction (Standley, 1986). Music has been found to be valuable in enhancing the immediate environment, providing a diversion, and lessening the impact of potentially disturbing sounds as an anxiolytic for pediatric patients (Klein & Winkelstein, 1996; Pfaff, Smith & Gowan, 1989), a wide variety of surgical patient experiences (Augustin & Hains, 1996; Kaempf & Amodei, 1989; Moss, 1988; Steelman, 1990; Stevens, 1990), coronary care patients (Bolwerk, 1990; White, 1992), and for those experiencing childbirth (Durham & Collins, 1986).

Pain Management. Music has also been used frequently as an adjunct to pain management with a variety of patients. Music is proposed to be effective for pain management via distraction, enhancing patient control, improving mood, and by facilitating the release of endorphins, the body's "natural painkillers" (Beck, 1991). Music has been used with varying success for acute pain management (Good, 1995), chronic pain management (Schorr, 1993), and for cancer-related pain (Beck, 1991).

Stress Reduction and Relaxation. Music has been employed as a method for reducing stress and physiologic arousal in a variety of settings. In the neonatal intensive care unit (NICU), music has been played for intubated babies as an effective means for minimizing their stress arousal in this setting (Burke, Walsh, Oehler, & Gingras, 1995; Collins & Kuck, 1991). Music of a soothing nature has been found to be an effective stress-reducing intervention for ventilator-dependent ICU patients (Chlan, 1995).

Music has also been found to be an effective method of promoting relaxation. Intensive care patients (Updike, 1990) and coronary care patients (Guzzetta, 1989) have demonstrated a generalized relaxation response following music intervention.

Stimulation. Music can be used either to calm or stimulate patients. The type of music selected for purpose each will vary. Homebound elders with depressive disorders responded favorably to a program of self-selected relaxing music listening; the result of the program was less depression (Hanser & Thompson, 1994). Using classical and new age music to calm patients has been successful with community-based elders who had suffered sleep disturbances (Mornhinweg & Voignier, 1995). Classical and popular music has been tested as a means of stimulation for brain-injured, comatose patients, although it was found to be less effective than taped voices of family and friends (Jones, Hux, Anderson, & Knepper, 1994).

Music Thanatology. An emerging area for the use of music in health care is *music thanatology,* a palliative modality employing prescriptive music to tend the complex physical and spiritual needs of the dying (Schroeder-Sheker, 1994). Music therapists partake in bedside vigils serving the dying in homes, hospitals, and hospice settings. They have served oncology patients, those with end-stage respiratory illness, degenerative diseases, and those with AIDS (Schroeder-Sheker, 1994). Nurses working with dying patients could facilitate referrals to persons providing this service.

Precautions in Use

Adaptation occurs if the auditory system is continually exposed to the same type of stimulus (Farber, 1982). Neural adaptation can occur after 3 minutes of continuous exposure, resulting in music no longer providing the stimulating or calming influence that was intended.

Use of stimulation, such as music, in Phase I following head injury may increase intracranial pressure. Music of a stimulating quality should be delayed until the autonomic nervous system has stabilized. Quiet music may be used to induce relaxation and block the irritating sounds from the environment. However, the patient's individual response to music should always be monitored.

Careful control of volume is essential. Permanent ear damage results from exposure to high frequencies and volumes. Decibels higher than 90 dB cause discomfort (Idzoriek, 1982). Fatigue occurs more frequently when stimulation is at higher frequencies (Farber, 1982).

Initiating music as an intervention without first assessing the patient's likes and dislikes may produce deleterious effects. Because of music's effect on the limbic system, it can bring about intense emotional responses. Therefore, assessment of musical preference is essential prior to intervention.

Before using music for therapeutic purposes, nurses need to have some knowledge of music and the effects that particular types of music can produce. Give thought to the type of music to use, when to use it, and for how long. Simply placing a radio at a patient's bedside does not constitute music therapy.

FURTHER RESEARCH

While the numbers of experimental and quasi-experimental studies examining the effects of music as a nursing intervention are increasing, many reports still contain only anecdotal information. Findings from published studies are inconsistent with regard to whether music intervention had the intended effects. It is likely that some of the nonsignificant results may be due to small samples sizes, or to a variety of individual differences among subjects not previously considered, such as prior experience with music (Hanser, 1988).

Studies reported from the music therapy discipline are helpful to nurses, yet research is needed from a nursing perspective in order to establish parameters for its use as a nursing intervention to promote health and well-being. Standley's (1986) meta-analysis provides an excellent overview of studies in the health sciences. Hanser (1985, 1988) provides an excellent overview and suggestions for further research in the area of music for stress reduction.

Identified areas of research from a nursing perspective that are needed in order to address the inconsistency of findings and to build a knowledge base for nursing practice are as follows:

1. The emerging field of psychoneuroimmunology is ripe for investigating the effects of music on salient immune measures. What are the effects of various types of music listening for patients in clinical settings on their immune functions and stress hormone levels (e.g., salivary cortisol)?

2. Consideration of individual differences in response to music also requires study. What are the influences of individual difference variables to music intervention outcomes (e.g., personality traits, sex differences, age, previous experience with music, influence of imagery)?

3. Standley (1986) has stated that music is the most effective intervention for anxiety reduction. In addition to anxiety reduction, what other uses may be successfully addressed?

4. Little is known about prescribing music for intervention. What is the most efficacious music prescription? (When, how much, how often, and what type of music?)

5. A majority of nursing research studies testing the effects of music intervention have employed designs restricted to immediate or short-term effects of the intervention. Intervention studies have not addressed the long-term effects of the intervention. Therefore, longitudinal studies are needed to determine what, if any, are the long-term or carryover effects of music intervention?

6. Little is known about the effects of music intervention as an adjunct to medication administration. Is music an effective adjunct to administration of pain medications and/or sedatives? Is music therapy effective in reducing the amount and frequency of medication administration?

While intervention research is very labor intensive and time consuming, there is a need for larger studies on music intervention, such as multicenter clinical trials with measurement of sensitive and appropriate variables. Also, findings from earlier works that utilized smaller samples need to be replicated or combined in a meta-analysis. Through the formation of research teams led by nurses, perhaps the needed research can be conducted testing the effects of music as an independent nursing intervention.

REFERENCES

Alvin, J. (1975). *Music therapy.* New York: Basic Books.

Augustin, P., & Hains, A. (1996). Effect of music on ambulatory surgery patients' preoperative anxiety. *AORN Journal, 63,* 750–758.

Bartlett, D., Kaufman, D., & Smeltekop, R. (1993). The effects of music listening and perceived sensory experiences on the immune system as measured by interleukin-1 and cortisol. *Journal of Music Therapy, 30*(4), 194–209.

Beck, S. (1991). The therapeutic use of music for cancer-related pain. *Oncology Nursing Forum, 18,* 1327–1337.

Bolwerk, C. (1990). Effects of relaxing music on state anxiety in myocardial infarction patients. *Critical Care Nursing Quarterly, 13*(2), 63–72.

Bonny, H. (1986). Music and healing. *Music Therapy, 6*(1), 3–12.

Burke, M., Walsh, J., Oehler, J., & Gingras, J. (1995). Music therapy following suctioning. *Neonatal Network, 14*(7), 41–49.

Chlan, L. (1995). Psychophysiologic responses of mechanically ventilated patients to music: A pilot study. *American Journal of Critical Care, 4*(3), 233–238.

Collins, S., & Kuck, K. (1991). Music therapy in the neonatal intensive care unit. *Neonatal Network, 9*(6), 23–26.

Cook, J. (1981). The therapeutic use of music: A literature review. *Nursing Forum, 20*(3), 253–266.

Cook, J. (1986). Music as an intervention in the oncology setting. *Cancer Nursing, 9*(1), 23–28.

Courtright, P., Johnson, S., Baumgartner, M., & Webster, J. (1990). Dinner music: Does it affect the behavior of psychiatric inpatients? *Journal of Psychosocial Nursing, 28*(3), 37–40.

Durham, L. & Collins, M. (1986). The effect of music as a conditioning aid in prepared childbirth education. *Journal of Obstetric, Gynecologic, and Neonatal Nursing, 15*(3), 268–270.

Farber, S. (1982). *Neurorehabilitation.* Philadelphia: Saunders.

Gerdner, L., & Swanson, E. (1993). Effects of individualized music on confused and agitated elderly patients. *Archives of Psychiatric Nursing, 7*(5), 284–291.

Good, M. (1995). A comparison of the effects of jaw relaxation and music on postoperative pain. *Nursing Research, 44*(1), 52–57.

Guzzetta, C. (1989). Effects of relaxation and music therapy on patients in a coronary care unit with presumptive acute myocardial infarction. *Heart & Lung, 18,* 609–616.

Guzzetta, C. (1995). Music therapy: hearing the melody of the soul. In B. Dossey, L. Keegan, C. Guzzetta, & L. Kolkmeier. *Holistic Nursing* (pp. 670–698). Gaithersburg, MD: Aspen.

Hanser, S. (1985). Music therapy and stress reduction research. *Journal of Music Therapy, 22*(4), 193–206.

Hanser, S. (1988). Controversy in music listening/stress reduction research. *The Arts in Psychotherapy, 15*(2), 211–217.

Hanser, S., & Thompson, L. (1994). Effects of a music therapy strategy on depressed older adults. *Journal of Gerontology, 49*(6), 265–269.

Herth, K. (1978). The therapeutic use of music. *Supervisor Nurse, 9*(10), 22–23.

Hoskyns, S. (1982, June). Striking the right chord. *Nursing Mirror, 154,* 14–17.

Idzoriek, P. (1982). *Comparison of auditory and strong tactile stimuli on responsiveness.* Unpublished Plan B Project. Minneapolis, MN: School of Nursing, University of Minnesota.

Janelli, L., Kanski, G., Jones, H., & Kennedy, M. (1995). Exploring music intervention with restrained patients. *Nursing Forum, 30*(4), 12–18.

Jones, R., Hux, Morton-Anderson, A., & Knepper, L. (1994). Auditory stimulation effect on a comatose survivor of traumatic brain injury. *Archives of Physical Medicine and Rehabilitation, 75*(1), 164–171.

Kaempf, G., & Amodei, M. (1989). The effect of music on anxiety. *Association of Operating Room Nurses Journal, 50*(1), 112–118.

Klein, S., & Winkelstein, M. (1996). Enhancing pediatric health care with music. *Pediatric Health Care, 10*(1), 74–81.

Mason, C. (1978). Musical activities with elderly patients. *Physiotherapy, 64*(3), 80–82.

Mavely, R., & Mitchell, G. (1994). Consider karaoke. *Canadian Nurse, 90*(1), 22–24.

Miluk-Kolasa, B., Obminski, A., Stupnicki, R., & Golec, L. (1994). Effects of music treatment on salivary cortisol in patients exposed to presurgical stress. *Experimental and Clinical Endocrinology, 102*(2), 118–120.

Moore, R., Staum, M., & Brotons, M. (1992). Music preferences of the elderly: Repertoire, vocal ranges, tempos, and accompaniments for singing. *Journal of Music Therapy, 29*(4), 236–252.

Moranto, C. (1993). Applications of music in medicine. In M. Heal, & T. Wogram. (Eds.), *Music therapy in health and education* (pp. 153–174). London: Kingsley.

Mornhinweg, G., & Voignier, R. (1995). Music for sleep disturbance in the elderly. *Journal of Holistic Nursing, 13*(3), 248–254.

Moss, V. (1988). Music and the surgical patient. *Association of Operating Room Nurses Journal, 48*(1), 64–69.

Munro, S., & Mount, B. (1978). Music therapy in palliative care. *Canadian Medical Association Journal, 119,* 1029–1034.

Nightingale, F. (1969). *Notes on Nursing.* New York: Dover. (Original published 1860).

Pfaff, V., Smith, K., & Gowan, D. (1989). The effects of music-assisted relaxation on the distress of pediatric cancer patients undergoing bone marrow aspirations. *Children's Health Care, 18*(4), 232–236.

Sambandham, M. & Schirm, V. (1995). Music as a nursing intervention for residents with Alzheimer's disease in long-term care. *Geriatric Nursing, 16*(2), 79–83.

Schorr, J. (1993). Music and pattern change in chronic pain. *Advances in Nursing Science, 15*(4), 27–36.

Schroeder-Sheker, T. (1994). Music for the dying: a personal account of the new field of music thanatology. *Journal of Holistic Nursing, 12*(1), 83–99.

Standley, J. (1986). Music research in medical/dental treatment: meta-analysis and clinical applications. *Journal of Music Therapy, 23*(2), 56–122.

Steelman, V. (1990). Intraoperative music therapy. *AORN Journal, 52*(5), 1026–1034.

Stevens, K. (1990). Patients' perceptions of music during surgery. *Journal of Advanced Nursing, 15*(6), 1045–1051.

Thaut, M. (1990). Physiological and motor responses to music stimuli. In R. Unkefer (Ed.), *Music therapy in the treatment of adults with mental disorders: theoretical bases and clinical interventions* (pp. 33–49). New York: Schirmer.

Updike, P. (1990). Music therapy results for ICU patients. *Dimensions of Critical Care Nursing.* 9(1), 39–45.

White, J. (1992). Music therapy: an intervention to reduce anxiety in the myocardial infarction patient. *Clinical Nurse Specialist, 6*(2), 58–63.

Woolf, H. (Ed.) (1979). *New collegiate dictionary.* Springfield, MA: G & C Merriman.

22

Prayer

Marilyne Gustafson

Prayer is an intimate conversation or dialog between an individual and God or a higher being. It is a practice common to all faiths and practiced by persons in practically all societies. In addition to its importance as an element in all organized religions, prayer is one of the oldest forms of healing therapies. For patients, prayer is a potential resource to meet spiritual needs, an activity often used as a spiritual coping strategy.

Spiritual needs of clients have begun to be addressed in the nursing literature. The nursing diagnosis of "spiritual distress" as well as research on spiritual well-being and spiritual needs provide the nurse with information on which to build an approach to the consideration of prayer as an independent nursing intervention.

DEFINITION

Prayer is defined as a solemn and humble approach to a divinity in word or thought, usually involving petition, beseeching, supplication, confession, praise, and thanksgiving. In the conversation or dialog with a divinity (sometimes called the Almighty or God), there is often the concept of communion or relationship. Relationship is central to many people and is often described as giving meaning or perspective to life as well as affirmation of the presence and power of God.

Prayer is viewed by many as a natural and necessary result of the spiritual aspect of humankind (Carson, 1989; Fish & Shelly, 1987). Thus, it is viewed as a source of strength to the person and thereby as a positive coping strategy which supports individuals when they are ill (Sodestrom & Martinson, 1987). Another definition of prayer is that it is a set form of words, such as a formula for supplication, addressed to God or the object of worship; prayer books contain prayers of this nature.

This chapter will provide a nursing framework in which to view prayer as spiritual support that respects the diversity of belief systems and cultures of individuals. This perspective will assist the nurse to intervene independently and/or collaborate with the patient, the family, and others concerned with spiritual needs.

Although research studies will be used to document pertinent findings in this area of study, a principle of importance is that "the value of prayers or spiritual rituals to the believer is not affected by whether or not they can be scientifically 'proved' to be beneficial" (Carpenito, 1983, p. 453). Prayer is a practice common to all faiths, however, faith is highly personal and generally not examined scientifically. Scientific findings and concepts regarding faith can help the nurse become informed and more comfortable in addressing spiritual needs. Appropriate assessment of spiritual needs, including religious needs and practices, can lead to the promotion, maintenance, and restoration of spiritual wholeness.

SCIENTIFIC BASIS

Nurses have begun to study prayer, which can be used as a coping strategy to meet spiritual needs. The Stallwood-Stoll model is a conceptual model of the nature of human beings that includes a spiritual component (Stallwood & Stoll, 1975). The spiritual, or transcendent, component is viewed as distinct from the biophysical and psychosocial components. The authors believe that nursing reflects an awareness that a human being is not simply a biological organism but also a psychosocial and spiritual being. Religion is the institutionalized form for the satisfaction of spiritual needs and thus comes under the larger component of spirituality. Spiritual needs are defined as any factors necessary to establish and maintain a person's dynamic personal relationship with God, as defined by that individual. Stallwood and Stoll (1975) stated that each person has a basic need for this relationship, wherein one experiences forgiveness, love, hope, trust, and meaning and purpose in life.

Prayer in nursing texts is included under the headings "spiritual care" (Fish & Shelly, 1987; Shelly, 1982) and "spiritual dimensions of nursing practice" (Carson, 1989). Numerous journal articles suggest prayer as an effective intervention for a variety of situations and patient populations (Carson & Huss, 1979; Piles, 1990; Stoll, 1979).

The need for prayer was the most frequent response in a study by Hess (cited in Shelly, 1982) to the question "Were you aware of having a spiritual need at any time during your hospitalization?" The patients' responses centered around the need to pray personally, to be prayed for or to pray with another person. Direct statements by the patients included: "I can't pray, my prayers aren't heard"; "I couldn't have gotten along without prayer"; "I prayed constantly because I was sure I was dying" (p. 158).

"Spiritual distress" is a nursing diagnosis approved by the North American Nursing Diagnosis Association (Kim, McFarland & McLane, 1987). In 1973 the category was termed "alteration in faith in God." In 1978 it was expanded to three categories of spirituality: "spiritual concern," "spiritual distress," and "spiritual despair." In 1980, the Fourth National Conference reconsolidated the condition to spiritual distress. In addition, many others (Carson, 1989; Fish & Shelly, 1987; Messner & Ward, 1989) concur with use of the diagnosis. Spiritual distress is defined as distress of the human spirit—a disruption in the life principle which pervades a person's entire being and which integrates and transcends one's biological and psychological nature (Kim et al., 1987). The defining characteristics include those of being unable to participate in usual religious practice, such as solitary praying, meeting to pray with others, and finding others to pray for or with the patients. Discussing principles and rationale for the diagnosis of spiritual distress, Carpentio (1983) states the value of prayers to the believer is not affected by whether or not they can be scientifically proven to be beneficial.

INTERVENTION

The need for a research base for nursing practice is no less important in the use of prayer than for other interventions. Research that includes a study of prayer is often seen in relationship to terms such as spirituality, spiritual needs, and spiritual distress. The use of research instruments and good assessment will provide important data on which to plan an appropriate nursing intervention. Ellerhorst-Ryan (1989) reviewed research instruments dealing with spirituality. Moberg, a sociologist, pioneered some of the early work focused on religiosity and spiritual well-being (SWB). Moberg worked with the White House Conference on Aging and has written extensively on religiosity, spirituality, SWB, and the elderly. In Moberg's Indexes of Spiritual Well-Being (1979), one of the questions is "How often do you pray privately?" The spiritual well-being scale developed by Ellison (1983) is a 20–item Likert scale that is shorter than the Moberg index. One of the items is, "I don't find much satisfaction in private prayer with God." Both the Moberg index and the Ellison scale have been used in several nursing studies. Stoll, a nurse author, used the Ellison scale in her research. Based on her experience, she suggested 13 questions and guidelines specific to the roles of prayer to be used for spiritual assessment (Stoll, 1979).

Carson (1989), Fish and Shelly (1987), and Stoll (1979) all emphasize the need for assessment data to determine the patient's beliefs and values regarding prayer. One of Stoll's questions is, "Has being sick made any difference in your practice of praying?" Carson (1989) suggests observations on nonverbal behavior (e.g., "Does the client pray during the day?") and verbal behavior ("Does the client talk about prayer, hope . . . ?") to determine the value of prayer in a patient's life. Since prayer can be very private, the nurse may not be aware of the behavioral changes resulting from prayer.

Carpenito (1983) indicates that spiritual distress is related to the inability to practice spiritual rituals. Objective data to support this might be that the patient is unable to say prayers or meditate or cannot assume a normal position for prayer or meditation. Before intervening she suggests assessing causative and contributing factors and limitations related to disease process or treatment regimen (e.g., cannot kneel to pray due to traction, cannot vocalize prayers due to laryngectomy).

Carson (1989) provided four guidelines about prayer for the nurse:

1. Prayer or any spiritual intervention is *never* used out of intuition but follows a careful assessment that reveals the presence of a spiritual need.
2. Prayer is *never* to be used as an activity or substitute for the nurse's time and presence with the client.
3. Prayer is *never* used to meet the nurse's needs but only to facilitate the client's relationship with God.
4. Prayer is not used to communicate a magical view of God that conveys a false sense of hope and expectation. (p. 169)

The Chadwich study (cited in Fish & Shelly, 1987) assessed the awareness and preparedness of nurses to meet spiritual needs. It showed that 75% of the nurses surveyed reported they would feel comfortable with either reading the Bible or praying with a patients, but 50% of them had never read the Bible or prayed with a patient. The comfort of the nurse in utilizing this intervention is critical. The nurse planning to use prayer as an intervention will do well to assess the appropriateness of prayer in a given situation by asking if it is meeting the patient's need or her own needs. If it is the latter, it would be better for the nurse to pray privately and not assume that this prayer reflects therapeutic use of self. Thoughtful assessment and concern for the client's needs must be paramount. A difference in religious faiths between the client and the nurse is discussed in the section on precautions.

Technique

Prayer may be conversational, spontaneous, silent, spoken, formal, written, or memorized. Aspects of petition, request, or praise may be included. Prayer may also be a part of a ritual and/or related to objects such as a prayer book or a rosary. The patients' wishes regarding prayer need to be ascertained and respected, since the purpose of prayer is to help them in their relationship to God, as they perceive God. Therefore, the form which the prayer takes is not what is important but rather the relationship that is involved. Further prayer should be viewed as providing strength and peace and not as increasing anxiety or offending the person.

The most appreciated prayers usually include simple, informal expressions of the patient's spiritual needs, hopes, and fears to God and a recognition of God's power. For those accustomed to using more formal prayers, spontaneous prayers may seem disrespectful. In the Christian tradition, the Lord's Prayer is familiar and meaningful to many. Children may have memorized table and/or bedtime prayers which are familiar to them. Roman Catholic patients may appreciate having a nurse of the same faith pray the rosary with them. For Jewish patients, prayers to the God of Abraham, Isaac, and Moses are appropriate.

Luna (1989) described the prayer needs of Muslims. She suggests that elderly Muslims place great importance on the performance of obligatory prayer along with the ritual cleansing or ablutions which are required according to Islamic tradition. The nurse would assess the client's wishes regarding prayer and the desired frequency. If prayer is desired, the nurse could use the intervention mode of cultural care accommodation by proving a basin of water and/or finding a quiet place for the client to carry our the ritual. For many Muslims, observing and performing the religious obligation of prayer is an important cultural expression for maintaining health and preventing illness.

Timing and When to Pray

The timing of prayer with a patient is important. Fish and Shelly (1987) suggest that (a) adequate communication in the relationship exists, (b) signs of the patient's concern (e.g., high anxiety, statement about being separated from the faith or worship community) have been clearly indicated, and (c) prayer is not seen as a way of ending a conversation.

The idea of referring the patient to the clergy is deliberately omitted from this discussion, but at times it may be the most appropriate intervention. However, too often referral to the clergy has been the immediate and first approach used by nurses without the nurse giving consideration to the use of prayer as a nursing intervention. This does not mean that the nurse should ignore an opportunity to join clergypersons in a group time of prayer (Saylor, 1972).

Measurement of Outcomes

As stated in the section on the scientific basis, the subjective nature of one's beliefs and faith make finding instruments to measure spiritual distress and the effectiveness of the intervention of prayer difficult but not impossible. The purpose for which the prayer was made will dictate the effectiveness from the patient's standpoint; however, some measures which have been reported have been increased peace or peacefulness, decreased anxiety and less feeling of anger, an increased sense of well-being, and more positive outlook about life changes (Carson, 1989).

USES

The universality of prayer needs no further documentation. The general uses of prayer apply to many age groups and many nursing and medical diagnoses. Carpenito (1983) states that "an individual is a spiritual person even when disoriented, confused, emotionally ill, delirious, or cognitively impaired" (p. 452). In a study of stress identification and coping patterns in patients with hemodialysis, Baldree, Murphy, & Powers et al. (1982) found that praying was a commonly acknowledged coping strategy. Sodestrom and Martinson (1987) studied patients with cancer and reported that the most frequently used coping strategies were personal prayer and asking others to pray for them. Bearon and Koening (1990) asked 40 adults (ages 65–74) about God's role in health and illness and their use of prayer in response to recent physical symptoms. Most held a belief in a benevolent God but were not clear about God's role in health and illness; over one-half had prayed about at least one physical symptom. Symptoms discussed with a physician or for which drugs were taken were more likely to be prayed about that were other symptoms, suggesting that prayer may be used for symptoms seen as serious. The use of prayer and seeking medical help did not seem to be mutually exclusive.

Referring to the use of prayer for patients with psychiatric and mental health needs, Carson (1980, 1989) and Shelly and John (1983) suggest that prayer is appropriate with this group of patients. In a study by Carson and Huss (1979), major changes occurred in psychiatric clients who were offered opportunities for prayer. Increased abilities to express feelings of anger and frustration and to have a more positive outlook about possible changes in their lives, and a decrease in somatic complaints occurred.

Prayer is an appropriate intervention for patients with chronic illness. Referring to chronic illness as a long, unpredictable, and uncertain journey unique to each person, Stoll (cited in Carson, 1989) includes prayer as one of the five practical coping strategies. Prayer was found to be helpful to patients on hemodialysis (Baldree et al., 1982). Populations for whom prayer has been used are found in Table 21.1.

TABLE 22.1 Uses of Prayer

Condition or Population	Source
Cancer	(Sodestrom & Martinson, 1987)
Children	(Betz, 1981; Carson, 1989; Foster, Hunsberger, & Anderson, 1989; Shelly, 1982)
Chronic illness	(Baldree et al., 1982; Carson, 1989)
Community settings	(Burkhardt & Nagei-Jacobson, 1985)
Coronary care units	(Byrd, 1988)
Death	(Carson, 1989)
Dying	(Amenta & Bohet, 1986; Carson, 1989)
Elderly	(Bearon & Koening, 1990; Carson, 1989; Moberg, 1979)
Healing	(Shlemon, 1976)

Precautions

Although prayer may be a very natural activity for both the patient and the nurse, it may be viewed by the patient as an unusual activity for the nurse in the role of healer.

Because of the highly personal nature of faith, spirituality, religious beliefs, and practices, the nurse must assess the patient's need for prayer as well as her own beliefs and comfort in using this nursing intervention. Carpenito (1983) states that in order to assist people in spiritual distress, the nurse must know certain beliefs and practices of the various spiritual groups found in this country. Carson (1989) and Carpenito (1983) provide excellent observations that capture the essence of the beliefs and practices of many faiths. Knowledge about other faiths and religions is becoming more imperative in a culturally pluralistic society. Prayer used improperly may offend, increase anxiety, or be a threat, reawakening anger or painfully negative, self-deprecating memories. Again, if it has been used to meet the nurse's and not the patient's need, it is inappropriate.

The nurse should be prepared to have a patient request a prayer that the nurse may view as manipulating God or being magical. The wise nurse must consider her own beliefs about requests that raise questions in her mind. Prayers for healing and for what might be considered "impossible" or miraculous are examples of possible requests which the nurse needs to thoughtfully consider before intervening.

RESEARCH QUESTIONS

The majority of the books and articles on the use of prayer are written from a Judeo-Christian perspective. Many of the instruments used by nurses have been originated in sociology and psychology and do not necessarily reflect a nursing perspective. Nurses have studied prayer in their investigations of spirituality. However, the area of spirituality, spiritual needs, and prayer as a coping strategy is just beginning to be studied in nursing.

The following are questions that could contribute to improved use of prayer as a nursing intervention:

1. How can we evaluate and adapted instruments from other disciplines to measure the use of prayer as a nursing intervention?
2. What is the relationship of spiritual diagnoses indicators (such as defining characteristics) to the use of prayer as an intervention?

3. What are the factors that help or hinder nurses in the process of cooperating with patients in the use of prayer?
4. What are some of the cross-culturally significant or divergent aspects of prayer related to its use as an intervention? Most studies that have been conducted thus far have been done from a Judeo-Christian perspective.

REFERENCES

Amenta, M., & Bohet, N. (Eds.). (1986). Spiritual concerns. In *Nursing care of the terminally ill* (Pp. 115–161). Boston: Little Brown.

Bacon, J. (1995). Healing prayer: The risks and rewards. *Journal of Christian Nursing, 12,* 14–17.

Baldree, K., Murphy, S., & Powers, M. (1982). Stress identification and coping patterns in patients on hemodialysis. *Nursing Research 31,* 107–112.

Bearon, L. & Koening, H. (1990). Religious cognition and use of prayer in health and illness. *The Gerontologist, 30,* 249–253.

Betz, C. (1981). Faith development in children. *Pediatric Nursing, 8(2),* 36–41.

Burkhardt, M., & Nagei-Jacobson, M. (1985). Dealing with spiritual concerns of clients in the community. *Journal of Community Health Nursing, 2,* 191–198.

Byrd, R. (1988). Positive therapeutic effects of intercessory prayer in a coronary care unit population. *Southern Medical Journal, 81,* 826–829.

Byrd, R., & Sherill, J. (1995). The therapeutic effects of intercessory prayer. *Journal of Christian Nursing, 12,* 21–23.

Carpenito, L. (1983). *Nursing diagnosis: Application to clinical practice.* Philadelphia: Lippincott.

Carson, V. (1980). Meeting the spiritual needs of hospitalized psychiatric patients. *Perspectives in Psychiatric Care, 18,* 17–20.

Carson, V. (1989). *Spiritual dimensions of nursing practice.* Philadelphia: Saunders.

Carson, V., & Huss, K. (1979). Prayer—an effective therapeutic teaching tool. *Journal of Psychiatric Nursing and Mental Health Services, 17,* 34–37.

Ellerhorst-Ryan, J. (1988). Measuring aspects of spirituality. In M. Frank-Stromberg (Ed.), *Instruments for clinical nursing research* (pp. 141–149). Norwalk, CT: Appleton & Lange.

Ellison, C. (1983). Spiritual well-being: Conceptualization and measurement. *Journal of Psychology and Theology, 11,* 330–340.

Ellison, C. (1995). Race, religious involvement and depression symptomatology in a southeastern U.S. community. *Social Science & Medicine,* *40,* 1561–1572.

Emblen, J., & Halstead, L. (1993). Spiritual needs and interventions: Comparing the views of patients, nurses and chaplains. *Clinical Nurse Specialist* , *7,* 175–182.

Fish, S., & Shelly, J. (1987). *Spiritual care: The nurse's role.* Downers Grove, IL: InterVarsity.

Fish, S. (1995). Can research prove that God answers prayer? *Journal of Christian Nursing, 12,* 24–28.

Foster, R., Hunsberger, M., & Anderson, J. (1989). *Family centered nursing care of children.* Philadelphia: Saunders.

Kim, M., McFarland, G., & McLane, A. (1987). *Pocket guide to nursing diagnosis.* St. Louis: Mosby.

Luna, L. (1989). Transcultural nursing care of Arab-Muslims. *Journal of Transcultural Nursing 1,* 22–26.

Messner, R., & Ward, D. (1989). The patient with a spiritual need. In S. Lewis, R.

Grainger, W. McDowell, R. Gregory, & R. Messner (Eds.), *Manual of psychosocial nursing interventions: Promoting mental health in medical-surgical settings* (pp. 259–269). Philadelphia: Saunders.

Moberg, D. (1979). The development of social indicators of spiritual well-being for quality of life research. In D. Moberg (Ed.), *Spiritual well-being sociological perspectives* (pp. 4–6). Washington, DC: University Press.

Piles, C. (1990). Providing spiritual care. *Nurse Educator, 15,* 36–41.

Saylor, D. (1972). Let us: Pray, work together. *Nursing '72, 2,* 5.

Shelly, J. (1982). *The spiritual needs of children.* Downers Grove, IL: InterVarsity.

Shelly, J., & John, S. (1983). *Spiritual dimensions of mental health.* Downers Grove, IL: InterVarsity.

Shelly, J., & Fish, S. (1995). Praying with patients: Why, when and how. *Journal of Christian Nursing, 12,* 9–13.

Shlemon, B. (1976). *Healing prayer.* Notre Dame, IN: Ave Maria.

Sodestrom, K., & Martinson, I. (1987). Patient's spiritual coping strategies: A study of nurse and patient perspectives. *Oncology Nursing Forum, 14,* 41–46.

Stallwood, J., & Stoll, R. (1975). Spiritual dimension of nursing practice. In I. Beland & J. Possos (Eds.), *Clinical nursing* (pp. 1086–1093). New York: MacMillan.

Stoll, R. (1979). Guidelines for spiritual assessment. *American Journal of Nursing, 79,* 1574–1577.

Stoll, R. (1989). Spirituality and chronic illness. In V. Carson (Ed.), *Spiritual dimensions of nursing practice* (pp. 180–216). Philadelphia: Saunders.

23

Humor

Kevin Smith

> *"A merry heart doeth good like a medicine,*
> *but a broken spirit drieth the bones."*
> Proverbs 17:22

Throughout history, many have accorded a beneficial effect to joy and mirth. Greek philosophers including Plato and Aristotle wrote treatises on humor (McGhee, 1979). Medieval physician Joubert wrote a treatise in 1560 describing the physical benefits of humor and how joy and sorrow were experienced in the heart, not the mind. Kant, in 1790, described physical effects of humor, a talent he believed enabled one to look at things from a different perspective (Haig, 1988). Henri de Mondville, the famous medieval surgeon, said, "Let the surgeon take care to regulate the whole regimen of the patient's life for joy and happiness, The surgeon must forbid anger, hatred, and sadness in the patient. Remind him that the body grows fat from joy and thin from sadness" (Walsh, 1928). In medieval physiology, the definition of the word *humor* is "moisture" or "vapor." Humor referred to the four principal fluids of the body: blood, phlegm, choler (yellow bile), and melancholy (black bile). A proper balance of the four was called "good humor," and a preponderance of any one made a bad compound called "ill humor." (Robinson, 1991).

The benefit of using humor and laughter to improve our ability to cope with difficulties and to stay healthy has become a popular notion. Interest in this area has increased since Norman Cousins's account of the use of laughter in his recovery from a painful collagen disorder (1979). The notion that humor and laughter positively influence health and the scientific work that will be reviewed here to support this notion have significant implications for nurses and others providing health care. Nursing journal articles continue to address many facets of humor, such as laughter and stress management

(Paquet, 1993; Woodhouse, 1993), humor as a nursing intervention (Hunt, 1993; Mornhinweg & Voignier, 1995), humor and the older adult (Herth, 1993), humor and healing (Macaluso, 1993), and the positive physiologic effects of humor (Lambert & Lambert, 1995). Humor organizations and publications continue to grow and expand, humor workshops are being offered to nurses and other health care providers, and many continuing education offerings and events are incorporating humorous presentations or activities.

Humor can be used as a specific independent nursing intervention or can be incorporated into other nursing interventions. Using humor as part of other nursing interventions can be considered a parallel intervention. The goals in using humor as an intervention are to enhance the well-being of the client, to enhance the therapeutic relationship between the nurse and the client, and to bring hope and joy to the situation. Virtually anyone can develop the requisite skills needed to use humor as an intervention.

DEFINITION

> *Humor is the good-natured side of truth.*
> Mark Twain

Nurse and humor expert, Vera Robinson (1978) describes the phenomenon of humor as "any communication which is perceived by any of the interacting parties as humorous and leads to laughing, smiling or a feeling of amusement" (p. 193). The American Heritage dictionary (1976, p. 641) defines *humor* as "the quality of being laughable or comical," and "the ability to perceive, enjoy, or express what is comical or funny." Humor can be the process of either producing or perceiving the comical. What we personally define or perceive as funny and the physical manifestations of humor are extremely variable between individuals. However, there are predictable laughter stimuli and responses.

Why do we laugh?

There are many different reasons why we laugh. Sometimes our laughter response is simply for the fun of it and other times it is for more important reasons. Four basic theories or situations that commonly invoke a laughter response will be presented: surprise, superiority, incongruity, and release.

Surprise. Good humor or a good joke catches you off guard. It surprises you and this in itself causes you to laugh. Another type of surprise humor is shock humor. This could be a startling or loud punch line or maybe something taboo or vulgar. This type of humor has caused most of our mothers to say, "Please do not encourage him/her." Shock humor is not recommended in clinical or therapeutic settings.

Superiority. The superiority theory of laughter (Robinson, 1991; Gruner, 1978) describes situations in which we laugh because we feel superior to an individual or a group. We are laughing at inferiority, stupidity, or the misfortunes of others. In its most simple form this could be slapstick humor. A more sophisticated form would be political satire. It has been suggested that the essential affect of humor is derived from a sense of mastery or ego strength (Lefcourt & Martin, 1986).

Incongruity. Another theory of laughter or stimuli for laughter is incongruity. Schafner (1981) concisely describes this theory by saying, "Laughter is the result of a perception of an incongruity in a ludicrous context." For example, a man walks into a psychiatrist's office with a duck on his head. The duck says, "Doc, you got to help me get this guy off my tail." You have two ideas which are juxtaposed in an impossible or absurd situation. The incongruity theory was advocated by the philosophers Kant, Schopenhauer, Spencer, and others. They emphasized the importance of a sudden surprise, shock, conflict of ideas, or incongruity that triggers laughter (Liechty, 1987). Asimov (1992) says that incongruities put the listener, for a brief moment, in a fantasy world. This suspension of reality has the listener ready for the crowning bit of fantasy, or the punch line, which will result in laughter.

Release. The basic premise of the release theory, as a laughter stimulus, is that humor and laughter help us to release our tensions and anxieties. Freud (1905/1960) viewed humor as a coping tool that allows individuals to reduce tension by expressing hostile or obscene impulses in a socially acceptable manner. Morreall (1983) calls this the *relief theory* and says humor that produces laughter is a method of venting nervous energy. This release type of laughter is often enhanced in group situations where many are sharing the same anxiety.

Styles of Humor

Two general styles of humor will be described, spontaneous and formal. Most of the humor that we use on a daily basis with our staff and patients is of the spontaneous type. This is situational humor that arises out of the normal absurdities of our day. This type of humor is also a very effective communication tool when used to "break the ice" with patients or co-workers. Your attempt to lighten up the situation also shows a sign of caring and allows for a free exchange of other thoughts, feelings and emotions. On the other hand, examples of formal humor, or "premeditated acts of humor" (Smith, 1995), include the sharing of jokes, cartoons, humorous articles or stories, novelty toys or gag-gifts, and practical jokes. Formal humor, like most forms of humor, is usually only effective when it is relevant to the situation in which it is presented. Other more specific humor styles include self-deprecating humor, puns and plays on words, ethnic humor, sarcastic humor, and gallows humor.

> *I couldn't be two faced. If I had two faces, I wouldn't wear this one.*
>
> Abraham Lincoln

Self-deprecating humor may be the most effective and powerful humor tool that you can develop and use. Showing that you can laugh at yourself demonstrates that you are a normal human being with weaknesses while at the same time displaying a level of confidence, self-awareness and self-esteem. Ronald Reagan used this type of humor effectively: When he was being taken to the operating room after an assassination attempt, he quipped, "I hope my surgeon is a Republican." Paulsen (1989) says that gently poking fun at yourself acts as a social lubricant. It shows that the person is at ease with the situation and others can feel the same way. On the other hand, we are suspicious or afraid of those without any sense of humor.

Puns and plays on words are simple and straightforward humor styles. Some consider puns to be the lowest form of humor. However, pun enthusiasts include Asimov and Freud. When using puns, do not expect laughs, expect groans. For example, "With friends like you, who needs enemas?" Ethnic humor is usually regional. Using your own ethnicity or profession as the target of the joke is the most acceptable approach. Sarcastic humor is even more risky. Sarcasm can be perceived as very negative and can make others uncomfortable. Overheard sarcasm can make a patient or anyone think that they are the targets of the sarcastic comments. Freud (1905/1960) noted that people make jokes about tragedy and death, which he called *gallows humor*. This is usually a grim type of humor, typically seen when people are faced with considerable stress among hospital staff. Freud theorized that jokes allow us to express unconscious aggressive or sexual impulses. Obrdlik (1942) asserted that the phenomenon of gallows humor has a definite social purpose. It provides a psychological escape and strengthens the morale of the group and in some situations undermines the morale of the oppressors. Victor Frankl, a psychiatrist and concentration camp survivor, states in *Man's Search for Meaning* (1963) that "Humor, more than anything else in the human makeup affords an aloofness and an ability to rise above any situation, if only for a few seconds." Hostage survivor Terry Anderson (1996) and his cell mates used humor as a coping mechanism. "Sometimes we would laugh at ourselves, sometimes at one another and sometimes at the guards." Gallows humor is frequently used in situations where individuals are under significant stress, such as emergency rooms, intensive care units, operating rooms, and morgues.

SCIENTIFIC BASIS

Many of the positive physiological effects of humor and laughter have been studied. Humor is considered the stimulus and laughter the response. This behavior creates a cascade of physiological changes in the body. William Fry (1971) studied the effects of mirthful laughter on heart rate and oxygen saturation level of peripheral blood and respiratory phenomena. He found that both the arousal and cathartic effects are paralleled in the physiological. Laughter, in contrast to other emotions, involves extensive physical activity. Laughter increases respiratory activity and oxygen exchange, increases muscular activity and heart rate, and stimulates the cardiovascular system, the sympathetic nervous system, and the production of catecholamines. The arousal state is followed by the relaxation state in which respiration rate, heart rate, and muscle tension return to normal levels. Although the oxygen saturation of peripheral blood is not affected during this relaxation state; blood pressure is reduced, and a state similar to the impact of hearty exercise exists.

Another circulatory study (Fry & Savin, 1988) investigated effects of humor on arterial blood pressure using direct arterial cannulization. There were increases in systolic and diastolic blood pressure directly related to the intensity and length of laughter. Blood pressure decreased immediately after the laughter to below the prelaughter baseline.

Many studies have found that humor and laughter increase levels of salivary immunoglobulin A (S-IgA), a vital immune system protein, the body's first line of defense against respiratory illnesses. In a controlled study, Dillon, Minchoff, and Baker (1985) demonstrated increased levels of S-IgA in college students who were exposed to a humorous video. Martin and Dobbin (1988) measured subjects' sense of humor and stress levels through self-report and S-IgA levels. They demonstrated that subjects with low scores on the humor scales showed a greater negative relationship between stress and S-IgA than did subjects with high humor scores. "Individuals with a strong sense of humor, as compared to their more serious counterparts, appear to experience both less disturbance in mood and less impairment in immune functioning following stressful experiences." Stone, Valdimarsdottir, Jandorf, Cox, & Neale (1987) demonstrated that the S-IgA response level was lower on days of negative mood and higher on days of positive mood. Another controlled study by nurse researchers Lambert and Lambert (1995) produced similar findings with S-IgA levels in well fifth grade students.

Lee Berk (Berk, Tan, & Fry, 1989; Berk, Tan, Napier, & Eby, 1989) at Loma Linda University School of Medicine's Department of Clinical Immunology investigated the effect of laughter on the neuroendocrine system, stress hormones, and immune parameters. There is a complex autonomic response with each catecholamine, suggesting that laughter may be an antagonist to the classical stress response. The laughter response stimulates moderate exercise that is eustress (i.e., good stress) rather than distress. Berk and his colleagues demonstrated that laughter lowers serum cortisol levels, increases the amount of activated T-lymphocytes, and increases the number and activity of natural killer cells. Essentially, the laughter stimulates the immune system, counteracting the immunosupressive effects of stress. The study of interactions among behavioral, neural and endocrine, and immune processes of adaptation has been termed *psychoneuroimmunology* (Moyers, 1993).

Psychological perspectives

Humor has been considered an adaptive or coping mechanism. Freud (1905/1960) regarded humor and laughter as one of the few socially acceptable means for releasing pent-up frustrations and anger, a cathartic mechanism for preserving psychic or emotional energy. Humor and laughter alter our perspective in various situations. Laughter can counteract negative emotions, allow us to transcend our predicaments, conquer painful circumstances, and help to cope with difficulties. By focusing our energy elsewhere, humor can diffuse our difficult events (Klein, 1989). The use of humor, more than distraction, has been shown to reduce threat-induced anxiety (Yovetich, Dale, & Hudak, 1990). The psychological impact of humor and laughter has led to much study related to the use of humor in managing psychiatric patients (Rosenheim & Golan, 1986; Saper, 1988, 1990). Moody (1978) has studied and incorporated approaches using positive emotions and humor for dealing with the fear, anxiety, and pain that go along with cancer and other chronic conditions. Schulz and colleagues (1996), in a study of 238 patients with cancer, demonstrated that endorsement of a pessimistic life orientation is an important risk factor for mortality.

INTERVENTION

Perhaps the only thing in life more enjoyable than laughing is helping others enjoy to laugh!

Roger Bates (1995)

As a caregiver, you can use humor judiciously to "connect" with your patients, express caring and understanding, and can enhance patients' ability to cope and their feelings of well-being. "Humor plays an important role in our feeling of well-being, as it provides an effective means of communicating a range of ideas, feelings, and opinions. Additionally, a sense of humor adds immeasurably to ones enjoyment of life and, especially, the company of others. These aspects of humor ensure that any disruption of a person's ability to understand or produce humor will have a marked effect on his/her quality of life" (Brownell, 1988, p. 17).

So what do we actually do when it comes to using humor as an intervention? There are many approaches, techniques, and tools. A first step in deciding how and when to use humor is to do a humor assessment, first of yourself, then your patient. You would never give an intramuscular injection or perform a patient assessment without thinking about what skills you need to use, what the process requires, and whether or not this intervention is in the best interest of your patient. In a study by

TABLE 23.1 Humor Assessment Interview Guide.

1. When you think of humor, what kinds of images or thoughts come to mind?
2. Was humor a part of your life when you were younger?
3. Is humor still part of your life?
4. How has humor been helpful or not helpful at this time in your life?
5. If humor is helpful, what do you do to maintain humor in your life?
6. Are there certain times when you appreciate humor more than other times?
7. When is humor a negative experience?
8. What types of activities do you find amusing or enjoyable?

From Herth, K. A., Humor and the older adult. *Applied Nursing Research 6*, 147. Used with permission.

TABLE 23.2 Eight Steps for Developing Your Sense of Humor

1. Gain an awareness and knowledge of the benefits of humor. Adopting a humorous outlook takes both a change in attitude and behavior.
2. Identify inappropriate humor. Avoid it. This is any type of humor that can be perceived as offensive to others. Humor should not be divisive.
3. Get to know what amuses you. What type of humor works for you on the job? What feels comfortable for you? Never tell a joke or a story unless you like it yourself and think it is really funny. It must be genuine.
4. Do a humor history on yourself. List favorite jokes, comedians, styles of humor, humorous situations that happened to you, TV shows and movies.
5. Keep a file of humorous anecdotes, stories, jokes, cartoons.
6. You need to be somewhat of a risk taker to start using humor or to use it more. Working humor into your routine is a process and not an event.
7. Allow yourself to be silly.
8. Surround yourself with people who have a humorous, positive outlook, and most of all, learn to laugh at yourself.

Herth (1993), a humor interview guide was developed to explore older adults' perceptions of humor (see Table 23.1). This may be adapted clinically or for research. To assess your own sense of humor, first think about what type of humor seems most natural for you. Are you the spontaneous type? Do you like more formal approaches? Are you comfortable sharing humor? Like all skills, you can always work on improving your sense of humor. Eight steps for developing your sense of humor are outlined in Table 23.2. Strickland (1993) says that the first and largest barrier to using humor is the fear of appearing foolish—of losing control over ourselves or our image.

The Technique of Humor Assessment and Intervention. Part of doing a humor assessment on your patient is to make a determination about what type of humor is appropriate or inappropriate. This determination is quite subjective and variable. Humor that is divisive in any way should be avoided. If your nursing assessment detects a problem with communication, anxiety, grieving, powerlessness or social isolation, humor may be an effective intervention (Hunt, 1993). The nurse may need to assess the patient's and family's prior use of humor and whether they currently appreciate and value humor and laughter (Bellert, 1989; Davidhizar & Bowen, 1992). Other factors to consider include the timing, the receptiveness of others to humor, and the content of the humor being used (Leiber, 1986). Spontaneous comments regarding a neutral topic such as the weather, equipment, or something about yourself can help you to see if the individual is open to humor. Their readiness for humor may or may not be apparent. Some of the intimate procedures the patient must face provoke anxiety.

Measurement of effectiveness

Physical responses to a humor intervention are the first indicators of effectiveness. According to Black (1984), there are multiple physical manifestations of the laughter response, from smiling to belly laughter, with all the associated objective physiological responses. Other positive responses need to be assessed such as relief of symptoms, affect (i.e., facial expression), degree of involvement in activities or with others, and strengthening of the relationship between caregiver and client. These assessments are subjective, yet valuable. The nurse can use other intuitive means for assessing the patient's response.

Lefcourt and Martin (1986) developed the Situational Humor Response Questionnaire (SHRQ) for determining an individual's response to particular types of humor. The SHRQ has been used in numerous studies and has been validated as effectively measuring humor. Many factors, such as development or culture, influence an individual's response to humor. Some individuals will merely smile at a joke they view as funny whereas others may produce a hearty belly laugh at most any humorous incident. Therefore, the nurse needs to be cued into the variations and subtleties of patient responses.

Ackerman, Henry, Graham, and Coffey (1994) developed a model for incorporating humor into the health care setting and described the steps one should take to create a humor program. They made humorous materials available to patients by bringing the "chuckle wagon" humor cart to patients' rooms. In addition, a nursing humor resource center was developed to assist nurses to incorporate humor into their patient care. A patient satisfaction evaluation tool was developed to assess the patients' response to the humor cart. Informal verbal evaluations were conducted with the nurses who used the humor resource materials. Appendix A lists several humor reference books, humor resource organizations, and newsletters for nurses and others.

USES

Whether the topic is bedpans or enemas, humor can provide a way to help manage or overcome shame and tension in embarrassing situations (Robinson, 1974). The nurse-patient relationship can be enhanced by giving patients the opportunity to gain control over their own healing and wellness and allowing them to explore new coping skills (Hulse, 1994). Humor used by a patient may be a cover-up of real feelings. At times a patient's humorous manner may signal an unstated wish to talk about experiences and feelings (Simon, 1989).

Cogan, Cogan, Waltz & McCue (1985) studied the effects of laughter and relaxation on discomfort thresholds. In a group of volunteers, tolerance levels of physical discomfort were measured after members of the group either listened to a laughter inducing narrative, heard an uninteresting narrative tape, or had no intervention. Patient discomfort thresholds increased (patients could handle more pain) in the laughter-inducing condition. Laughter, and not simply distraction, reduces discomfort sensitivity, suggesting that laughter has the potential as an intervention strategy for the reduction of clinical discomfort. The effectiveness of a naturally occurring response such as laughter suggests that laughter might be particularly useful as a technique for reducing pain sensitivity in some circumstances. Situations involving short-term pain induction, as in some nursing treatments (e.g., injections) and situations involving pain during recovery (e.g., postsurgical pain), seem to be particularly appropriate for laughter effects. In such situations, it might well be worth taking laughter seriously as an intervention for the reduction of pain. There are many approaches and techniques that can be used for humor interventions in health care. (See Table 23.3).

Precautions

The timing of the use of humor in the clinical setting is crucial for its success. Leiber (1986) cautions that one must assess the patients'

**TABLE 23.3 Techniques and Activities for Humor
Interventions**

1. Humor rooms, humor carts, humorous videos.
2. Guest performers (comedians, magicians, clowns)
3. Wear a humorous item, silly button, neck tie
4. Display humorous photos of staff
5. Have a cartoon bulletin board with favorites from staff and patients displayed each week
6. Play music which encourages playful movement
7. Support and applaud the efforts staff and patients make regarding humor and positive attitudes

receptiveness to humor. What may be funny to a patient when feeling well, may not seem funny during an illness episode. Humor and laughter have no place in the height of a crisis, although it can be useful as the crisis subsides to help allay tension. Inside jokes amongst health care professionals can seem offensive or callous to outsiders who may overhear them. Goodman (1992) stated that laughing at others negates confidence and destroys teamwork whereas laughing with others builds confidence, brings people together, and pokes fun at our common dilemmas. Crane (1987) states that there are times when humor is contraindicated. Patients may use inappropriate or sexually aggressive remarks under the pretense of a joke. Further assessment may be indicated to determine the underlying reason for the aggressive verbal behavior. Ziv (1984) describes the use of humor as a defense mechanism for dealing with our anxieties. As a provider of patient care, one must be sensitive to the fact that the use of humor could be an attempt on the part of patients to avoid facing more serious issues or feelings. Recognizing this situation may help you to understand the patients' feelings so that open and effective communication can occur.

RESEARCH QUESTIONS

The therapeutic use of humor by nurses has been and will continue to be an important aspect of providing patient care. Awareness of the importance of humor is increasing, as demonstrated by the plethora of articles published in support of humor as an intervention, numerous scientific studies regarding nursing humor interventions, and the increase in humor education through humor workshops and publications. Nurses need to be knowledgeable regarding the importance of humor, the types of humor that are most useful and helpful for patients, and the most effective ways to use humor. In addition, we need to gain a better understanding of how humor, laughter, and positive emotions benefit the physiology and potential healing capacity of individuals. Nurses can use this same information to incorporate humor into their lives to make their work and personal life more enjoyable and to help them become more effective providers of care. The following are some areas where more definitive data are needed:

1. Development of effective humor assessment tools is warranted. Tools are needed that can be easily incorporated into other assessments and allow for variations in age and patient background.
2. Further substantiation of of the physiological effects and benefits of humor is needed.
3. What types of humor interventions (such as spontaneuous humor, videos, books, individual, groups) are most effective with various patient populations?
4. How can nurses become better educated regarding effective use of therapuetic humor and how can their effectiveness be measured?
5. How do the dynamics of a nurse-patient relationship change when humor is used?
6. How can nurses, and particularly nursing leaders, foster and support an environment in which the exchange of humor between staff and patients is welcome and encouraged?

APPENDIX A

Additional Reading

Allen, Steve. (1987). *How to be funny: Discovering the comic in you.* New York: Mcgraw-Hill.

Barreca, R. (1991). *They used to call me Snow White . . . but I drifted: Women's strategic use of humor.* New York: Viking.

Bates, Roger. (1995). *How to be funnier happier, healthier and more successful too!* Minneapolis: Trafton.

Cousins, Norman. (1979). *Anatomy of an illness.* New York: Norton.

Klein, Allen. (1989). *The healing power of humor.* Los Angeles: Tarcher.

Moody, Raymond. (1978). *Laugh after laugh.* Jacksonville, FL: Headwaters.

Paulson, Terry. (1989). *Making humor work: Take your job seriously and yourself lightly.* Los Altos, CA: Crisp.

Robinson, Vera. (1991). *Humor and the health professions* (2nd ed.). Torofare, NJ: Slack.

Humor Resources

American Association for Therapeutic Humor. Bi-monthly newsletter, conferences, bibliographies, networking. AATH, 222 Meramec, Suite 303, St. Louis, MO 63105. Ph.: (314) 863-6232.

Humor and Health Letter. Bimonthly newsletter about laughter research and applications of humor. P.O. Box 16814. Ph.: Jackson, MS 39236–6814 (601) 957-0075.

Journal of Nursing Jocularity. Humorous quarterly publication, written by nurses, for nurses, about the funny side of the nursing/medical profession. Subscriptions: 5615 West Cermak Road, Cicero, IL 60650-2290. Doug Fletcher, RN, publisher, P.O. Box 40416, Mesa, AZ 85274. Ph.: (602) 835-6165 or e-mail 73314.3032@compuserve.com.

The Fellowship of Merry Christians. *The Joyful Noiseletter,* books, cards, tapes, church-related humor for ministers and others. P.O. Box 668, Kalamazoo, MI 49005-0668.

The Humor Project. *Laughing Matters* publication four times/year. Dr. Joel Goodman, seminars, HUMOResources catalog for books, videos, audiotapes, etc. 110 Spring Street Saratoga Springs, NY 12866. Ph.: (518) 587-8770.

Whole Mirth Catalog. Access to many humorous items, toys, gags, books. 1034 Page Street, San Francisco, CA 94117.

REFERENCES

Ackerman, M., Henry, M., Graham, K., & Coffey, N. (1994). Humor won, humor too: A model to incorporate humor into the health care setting (revised). *Nursing Forum, 29*(2), 15–21.

American heritage dictionary of the English language. (1976). Boston: Houghton Mifflin.

Anderson, T. (1996). Interview with J.R. Dunn. *Humor and Health Journal, 5*(4), 1–5.

Asimov, A. (1992). *Asimov laughs again.* New York: HarperCollins.

Bates, R. (1995). *How to be funnier, happier, healthier, and more successful too!* Minneapolis: Trafton.

Bellert, J. L. (1989) Humor. A therapeutic approach in oncology nursing. *Cancer Nursing, 12*(2), 65–70.

Berk, L., Tan S., & Fry W. (1989). Neuroendocrine and stress hormone changes during mirthful laughter. *American Journal of Medical Sciences, 298*(6), 390–396.

Berk, L., Tan, S., Napier, B., & Eby, W. (1989). Eustress of mirthful laughter modifies natural killer cell activity. *Clinical Research, 37*(1), 115A.

Black, D. (1984). Laughter. *Journal of the American Medical Association, 25*(21), 2995–2998.

Brownell, H. (1988). Neuropsychological insights into humor. In J. Durant & J. Miller (Eds.), *Laughing matters: A serious look at humor* (p. 17). New York: Longman.

Cogan, R., Cogan, D., Waltz, W., & McCue, M. (1987). Effects of laughter and relaxation on discomfort thresholds. *Journal of Behavioral Medicine, 10,* 139–144.

Cousins, N. (1979). *Anatomy of an illness.* New York: Norton.

Crane, A. L. (1987). Why sickness can be a laughing matter. *RN, 50,* 41–42.

Davidhizar, R., & Bowen, M. (1992). The dynamics of laughter. *Archives of Psychiatric Nursing, 6*(2), 132–137.

Dillon, K., Minchoff, B., & Baker, K. (1985). Positive emotional states and enhancement of the immune system. *International Journal of Psychiatry in Medicine, 15*(1), 13–17.

Frankl, V. (1963). *Man's search for meaning.* New York: Washington Square.

Freud, S.(1960). Jokes and their relation to the unconscious. New York: Norton. (Originally: *Der Witz und seine Beziehung zum Unbewussten.* Leipzig and Vienna: Durticke, 1905)

Fry, W. (1971). Mirth and oxygen saturation of peripheral blood. *Psychotherapy and Psychosomatics, 19,* 76–84.

Fry, W. F., & Savin, M. (1988). Mirthful laughter and blood pressure. *Humor, 1,* 49–62.

Gaberson, K. (1991). The effect of humorous distraction on preoperative anxiety. *Association of Operating Room Nurses Journal, 54*(6), 1258–1264.

Haig, R. A. (1988). *The anatomy of humor. Biopsychosocial and therapeutic perspectives.* Springfield, IL: Thomas.

Goodman, J. (1992). Laughing matters: Taking your job seriously and yourself lightly. *Journal of the American Medical Association 267*(13), 1858.

Gruner, C. (1978). *Understanding laughter. The workings of wit and humor.* Chicago: Nelson Hall.

Herth, K. A. (1993). Humor and the older adult. *Applied Nursing Research, 6*(4), 146–153.

Hulse, J. (1994). Humor: A nursing intervention for the elderly. *Geriatric Nursing, 15*(2), 88–90.

Hunt, A. H. (1993). Humor as a nursing intervention. *Cancer Nursing,* *16*(1), 34–39.

Klein, Allen, (1989). *The healing power of humor.* Los Angeles: Tarcher.

Lambert, R., & Lambert, N. K. (1995). The effects of humor on secretory immunoglobulin A levels in school-aged children. *Pediatric Nursing,* *21*(1), 16–19.

Lefcourt, H. M., & Martin, R. A. (1986). *Humor and life stress: Antidote to adversity.* New York: Springer-Verlag.

Leiber, D. B. (1986). Laughter and humor in critical care. *Dimensions in Critical Care Nursing,* *5*(3), 162–170.

Liechty, R. D. (1987). Humor and the surgeon. *Archives of Surgery, 122,* 519–522.

Macaluso, M. C. (1993). Humor, health and healing. *American Nephrology Nurses Association Journal, 20*(1), 14–16.

Martin, R., Dobbin J. (1988). Sense of humor, hassles, and immunoglobulin evidence for a stress-moderating effect of humor. *International Journal of Psychiatry in Medicine, 18*(2), 93–105.

McGhee, P. (1979). *Humor, it's orgin and development.* San Francisco: Freeman.

Moody, R. A. (1978). *Laugh after laugh.* Jacksonville, FL: Headwaters.

Mornhinweg, G., & Voignier, R. (1995). Holistic nursing interventions. *Orthopedic Nursing 14*(4), 20–24.

Morreall, J. (1983). *Taking laughter seriously.* Albany: State University of New York Press.

Moyers, B. (1993). *Healing and the mind.* New York: Bantam.

Obrdlik, A. (1942). Gallows humor: A sociological phenomenon. *American Journal of Sociology, 47,* 709–716.

Paquet, J. (1993, November/December). Laughter and stress management. *Today's O.R. Nurse,* pp. 13–17.

Parfitt, J. M. (1990). Humorous preoperative teaching: Effect of recall of postoperative exercise routines. *American Association of Operating Room Nurses Journal, 52*(1), 114–120.

Paulsen, T. (1989). *Making humor work. Take your job seriously and yourself lightly.* Los Altos, CA: Crisp.

Robinson, V. M. (1991). *Humor and the health professions* (2nd ed.). Thorofare, NJ: Slack.

Robinson, V. (1978). Humor in nursing. In C. Carlson & B. Blackwell (Eds.), *Behavioral concepts and nursing interventions.* Philadelphia: Lippincott.

Robinson, V. (1974). The tactful use of humor in nursing. *RN, 37*(10), 38–39.

Rosenheim, E., & Golan, G. (1986). Patients' reactions to humorous interventions in psychotherapy. *American Journal of Psychotherapy, 40*(1), 110–124.

Saper, B. (1988). Humor in psychiatric healing. *Psychiatric Quarterly, 59*(4):, 306–319.

Saper, B. (1990). The therapeutic use of humor for psychiatric disturbances in adolescents and adults. *Psychiatric Quarterly, 61*(4), 261–272.

Schaefner, N. (1981). *The art of laughter.* New York: Columbia University Press.

Schulz, R., Bookwala, J., Knapp, J., Scheier, M., & Williamson, G. (1996). Pessimism, age, and cancer mortality, *Psychology and Aging, 11*(2), 304–309.

Simon, J. M. (1989) Humor techniques for oncology nurses. *Oncology Nursing Forum, 16,* 667–670.

Smith, K. L. (1995, May 5). *Medicinal mirth: The art and science of therapuetic humor.* Presentation to North Memorial Hospice and Home Care, 3300 Oakdale, Minneapolis, MN 55422.

Stone, A., Valdimarsdottir, H., Jandorf, L., Cox, D., & Neale, J. (1987). Evidence that IgA antibody is associated with daily mood. *Journal of Personality and Social Psychology, 52,* 988–993.

Strickland, D. (1993, November/December). Seriously, laughter matters. *Today's O.R. Nurse,* pp. 19–24.

Walsh, J. J. (1928). *Laughter and health.* New York: Appleton.

Woodhouse, D. K. (1993). The aspects of humor in dealing with stress. *Nursing Administration Quarterly, 18*(1), 80–89.

Yovetich, N. A., Dale, A., & Hudak, M. (1990). Benefits of humor in reduction of threat induced anxiety. *Psychological Reports, 66,* 51–58.

Ziv, A. (1984). *Personality and sense of humor.* New York: Springer-Verlag.

24

Animals in Health Care

Kirsten James

I saw a child who couldn't walk,
sit on a horse, laugh and talk,
Then ride it through a field of daisies
and yet he could not walk unaided.
I saw a child, no legs below,
sit on a horse, and make it go
through woods of green
and places he had never been
to sit and stare,
except from a chair.
I saw a child who could only crawl
mount a horse and sit up tall.
Put it through degrees of paces
and laugh at the wonder in our faces.
I saw a child born into strife,
Take up and hold the reins of life
and that same child was heard to say,
Thank you God for showing me the way.

—"I Saw a Child," John Anthony Davies

Humans have a long history of therapeutic association with animals. Animals have been—and still are—used for protection, companionship, work and to engender caring and responsibility in our children. The role of animals in human health care has received greater attention in Western medical circles in recent years, with a number of research studies indicating that there are clear health benefits when animal interaction occurs (McCormack, 1993).

This healthy association is not just related to pet ownership and pet therapy; the use of animals for deliberate therapeutic purposes is a well-known practice with a long history. The uses of horses include riding for the disabled, and hippotherapy. In more recent years, dolphins have participated in therapy for humans.

Mind/body medicine, or psychoneuroimmunology, values pleasurable activities because they can be scientifically proven to enhance health. Therefore, the role of animal observation in settings such as zoos, reservations, sanctuaries, and through bird and whale-watching, should not be overlooked as ways in which animals positively impact our health.

The therapeutic use of pets was first introduced by the Quakers in England in 1792, but it wasn't until the 1980s that the first World Congress on Pet Therapy was held in that same country. Since then, a number of societies have been established such as the North American Association of Pet Facilitated Therapists and the charitable organization, Pets as Therapy (PAT) in the United Kingdom (Berrisford, 1995).

Approximately 66% of Australian households own a pet, which is the highest in the world per capita (Australian Companion Animal Council, 1995). The United States ranks closely with an estimated 28 million households with cats and 34 million households with dogs (American Pet Products Manufacturers Association, 1994).

Whether the creatures be furry, hairy, slippery, or feathered, these companions are now being recognized as contributing to the well-being of their owners on both a psychological and physiological level (Anderson, 1996; Padus, 1992).

SPECIFIC DEFINITION

According to Berrisford there are many definitions of pet therapy. It has become "a generic term that includes visitation, possession, attempts at milieu therapy and using an animal as an active participant in psychotherapy" (Berrisford, 1995, p. 86).

In many countries, the presence of animals in either a residential or visiting capacity is on the increase in a variety of Western health care settings, such as hospital wards, hospices, nursing homes, rehabilitation centers and psychiatric institutions (Cusack & Smith, 1984; Padus, 1992; Sylvester, 1988). Dogs, cats, birds, and fish are the most common creatures in residence because they are relatively easy to keep and maintain, but if having animals live in is not possible, some health care agencies have adopted a compromise. They engage volunteer pet visitors who bring in their trained and registered animals (usually dogs) on a regular basis for patients and residents. Caring for the animal, touching it, taking it for walks, and talking to it are commonly accepted ways that humans interact with pets; these simple interactions are what makes the pets therapeutic (Dillow, 1996).

SCIENTIFIC BASIS

Pet ownership has been associated with positive health outcomes in a number of studies. In a 1980 study of 96 people with heart disease, psychiatrist Erika Friemann of the University of Pennsylvania found that after being released from the coronary care unit, pet owners had a higher survival rate one year later than petless patients with comparable disease (Spiegal, cited in Goleman & Gurin, 1995). Likewise, UCLA psychologist Judith Siegal found in her 1990 study of 345 elderly pet owners, that they went to physicians fewer times in the course of a year than a group of petless counterparts (Spiegal, cited in Goleman & Gurin, 1995).

The report of a 1992 survey of 5,741 people attending the cardiovascular risk clinic at the Baker Medical Research Institute in Melbourne, Australia, contained some noteworthy findings. Systolic arterial pressure and serum triglyceride levels were significantly lower in pet owners than in non-owners, averaged across all ages studied (20–60 years) and both sexes. In men between 20 and 60 years, plasma triglyceride and plasma cholesterol levels were lower in pet owners. In women between 40 and 60 years, the pet owners had significantly lower systolic arterial pressures and serum triglyceride levels. The results were not confounded by variables such as differences in body mass, lifestyle, or socioeconomic status between pet owners and non-owners (Anderson, Reid, & Jennings, 1992).

A recent American study followed up a group of patients with asymptomatic ventricular arrhythmias after myocardial infarction, finding that only 1% of dog owners died in the following year, compared to 7% of the non-owners (Friedmann & Thomas, 1995, cited in Anderson, 1996). A similar study by Bricklin in 1990 found that heart attack survivors who were pet owners live longer than those who don't (cited in McCormack, 1993).

People often satisfy their tactile needs with pets. Studies have proven the value of pet therapy where traditional forms of therapy have failed. Corson and colleagues at Ohio State University used dogs of various breeds in the Department of Psychiatry to facilitate communication and expression in humans who had been long silent. They state that the attachment the humans develop with the dogs is probably related to the animal's ability to offer love and tactile reassurance without criticism (Montagu,1978). This unconditional love may be one of the main reasons we respond so well to pets. Cusack and Smith (1984) have described the love that animals give as open, straightforward, uncomplicated and unchanging. The authors go on to cite Corson, who observed that pets provide a means of nonverbal communication that is reassuring and comforting to the lonely and withdrawn elder.

It is also socially acceptable for people to dispense affection to pets in public—to demonstrate feelings via petting, stroking, hugging and kissing. The same activities may be frowned upon or misinterpreted by members of the public if undertaken between humans. This is of particular significance to the elderly, many of whom live in isolation and whose partners may have died.

There are numerous advantages to owning pets. Pets can provide incentive for elders to keep busy and active; as care providers, they can feel a sense of responsibility. Caring for animals as part of a daily routine also helps with reality orientation. Companion animals, especially dogs, also help people feel safer; for hearing or sight-impaired people, the trained dog can provide independence and security, while allaying anxiety and fear. It has even been suggested that people who owned dogs as children have healthier egos, greater trust and more self-esteem than those who have not (Cusack & Smith, 1984). According to Montagu (1978), child-battering and abusing parents who were themselves neglected and abused as children rarely report having had a childhood pet.

Research which looks at the health benefits of pet ownership and the corresponding impact on government health budgets has been undertaken in one Australian study. Based on the findings in the National People and Pets Survey (McHarg, Baldock, Heady, & Robinson, 1994) which revealed fewer doctor visits and less use of cardiovascular disease medications, Heady & Anderson (1995) calculated health care savings of hundreds of millions of dollars.

INTERVENTION

Riding for the Disabled (RDA) is an international organization which is dedicated to providing disabled people with the opportunity to participate in horseriding and other related activities, thereby promoting "fun, freedom and fitness" (RDA, 1996). Horses are used in other therapies as well.

In ancient Greece, Hippocrates (460–377 BC) wrote on "natural exercise," which included horse riding. Riding therapy uses functional riding skills to achieve specific therapeutic goals. It can be carried out by qualified riding instructors, but under consultation from a medical professional. It may also use specific exercises involving stretching, relaxation, strengthening, balance, coordination or movement patterns (Bailey, 1996). Hippotherapy is a specialized medical therapy whereby the horse influences the client, rather than the client controlling the horse. The client is placed in a number of positions and actively responds to the movement of the therapy horse. The therapist directs the horse's movement, analyzing the client's response and adjusting the treatment accordingly.

The hippotherapy team consists of the horse, a "side helper," and the horse expert, who is a qualified and specially trained physical or occupational therapist. The key goals of hippotherapy are to improve posture, balance, mobility, and function. Because it is specialized therapy, it is inappropriate to elaborate too much on hippotherapy here. However, in our role as health eductors, nurses should have broad knowledge and awareness of treatments and resources available.

Hippotherapy is indicated for the following common problems: abnormal tone and reflexes, asymmetry, poor postural control, impaired balance responses, impaired coordination, malalignment and decreased mobility. The primary medical conditions treated by hippotherapy include cerebral palsy, stroke, multiple sclerosis, traumatic brain injury, functional spinal curvature and first degree scoliosis (P. Bailey, personal communication, August, 1996). A number of reference texts and research papers are available on the therapy, and further information in North America can be obtained from the American Hippotherapy Association and the Canadian Therapeutic Riding Association.

Another form of interaction where the animals influence the client occurs with dolphins. Judith Muir, who has worked in this area for over 12 years, has witnessed countless examples of the profound effects that dolphins in their natural habitat can have on humans. She and her staff are qualified special needs teachers as well as divemasters. Although her company specializes in working with people who have disabilities and illnesses, it is acknowledged that politicians, celebrities and others are all affected by dolphins. The interaction induces a sense of well-being, and fears are often overcome. She believes that people respond to the energy, intelligence, and dynamism of the dolphins. Treatments or cures are never offered, but peoples lives are always touched and enhanced by being close to these extraordinary creatures.

The use of dolphins in health care appears to be largely anecdotal at this time, and further research is clearly indicated to support this form of therapeutic interaction. The same is true for visits to observational settings such as zoos and sanctuaries, for whale-watching trips, and other opportunities for interspecies contact. It is widely acknowledged that animals are a great source of enjoyment, which, in turn undoubtably stimulates endorphin release, but the importance of such settings and experiences to our health appears to be unacknowledged and largely unstudied to date.

Guidelines for Pet Therapy

For those contemplating the implementation of pet therapy in their workplace, the staff and administration need to decide whether they wish to have animals in residence, or in a visiting capacity. If the former is chosen, then the following guidelines, drawn from Berrisford (1995) and Sylvester (1988) are useful:

- A policy for residents, staff, and visitors on the subject is advisable.
- Responsibility for feeding, cleaning, training, exercising, and grooming needs to be considered. This may involve one staff member per animal, or a roster system may be organized.
- Costs of purchasing, vaccinating, and veterinary visits/check-ups, food, toys, grooming and bedding equipment, and other expenses need to be determined and sourced.
- Choice of animal(s) needs to be made. Choice may be determined by available space, type of patients/residents, layout of workplace, staff or patient allergies or dislikes to certain animals. Temperament assessment and training for the animals are also advisable.
- Although concern over disease risk is sometimes expressed, in fact, an animal that is clean, friendly and vaccinated has less chance of transmitting disease than a human. Routine handwashing, particularly at meal times, should be observed.
- Suitable insurance should be arranged to cover any unforeseen liabilities arising from accidents involving pets.
- Some hospices and nursing homes allow people to bring their own pets. Birds are usually no problem, and those with dogs are given a single room. Fish are even easier!

For those not desiring the ongoing or long-term responsibilities of resident pets, having an animal visit may be a good option. Kelly (personal communication, September, 1996) offers some basic guidelines for the introduction of a visiting dog in a health care setting:

- Assess the receptiveness of the patients by asking their opinions, and then checking their reactions.
- Keep the dog on a lead—this element of control provides a sense of reassurance and security.
- Some handlers encourage the patient to get to know the dog by feeding them a treat.
- Allow the dog to spend quality time with those patients who react positively, rather than persisting with someone who is indifferent.

Measurement of Outcomes

Pet therapy and pet ownership may result in both long-term and short-term outcomes. Outcomes are assessed relative to the various uses of pets and intended effects. For example, pet therapy is often used to help relieve tension, pain, and isolation. This is achieved through petting and holding; the warmth of the animal's body is soothing and comforting. It has also been used as a means of encouraging communication (Cusack & Smith, 1984; Sylvester, 1988). Interaction with pets can facilitate expression through affectionate touch and talk (Montagu, 1978) and can encourage exercise by providing a reason to go outside and a sense of purpose in caring for the animal (Padus, 1992; Sylvester 1988). The unconditional love that an animal can show to humans is another way that pets bring comfort.

There are also more easily measurable positive effects, such as lower blood pressure, serum cholesterol, quicker recovery from surgery and illness, and fewer doctor visits, cited in the studies on pet ownership (Friedmann & Thomas, 1995, cited in Anderson, 1996; Australian Companion Animal Council 1995; Anderson, Reid & Jennings, 1992; Padus, 1992).

USES

Populations in Which Animals Have Been Used

As indicated previously, there are numerous benefits and indications for pet therapy. To date, literature concerning the use of this therapy has been found related to clients, patients and/or residents in the following settings: hospitals, hospices, psychiatric institutions, rehabilitation facilities, and nursing homes.

Precautions

Some people do not like animals. There may be negative memory associations from past experience, allergy to dog hair or cat fur, or there may be no discernable reason. As for all complementary therapies, the preference of the individual needs to be respected and considered. Hygiene is, of course, an important consideration in health care, and naturally, this should be part of the care and maintenance plan of the pet therapy program. Common sense should prevail!

RESEARCH QUESTIONS

The effectiveness of pet therapy should continue to be monitored and studied, as an increasing number of health care centers are introducing animals into the patients' environment (Berrisford, 1995). Although there appears to be a general recognition in the community that animals can have a positive effect on our lives, it is an area which is underresearched in terms of specific health benefits. Nurses, working in a range of health care settings, may be able to pursue further scientific exploration. In the context of complementary care, here is a perfect opportunity to work with Mother Nature, and understand more clearly how we can facilitate healing and health and enhance quality of life by relatively simple, inexpensive, and pleasurable means. Possible research questions are:

1. What health benefits are to be gained from observing animals (e.g., in zoos, sanctuaries, whale-watching and so on)?
2. What is it about interaction (i.e., swimming) with dolphins that induces well-being in humans?
3. Are animals that can be touched more therapeutic in their effect than those that cannot be?

ACKNOWLEDGMENTS

The author is grateful for professional contributions to this article from her colleagues P. Bailey, Occupational Therapist, R.D.D.A., Victoria, Australia (Interview & notes); J. Kelly, Psychologist and Registered Nurse, Melbourne, Australia (Interview); and J. Muir, Special Education Teacher & Manager, Polperro Dolphins, Mornington Peninsula, Victoria, Australia.

REFERENCES

American Pet Products Manufacturers Association. (1994). *Pet owners survey*. Washington, D.C.: Author.

Anderson, W. P. (1996). The benefits of pet ownership. *The Medical Journal of Australia, 164*, 441–442.

Anderson, W. P., Reid, C. M., & Jennings, G. L. (1992). Pet ownership and risk factors for cardiovascular disease. *The Medical Journal of Australia, 157*, 298–300.

Australian Companion Animal Council. (1995). *The power of pets*. New South Wales, Australia: Author.

Berrisford, J. A. (1995). Implications of pet-facilitated therapy in palliative nursing. *International Journal of Palliative Nursing, 1*(2), 86–89.

Cusack, O., & Smith, E. (1984). *Pets and the elderly*. New York: Hayworth.

Dillow, K. A. (1996, March-April). Pets and the Elderly. *New Horizons*, pp. 5–6.

Goleman, D., & Gurin, J. (1995). *Mindbody Medicine*. Marrickville, NSW: Choice.

Heady, B., & Anderson, W.P. (1995). *Health cost savings: The impact of pets on Australian health budgets*. South Yarra, Victoria : Pet Information and Advisory Service.

McCormack, G. L. (1993). *Pain management—Mindbody techniques for treating chronic pain syndromes*. Tucson, AZ: Therapy Skill Builders.

McHarg, M., Baldock,C., Heady, B. W., & Robinson, A. (1995). *National people and pets survey*. Sydney, NSW: Urban Animal Management Coalition.

Montagu, A. (1978). *Touching* (2nd ed.). New York: Harper & Row.

Padus, E. (1992). *The Complete guide to your emotions and your health*. Emmaus, PA: Rodale.

Riding for the Disabled Association of Australia. (1996). *Riding for the disabled*. [Brochure]. Ascot Vale, Australia: Author.

Sylvester, J. (1988). Animal crackers. *Nursing Standard, 3*(13/14), pp. 28–29.

25

Contracting

Ruth Lindquist

Health behaviors and patient adherence to prescribed regimens and health practices are major concerns of health professionals. Considerable attention has been focused on ways to change health behavior or to increase adherence (Azrin et al., 1994; Higgins, Budney, Bickel, & Badger, 1994; Swain & Steckel, 1981). Although providing patients with information may help to change behaviors and improve adherence, education in and of itself is not sufficient. In fact, Swain and Steckel (1981) reported a higher dropout rate for persons with hypertension who had been in the patient education group than for those in the routine visit group. However, involving the patient in the plan of care and making the person more responsible for the outcomes of care have been found to increase adherence to recommended health practices and regimens (Steckel, 1982). Contracting is one method to increase patient responsibility for outcomes.

Contracting is an intervention in which the patient is involved in both the development and execution of the plan of care. Contracting may be effective in increasing compliance because it clarifies the specific responsibilities of both the health care professional and the patient for achieving agreed upon goals. In so doing, an appropriate degree of responsibility for attaining the outcome is transferred from the health care professional to the patient. Contracting is a strategy that has the potential for increasing congruence in values and priorities between the patient and the health professionals, leading to a mutually acceptable plan of care (Hayes & Davis, 1980).

Contracting helps persons to become integrally involved in their care and to take responsibility for their own care to the extent possible. This is often accomplished in a stepwise progression. Achievement of a desired goal may require many behavioral steps over considerable time to change behavior and then to maintain the behavioral change.

Contracting may be used as a primary intervention or as a supplemental intervention to accomplish behavioral performance towards the achievement of specific ends. Contracting has been used in a variety of settings with diverse populations. Although many studies on the effectiveness of contracting are found in other disciplines, relatively few studies have tested its effectiveness within the context of nursing. In her review of the research that had been conducted on the use of contracting within nursing, Boehm (1989) found 20 articles, with only 8 of these research based.

DEFINITION

A contract is a binding agreement between two or more persons or parties. A contract explicitly details the expectations, in terms of means, activities, outcomes, and responsibilities of each party towards goal attainment. Contracting rests on the premise that the nurse and patient are equal partners, but that each has different responsibilities for achieving the agreed upon goal (Zangari & Duffy, 1980). Contracts can be either written or verbal. However, only written contracts related to fostering health-related behaviors are addressed in this chapter.

Contingency contracting is a specific form of contracting. The element that differentiates contingency contracts from other types of patient contracts is reinforcement. Contingency contracting involves the selection, identification, and description of the desired behavior in measurable terms that are observable and acceptable to all parties involved, and provides for an exchange of some agreed upon form of reinforcement in return for performance of behaviors (Steckel, 1982).

SCIENTIFIC BASIS

Contingency contracting has its roots in operant conditioning, founded in the work of Skinner (Janz & Hartman, 1984). Contingency contracts are related to behavior modification. A premise of behavior modification is that the performance of a behavior depends on the consequences of that behavior. Kazdin (1980) stated that behavior change occurs only when the consequences contingent upon the performance of that behavior are altered. Positive or negative reinforcers can be used to bring about changes in that behavior. This chapter will focus on contingency contracts.

Classical conditioning, also called respondent conditioning, is one type of learning used by behavioralists. Pavlov's famous salivating dog investigations explored classical conditioning. A specific stimulus, also called a conditioned stimulus, automatically evokes a response. Some stimuli in the person's environment elicit reflex responses over which the person does not have control, for example, salivating when food is smelled. With classical conditioning, a person can be taught to respond to a neutral stimulus by pairing conditioned and unconditioned stimuli. Over time, the unconditioned, unpaired stimulus singly elicits the desired response.

Operant, or instrumental conditioning, is a second type of behavioral learning. The majority of human behaviors are voluntary and not reflexive. Voluntary behaviors occur spontaneously and are primarily controlled by their consequences. If behaviors can be controlled by changing their consequences, they are termed operants (Skinner, 1953). Operants can be increased or decreased by changing the events that follow them.

An overlap exists between classical and operant conditioning. It is now known that humans can control some of their reflex responses such as heart rate and blood pressure. Also, operant behaviors can be controlled by antecedent stimuli and not by just the consequences. Cues antecedent to the behavior may key the person to respond in a particular manner. These cues act to stimulate the response to occur. Most human behaviors are learned through a combination of respondent and operant conditioning (Steckel, 1982).

Reinforcement theory provides the basis for contingency contracts. Reinforcers are directly related to a behavior. Determined by the effect they have on a behavior; they may be called either positive or negative. Positive reinforcement results in an increase in the incidence of a behavior when it is followed by a favorable consequence. Likewise, negative reinforcement following a behavior results in a decrease in the incidence of that behavior.

Reinforcers are unique for each person. Observing the person's behavior and determining what activities occur in relation to each other is one way to identify reinforcers. The terms *reward* and *reinforcer* are often used interchangeably. However, the two terms are distinct and should not be used interchangeably. A reward is a pleasant consequence related to the goal and is not tied to the subsequent performance of the target behavior. Reinforcers are intimately linked to the targeted behavior. A reward may be written into the contract and be given when the goal is reached. Reinforcers are used to help achieve the goal.

Kazdin (1980) provided four considerations for maximizing the effectiveness of positive reinforcement: proximity of reinforcement to the event, magnitude or amount of reinforcement given, quality, and type pattern (schedule) of reinforcement. The closer the reinforcer is to the target behavior (behavior to be changed), the more likely it will produce the positive results. Delayed reinforcement can be used after the target behavior is learned and the focus is sustaining the behavior. Generally, the more frequent the reinforcer or the greater its size, the greater will be the response. Patient preference in the selection of the reinforcer helps assure that the quality or type of reinforcer will be effective. The schedule used in reinforcing the behavior can be *continuous* or *intermittent* and *fixed* or *random*. In continuous reinforcement, the person is reinforced each time the behavior is performed, whereas in intermittent reinforcement, the behavior may have to be executed a number of times before reinforcement occurs. When a fixed ratio of reinforcement is used, the person knows that after a specific number of performances, they will receive the reinforcer. No set pattern of reinforcement is used in the random ratio method. Random reinforcement is frequently used after the person has mastered the behavior and is being weaned from the reinforcer.

Fading is the term used to describe the process of weaning a person from the reinforcer while sustaining the desired behavior change. A fixed ratio of reinforcement may be used at first so that the person is receiving less reinforcement but knows when it will occur. This is followed by random reinforcement; the person knows that the behavior will be reinforced on some occasions but is not certain when this will happen. When the behavior has been sustained with less and less reinforcement, no reinforcement is given. However, follow-up is needed to determine if the behavior continues. Another technique is to move the reinforcement to the patient.

Sustaining behavior change is the ultimate hallmark of the success of a behavior change intervention. Relapse in behavior change is commonplace (Marlott & Gordon, 1979). Return to preintervention behavior or habit is a frequent result, and remains a challenge to caregivers and clients alike. Contingency contracts may be effective in sustaining positive behaviors and the goal that has been achieved. Other strategies for early identification of relapse and for regaining behavioral control may need to be anticipated, and employed if behavioral relapse occurs (Cummings, Gordon, & Marlott, 1980).

INTERVENTION

Establishing rapport with the patient precedes initiating a contract. The rationale for the contract and the technique are explained. Cooperation and involvement of the patient, and often the family or significant other, are essential to the success of this intervention. Indeed, in a program of outpatient behavioral treatment for cocaine dependence which involved behavioral contracts, the best single predictor of cocaine abstinence was whether a significant other participated in treatment (Higgins et al., 1994).

Steps in contingency contracting consist of (a) determining and defining the behavior along with its consequences and antecedent, (b) planning and writing the contract, (c) reviewing and signing the contract, and (d) evaluating the progress. These steps are described more fully below.

Techniques

When discussing a problem or concern with the patient, a number of related problems may emerge. Priorities need to be established as attention is focused on one behavior at a time. The patient determines which one has first priority. If a behavioral change is not deemed important by the patient, the chances for achieving the outcome are low. After the priority problem has been determined, goals are formulated. Frequently goals need to be broken down into smaller segments so that the behavior can be specifically defined. If they are not, confusion and misunderstanding may result. *Shaping behaviors* is the term given to breaking down the more complex behavior into smaller components and using them as building blocks of the ultimate target behavior. Each successive component is reinforced until the overall behavior is achieved; the behaviors form what is called a "chain." No behavioral step is too small to reinforce: Starting with the easiest change may encourage progress toward the ultimate goal (Steckel, 1982).

Behaviors are defined in very specific terms so that all parties know exactly what is being observed. The behavior should be so well defined that all persons will know it if they see it, without ambiguity.

Breaking down complex behaviors into smaller, clearly distinguishable segments helps recognition. Determination is made of the precise behavior and the context in which it occurs. This activity may be the basis for the first step in the process. An agreement is written stating that the patient will come to the next meeting with a description of the context in which the behavior occurs and the number of times it occurs. Several methods may be used for this assessment. Counters can be used to keep track of how often a behavior occurs. The novelty of the counter may assist the patient to focus on the behavior and become more aware of its frequency. Keeping a diary is another method that may be used for assessing the extent of the behavior. Establishing the baseline—the number of times that the behavior occurs in a day or week—is necessary so that progress can be measured.

Observations by family members or health professionals are helpful in assisting the person to identify consequences and antecedents of the target behavior. Antecedent behaviors serve as cues to the occurrence of the target behavior. Behaviors are frequently controlled by antecedents. Thoughts, feelings, places, or other persons are examples of antecedents (Steckel, 1982). Behaviors that are controlled by an antecedent are termed *strong stimulus control behaviors.*

Determining the consequences of the behavior is also part of the initial assessment. An accurate picture of the context of the behavior assists in establishing the terms of the contract. Reinforcers need to be related to the behavior. Ideas are obtained from the patient regarding reinforcers that would be effective. Observing the behavior to be changed and the context in which it takes place also may suggest possible reinforcers. If the patient has difficulty in identifying possible reinforcers, a list of possible and realistic reinforcers can be formulated and shared with the patient, but final selection always resides with the client.

Kazdin (1980) listed essential elements to be included in a contingency contract including: (a) a statement of the privileges each party expects to achieve from the contract, (b) specification of the selected and readily observable client behaviors, (c) explicitly stated sanctions for failure to meet the terms of the contrac, and (d) stated provisions for monitoring progress. A bonus clause (extra privileges) can be used to reinforce compliance with the terms of the contract. Details of a contingency are illustrated in Figure 25.1.

Dates of contract: September 1, 1997 to October 1, 1997

We agree to perform the following behaviors during the month of September: If Anne refrains from eating junk food snacks from the time of her arrival home from work until bedtime, Marci will spend one hour playing tennis with her twice a week. We will meet with Ms. Smith, to review progress and performance as scheduled September 30th.

Reward: If this is adhered to for a month, Marci will buy tickets for both to attend the Northwest Tennis Tournament on October 15.

Penalty: If Anne eats junk food during the week, she will clean the apartment on Saturday.

Anne will keep a log of her evening eating, which will be shared with Marci on Friday evening.

Signature:	*Anne Johnson*	*8/20/97*
Signature:	*Marci Maus*	*8/20/97*
Signature:	*Barbara Smith, RN*	*8/20/97*

FIGURE 25.1   Example of a written contract illustrating inclusion of the essential elements of contingency contracts: privileges, client behaviors, explicit sanctions, and provisions for monitoring.

Guidelines for Contingency Contracting

Table 25.1 details steps in the process of using contracting as an intervention. In each step the involvement of the client is obvious. Providing a copy of the contract to clients serves to remind them of their duties in relation to the contract. Suggest that the client place

TABLE 25.1   Guidelines for Contingency Contracting

1. Establish and select the problem of importance and priority to client and client's health.
2. Examine context and baseline "count" (frequency) of behavior; structure client examination and self-assessment of behavior through diary, count, etc. Client identifies antecedent and consequent reinforcers.
3. Formulate specific goal and subgoals. Break down goals into segments to identify specific behaviors in specific terms. Agree upon and select a starting point or the initial behavior to be changed. Select one that will permit initial success.
4. Establish reinforcer(s).
5. Develop a mutually agreeable plan for interaction.
6. Monitor progress; reevaluate and modify contract as necessary.
7. Deliver planned and scheduled reinforcers as per terms of the contract.
8. Plan maintenance and strategies for relapse.
9. Complete contract; provide closure.

the contract in a prominent place as aconstant reminder of the behavior to be changed.

Measurement of Outcomes

To permit a fair test of the use of contracts, it is best to err on the side
of giving too much time for reaching the goal rather than providing
for too short a time frame. Not seeing sufficient progress may be
discouraging for the patient. Times for reviewing the contract need to
be established and known to both parties. Flexibility in reaching a
goal is needed; unforeseen circumstances may arise that affect the
performance of agreed-upon activities. Or, an unrealistic time frame
may have been established initially.

Methods for keeping track of progress are used to determine if the
goal has been achieved; they also can serve to motivate the patient to
continue with the contract. Graphs are an easy way to depict progress
over time. Graphs also display the occurrence of plateaus. Providing
an explanation to the patient about the possibility of plateaus before
the contract begins helps decrease the discouragement associated with
this seeming lack of progress.

USES

Conditions/Populations

Contracts have been used in many settings, with many populations for
many diverse conditions. Table 25.2 lists conditions for which contracting has been used as an intervention. Two conditions, weight
reduction and adherence to therapeutic regimens, will be discussed
as examples of the use of contingency contracting as an intervention.

Weight Reduction

Weight loss and control are concerns of many persons in our society.
Countless programs for weight loss, using a variety of techniques,
exist. A frequently voiced complaint of program participants is that
after achieving their goal, they are unable to maintain the weight loss.
This discourages the person from enrolling in another program and
trying again. Too often programs focus only on weight loss and not
on changes in behavior and lifestyle that would sustain losses achieved.

TABLE 25.2   Examples of Health-related Uses of Contracting

Acquiring health behaviors (Hayes & Davis, 1980)

Adherence to diabetes mellitus regimen (Lowe & Lutzker, 1979; Morgan & Littell, 1988)

Compliance with medical regimens (Becker & Maiman, 1980; Koch, Giardina, Ryan, McQueen, & Hilgartner, 1993; Levendusky, Berglas, Dooley, & Landau, 1983)

Compliance with hypertension education (Swain & Steckel, 1981)

Coronary care unit patients (Ziemann & Dracup, 1989)

Physical activity (Miller, 1995)

Drug abuse treatment and rehabilitation (Azrin, et al., 1994; Calsyn et al., 1994; Higgins et al., 1994; Saxon, 1993)

Smoking cessation (Neisworth, 1972)

Suicide prevention (Twiname, 1981)

Prevention of unplanned pregnancy (Van Dover, 1986)

Psychiatric patients (Loomis, 1985)

Weight reduction (Jeffery, Bjornson-Benson, Rosenthal, Lindquist, & Johnson, 1984; Wing, Epstein, Marcus, & Shapira, 1981)

Anorexia nervosa (Solanto, Jacobson, Heller, Golden, & Hertz, 1994)

Jeffery and colleagues (1983) utilized a monetary contract in a group of 89 overweight men who were randomly assigned to one of six weight loss treatment groups as part of a 15-week behavioral weight reduction program. All participants agreed to lose 30 pounds and completed a monetary contract with deposits of varying amounts to be returned upon successful weight loss. The 6 groups varied in the amount of the deposit ($30, $150, or $300) and in the type of contract (either group or individual performance). Overall, the weight loss over the 15-week period was large. However, the groups that had contracts contingent upon group performance lost more weight than those having individual contracts. The amount of the deposit was only weakly related to short-term weight reduction. At 2-year follow-up (Jeffery et al., 1984), in the absence of effective maintenance program, weight losses as compared to baseline were modest. However, group contracts were still more effective in producing long-term weight loss than individual contracts. The weight loss reported at 2 years was not significantly different than other behavioral weight loss programs without monetary contracts.

Adherence to therapeutic regimens. Over 50% of all Americans have some chronic illness. Many have prescribed regimens to prevent complications, reduce symptoms, and control the progression of the pathology. Compliance with therapeutic regimens is extremely low. Although information about the regimen is helpful, this in itself is often not sufficient to ensure that the patient will adhere to the regimen. Contingency contracts offer a way to help persons incorporate the necessary practices or behavioral changes into their life and to maintain them over time.

Behavioral contracts have been employed in programs to increase adherence to drug regimens. Twenty-three patients with thalassemia (a genetically determined chronic anemia) ranging in age from 3 to 30 years, contracted to improve adherence to the use of subcutaneous desferrioxamine by increasing their number of days of its use over a 6-month period (Koch et al., 1993). Adherence to therapy was measured by empty vial counts. The use of the drug was positively reinforced by a behavioral reward system and careful monitoring. Contingency contracting was successful in 76% of the patients over the time of the study, with most of these patients maintaining adherence 2 months after the program. Investigators concluded that such behavioral strategies are efficacious in promoting adherence to therapy in chronic illness.

Precautions

Interventions employing contingency contracts may be time consuming. However, sufficient time must be allowed for patients to gain a clear understanding of what the contract requires. Patient acceptance is critical to the effectiveness of the process. If family or friends are to be involved, explanations also need to be given to them.

When care is given by a health care team, for example in the hospital setting, good communication and commitment to the plan and contract are important to the success of contracting. Because health professionals are accustomed to making decisions and implementing a plan of care without input from the patient, many may have difficulty including the patient as an equal partner. Inservice education for the staff may be necessary.

It may be necessary to include the contract in the chart. Because nurses have responsibility to protect patient rights, it is important for contracts to be nonbinding; patients can terminate the contract. Nurses must ensure that patients perceive them as voluntary so as not to induce unwanted anxiety.

FURTHER RESEARCH

Several reviews of the literature on contracting have been published (Boehm, 1989; Janz & Hartman, 1984). Notable in Boehm's review was the small number of studies in which the effectiveness of contracting had been tested in nursing. The following are some of the questions in nursing research might ask on contracts to productively add to our knowledge base:

1. Are there particular patient characteristics that suggest that contingency contracting would be an effective intervention to employ? Are there patient populations or conditions for whom contracts should not be used?
2. Are there occasions when negative reinforcers should be used as opposed to positive reinforcers? What are the effects of negative reinforcers on behavior, patient emotional well-being and participation? Since emphasis is placed on the positive reinforcement, attention to the use of negative reinforcers has been minimal.
3. Is group contingency more effective than individual contingencies in promoting behavior change? Jeffery et al. (1983) found that group contingencies were more effective in producing weight loss. Does this finding generalize to other health behaviors?
4. How might technology be used to cost-effectively monitor behavioral adherence or to deliver behavioral reinforcement in the context of contingency contracting?

REFERENCES

Azrin, N. H., McMahon, P. T., Donohue, B., Besalel, N. A., Lapinski, K. J., Kogan, E. S., Acierno, R. E., & Galloway, E. (1994). *Behavior Research & Therapy, 32,* 857–866.

Becker, M., & Maiman, L. (1980). Strategies for enhancing patient compliance. *Journal of Community Health, 6,* 113–135.

Boehm, S. (1989). Patient contracting. In J. Fitzpatrick, R. Taunton, & J. Benoliel (Eds.), *Annual review of nursing research. Vol. 7* (pp. 143–153). New York: Springer.

Calsyn, D. A., Wells, E. A., Saxon, A. J., Jackson, T. R., Wrede, A. F., Stanton, V., & Fleming, C. (1994). Contingency management of urinalysis results and intensity of counseling services have an interactive impact on methadone maintenance treatment outcomes. *Journal of Addictive Diseases, 13*(3), 47–63.

Cummings, C., Gordon, J. R., and Marlott, G. A. (1980). Relapse: Prevention and prediction. In W. R. Miller (Ed.), *Addictive behaviors: Treatment of alcoholism, drug abuse, smoking, and obesity,* (pp. 291–321). Oxford: Pergamon.

Hayes, W., & Davis, L. (1980). What is a health care contract? *Health Values: Achieving High Level Wellness, 4*(2), 82–89.

Higgins, S. T., Budney, A. J., Bickel, W. K., & Badger, G. J. (1994). Participation of significant others in outpatient behavioral treatment predicts greater cocaine abstinence. *American Journal of Drug and Alcohol Abuse, 20,* 47–56.

Janz, N. K., & Hartman, P. E. (1984). Contingency contracting to enhance patient compliance: A review. *Patient Education and Counseling, 5,* 165–178.

Jeffery, R. W., Gerber, W. M., Rosenthal, B. S., & Lindquist, R. A. (1983). Monetary contracts in weight control: Effectiveness of group and individual contracts of varying size. *Journal of Consulting and Clinical Psychology, 51*(2), 242–248.

Jeffery, R. W., Bjornson-Benson, W. M., Rosenthal, B. S., Lindquist, R. A., & Johnson, S. L. (1984). Behavioral treatment of obesity with monetary contracting: Two-year follow-up. *Addictive Behaviors, 9,* 311–313.

Kazdin, A. (1980). Behavior modification in applied settings. Homewood, IL: Dorsey.

Koch, D. A., Giardina, P. J., Ryan, M., MacQueen, M., & Hilgartner, M.W. (1993). Behavioral contracting to improve adherence in patients with thalassemia. *Journal of Pediatric Nursing, 8*(2), 106–111.

Levendusky, P., Berglas, S., Dooley, C., & Landau, R. (1983). Therapeutic contract program: Preliminary report on a behavioral alternative to the token economy. *Behavior Research and Therapy, 21,* 137–142.

Loomis, M. E. (1985). Levels of contracting. *Journal of Psychosocial Nursing, 23*(3), 9–14.

Lowe, K., & Lutzker, J. (1979). Increasing compliance to a medical regimen with a juvenile diabetic. *Behavior Therapy, 10,* 57–64.

Miller, N. H. (1995). Physical activity: One approach to the primary prevention of hypertension. *American Association of Occupational Health Nurses Journal, 43,* 319–326.

Morgan, B. S., & Littell, D. H. (1988). A closer look at teaching and contingency contracting with Type II diabetes. *Patient Education and Counseling, 12,* 145–158.

Marlott, G. A., & Gordon, J. R. (1979). Determinants of relapse: Implications for the maintenance of behavior change. In P. O. Davidson (Eds.), Behavioral medicine: Changing health lifestyles (pp. 410–452). New York: Brunner/Mazel.

Neisworth, J. (1972). Elimination of cigarette smoking through gradual phase-out of stimulus controls. *Behaviorally Speaking, 10,* 1–3.

Saxon, A. J., Calsyn, D. A., Kivlahan, D. R., & Roszell, D. K. (1993). Outcomes of contingency contracting for illicit drug use in a methadone maintenance program. *Drug & Alcohol Dependence, 31*(3), 205–214.

Skinner, B. (1953). *Science and human behavior.* New York: Free Press.

Solanto, M. V., Jacobson, M. S., Heller, L., Golden, N. H., & Hertz, S. (1994). Rate of weight gain of inpatients with anorexia nervosa under two behavioral contracts. *Pediatrics, 93,* 989–991.

Steckel, S. (1982). *Patient contracting.* Norwalk, CT: Appleton-Century-Crofts.

Swain, M., & Steckel, S. (1981). Influencing adherence among hypertensives. *Research in Nursing and Health, 4,* 213–222.

Twiname, B. (1981). No-suicide contract for nurses. *Journal of Psychiatric Nursing and Mental Health Services, 19*(7), 11–12.

Van Dover, L. (1986). Influence of nurse-client contracting on family knowledge and behaviors in a university student population. *Dissertation Abstracts International, 46,* 3787B.

Wing, R., Epstein, L., Marcus, M., & Shapira, B. (1981). Strong monetary contingencies for weight loss during treatment and maintenance. *Behavior Therapy, 12,* 702–710.

Zangari, M., & Duffy, P. (1980). Contracting with patients in day-to-day practice. *American Journal of Nursing, 80,* 451–455.

Ziemann, K.M., & Dracup, K. (1989). How well do CCU patient-nurse contracts work? *American Journal of Nursing, 89,* 691–692.

26

Groups

Merrie J. Kaas and Mary Fern Richie

Nursing's use of group work to improve the health of clients has been documented since the early 1960s (Burnside, 1986). Use of groups as a nursing intervention is congruent with nursing's concern for individuals, families, groups, and communities. Nurse-led groups have been developed to foster independence, promote health, and prevent illness for clients and their families, and for community consumers.

In this time of cost consciousness in the health care industry, health care professionals, including nurses, are expected to provide cost-efficient treatments with documented therapeutic outcomes. Group work with clients and families can be cost efficient while providing effective treatment for many individuals (Weiner, 1992). The purpose of this chapter is to provide practitioners with the basics for incorporating group work as an intervention into their practice. This chapter will review types of groups and group characteristics. It will also describe techniques for establishing, conducting, and evaluating a group, precautions and research questions.

DEFINITION

What is a group? We all belong to groups, but a group is more than a just collection of people. Forsyth (1990) defines a group as "two or more interdependent individuals who influence one another through social interaction" (p. 23). Groups have a number of common features which can change over time, including level of interaction among members, structure, variations in size, shared common goals, and degree of cohesiveness.

Groups are an agent of change. People join groups for a variety of reasons. Some individuals want to learn different skills in managing an illness; others want to understand their behavior and/or relationships. Still other people want personal support during a life change or loss of health status. Therapeutic groups help individuals achieve goals they cannot achieve alone by helping members increase their knowledge about themselves and others, clarifying the changes they want to make, and giving them the tools to make the changes (Corey & Corey, 1992). Yalom (1995) identified 11 curative factors that are operative in therapeutic groups: instillation of hope, universality, imparting information, altruism, development of socialization techniques, imitative behavior, learning interpersonal skills, group cohesiveness, and catharsis.

SCIENTIFIC BASIS

Practitioners use groups because they are efficient. Empirical data suggests that groups are as effective as other treatments with certain clients. Numerous techniques for implementing groups are described, but the choice of a specific technique is often based on pragmatism, rather than theory or research. Client and practitioner variables, and intervention techniques which contribute to positive outcomes are not well quantified.

Although much progress has been made in the empirical demonstration of the efficacy of group interventions, practitioners are still hesitant to use research methods to document the effectiveness of their group work. Dies and Dies (1993) suggest that this is changing because of internal and external pressures for integrating research and practice in group work. Empirical evidence that certain types of group interventions work better than others for clients with certain symptoms will influence practitioners to more closely match the type of group intervention with specific client needs. For instance, a recent experimental study found that cognitive-behavioral and social support group therapies resulted in less depression for cancer patients receiving radiation than no group intervention (Evans & Connis, 1995). In another study, Buccheri, Trygstad, Kanas, Waldron, and Dowling (1996) reported the effectiveness of group work for schizophrenic patients learning to manage their auditory hallucinations. Research findings from another experimental study indicated that cognitive group interventions and biofeedback group interventions significantly decreased hypertension as compared to no intervention (Achmon, Granek, Golomb, & Hart, 1989).

This integration of research and practice allows the practitioner to respond to clients and insurance companies who are seeking short-term, practical, cost-efficient, and expedient types of treatment. The incorporation of research instruments into clinical practice can also assist practitioners to improve their understanding of the client's diagnostic and treatment issues and enhance the quality of the therapeutic response to group interventions (Dies & Dies, 1993).

INTERVENTION

Groups established for the purpose of support and behavioral change will be discussed in this chapter. Establishing, conducting, terminating, and evaluating a group requires specific knowledge and skills. In this section, theories and concepts which provide the basis for these activities, along with strategies for operationalizing and evaluating them are discussed.

Techniques

It is difficult to describe a particular technique for the intervention group. Because the group leader sets the context of the group and facilitates the group process, group leadership skills are discussed first. Subsequently, the stages of group development are addressed and specific suggestions for evaluating the group process are given.

Group Leadership. The group leader's behavior and skills have a profound effect on the process of the group. According to Janosik (1982), the leader creates and maintains the group as a whole, while attending to the individual members' needs. Heiney and Wells (1989) identified three areas of focus for group leaders. First, the group leader structures the group. This includes identifying the objectives, selecting members, and establishing the parameters of the group sessions, as well as orienting the members to the group's purpose and goals, and summarizing the progress toward these goals. Table 26.1 presents guidelines for the planning process. Second, the group leader promotes the growth of the group by recognizing and monitoring the stages of group development. Third, the group leader identifies and manages group processes such as trust, power, conflict, scape-

TABLE 26.1   Guideline for Planning a Group as an Intervention

Rationale

What type of group is to be formed?

Whom is the group for?

Why is there a need for such a group?

Can the needs best be met via a group experience?

What are the basic assumptions underlying this experience?

What are your qualifications to lead the group?

Objectives

What are the general goals and purposes of the group?

Are specific outcomes measurable and attainable?

Practical Considerations

What recruitment, screening and selection procedures for membership will be used?

How many members will be in the group?

How often and for how long will the group meet?

Will new members be allowed to join the group once it has started?

How will the members be prepared for the group experience?

What ground rules will be established at the outset?

Procedures

What structure will the group have?

What techniques will be used?

What topics will be explored in the group?

Are these appropriate and realistic for the given population?

To what extent are the topics and structure determined by the group members and to what extent by the leader?

Evaluation

What evaluation procedures are planned? What follow-up procedures?

Are the measurement instruments valid and reliable?

Are the evaluation methods objective, practical, and relevant?

What do you expect to be the characteristics of the various stages of the group?

What might the problems be at each stage, and how will these be addressed?

Note. Adapted from *Groups: Process and Practice* (4th ed.), by M. S. Corey & G. Corey, 1992, Pacific Grove, CA: Brooks/Cole.

goating, resistance, decision making, and performance. The reader is referred to Corey and Corey (1992), Forsyth (1990), or Yalom (1995) for specific group leader functions at various stages of group development and for information on managing problem behaviors.

In some instances the use of a co-leadership model is preferable.

Having co-leaders allows one person to actively lead the group while the other attends to the group process. This model is also useful when a senior leader works with a novice leader who is learning group process and techniques. Co-leadership also provides for continuity if one person is unable to be present. Disadvantages of co-leadership include the possibility of competition and rivalry if group members become attached to one leader rather than the other. Therefore, considerable planning and debriefing at the conclusion of each session are needed if co-leadership is to be used successfully.

A final consideration with respect to group leadership relates to supervision/consultation. It is recommended that the group leader, particularly the novice, establish a relationship with an experienced person who can assist the group leader in processing the dynamics of the group, and provide constructive feedback regarding ways in which the group functioning and outcomes can be improved (Clark, 1994).

Process of Group Development. There are numerous theories concerning the number and type of stages of group development; and there is some debate whether stages actually typify group development (Forsyth, 1990). Nevertheless, most models include 5–6 basic stages of group development. The most noted group development model is Tuckman's 1965 5-stage model. (For a thorough description of this model, the reader is referred to Tuckman [1965] and Forsyth [1990].) We have included a pretreatment stage because the group leader is very involved in facilitating the group process before the group actually begins.

Pre-Treatment Stage. One goal of the pretreatment phase is the selection of group members. The importance of careful screening and selection for group membership cannot be overemphasized. Ideally, preliminary screening sessions can be held in which both the group leader and potential member can interview one another about the proposed group experience. The group leader can assess the degree to which the group would benefit the potential member, whether he/she understands the purpose of the group, and whether any contraindications for group participation exist. Audiotapes, videotapes, printed material, as well as interviews can facilitate the selection process and prepare potential members for the group experience, thereby improving member involvement in the group process (Dies & Dies, 1993).

Inclusion and exclusion criteria should be developed to guide the selection of group members. Utilizing research instruments that are brief, easily administered, and valid can assist the group leader to determine whether the potential member is appropriate for the group and can provide a measurement of individual change throughout the group experience. For example, Abraham, Neundorfer, and Currie (1992) studied the effects of cognitive-behavioral group therapy, focused visual imagery group therapy, and education-discussion groups on cognition, depression, hopelessness, and dissatisfaction with life in depressed nursing home residents. To be included in the groups, residents had to (a) score at least 11 on the Geriatric Depression Scale (Yesavage, Brink, Rose, & Lum, 1983), and (b) have significant hearing and vision, as well as verbal comprehension skills. Exclusion criteria were the presence of major cognitive impairment, use of antidepressant medications, and history of endogenous depression. Other instruments can be used to identify potential members' specific goals for therapy. Garfield (1986) reported that potential members who were able to articulate their problems and goals for group therapy are less likely to drop out of the group. Either an open-ended or a short answer questionnaire could be used to ask potential members about their purpose, goals, fears, and expectations.

Homogeneity or heterogeneity of membership is another factor to be considered in the selection of members. In most instances, for a specific population with given needs, a group comprising persons of that population would be more desirable than a heterogeneous group including persons with potentially unrelated needs. For example, Lovrin (1995) found that a group of children who had lost parents or siblings to AIDS were able to provide interpersonal support to one another because of the similarities in their intellectual, emotional, and social development. Beyers (1987/1988) noted that homogeneous groups develop cohesiveness more quickly, offer more immediate support to their members, and have better attendance.

The minimum and maximum numbers of members for a successful group has been debated (Sampson & Marthas, 1990), and depends upon several factors: age of the members, the experience of the leader, the type of group, and the problems to be explored (Corey & Corey, 1992). If the group size is too small, interaction and gain from others is lessened. On the other hand, a smaller group size is desirable with certain populations, for example, school-age children or cognitively impaired elderly. When the group becomes too large, subgroups tend to form, mitigating against the cohesiveness of the total group. Therapeutic exchange also is lessened in large groups as there is less time for each member to speak. In all, the group should have sufficient opportunity for interaction, be such that the group leader can maintain control, yet at the same time offer an experience in which a sense of the "group" exists. Declining attendance is not an unusual feature of the group intervention modality. For that reason, some group leaders may choose to start out with a slightly larger number of members. Group leaders may use contracts, postcard reminder mailings, and telephone calls to maintain the attendance of the group members.

The group leader must also decide whether membership will be open or closed. Open groups are marked by a changing membership. Closed groups are typically time limited and members are expected to attend until the group ends. Disadvantages of open groups include increased difficulty attaining cohesion because membership is in a constant flux, and an increased need to spend more time orienting new members to group ground rules and goals. Similarly, groups that have definite objectives to be accomplished in a predetermined time would find it difficult to function as an open group.

The number and frequency of sessions needed varies according to the purpose for which the group was established. Support groups offered to families of patients in intensive care units may be ongoing. Psychotherapy groups which offer the opportunity for more in-depth work and implementation of new behaviors over time often extend over months. Interpersonal learning education and psychoeducation groups typically run over 6–12 sessions with predetermined topics for each meeting. Although single group sessions are used infrequently, these do have value. For example, single sessions have been used successfully for preoperative teaching and discharge planning purposes. Length of time for group sessions is usually 1 to 2 hours, although they may run shorter for children or adults for whom attention spans are abbreviated or for whom restlessness is a problem. Beginning and ending each group session on time is critical. With most groups, it is recommended that a termination date be determined at the outset (Corey & Corey, 1992).

Forming Stage. Once the group leader has determined the group structure and selected the members, the place, and measurement tools, the group is ready to meet. Tuckman's (1965) model differentiates stages of group development based on the processes and tasks associated with each. The first stage, forming, is characterized by members feeling insecure and ambivalent about being in the group. Members question whether or not they want to be in or out of the group and how much they want to self-disclose. Orientation occurs during this stage as members exchange information and explore their commonalities. Interactions are tentative and polite. The general goals of the group leader during this stage of development are to teach the group members the basics of group membership, facilitate trust, and model therapeutic communication.

Storming Stage. As group members establish an initial level of trust and openness, resistance to disclosure develops and disagreement between members or with the group leader becomes more overt. Group members struggle with how close they want to get to others in the group and how much control they have in the group (Corey, 1995). Conflict is the central process in this stage, and is operationalized by criticism of others, poor attendance, and the development of subgroups. It is important to recognize that conflict in groups is inevitable, and should not be viewed as negative. Corey and Corey (1992) note that it is the avoidance of conflict that makes it destructive. They urge group leaders to avoid cutting off the expression of conflict, and facilitate a more direct expression of feelings and thoughts. Dies and Dies (1993) suggest that this is an opportune time to formally assess the members' concerns because it is at the storming stage that members tend to leave the group. They suggest using questionnaires that measure the group climate, cohesiveness, and individual willingness to disclose. These assessment measures could be administered between sessions and offer members an opportunity to express their concerns. The results from these measures could guide the group leader in structuring the group more effectively and might reduce the number of members that leave the group prematurely.

Norming Stage. As trust develops and conflicts are resolved, mutual caring and cohesion become evident. Roles and relationships are established, and a feeling of "we-ness" and camaraderie increases. When a cohesive group has developed, members feel free enough to express what they think and feel, they relate to others on a deeper level, and they are able and willing to do the work they originally came to accomplish. The group leader promotes cohesion by looking for and sharing commonalities among members, and positively reinforcing member behaviors that foster cohesion. Again, incorporating various research and/or assessment measures can contribute to the group's cohesiveness by focusing the discussion on cohesion among group members.

Performing Stage. Once cohesion exists, the group moves into the stage of performing, in which there is great emphasis on achieving goals. Members feel hopeful that they can change and are willing to work outside the group to make those changes. Member behaviors evident in this stage include decision making, group problem solving, and mutual cooperation. The group leader provides positive reinforcement for trying new behaviors and encourages members in their efforts. By sharing outcomes of the group process at this stage, the group leader can reinforce the progress of the group in working together (Dies & Dies, 1993). The group leader can also use research measures to assist the individual group members to chart their progress. Members can review the goals they identified in the pretreatment or forming stages and refocus their efforts in the performing stage.

Adjourning Stage. The final stage, adjourning, is characterized by a reduction in dependency, withdrawal, and regret (Forsyth, 1990; Tuckman, 1965). Because the termination period is vital to a successful group experience and may be difficult for some members, it is important that termination issues be brought up early in the group development. In this stage, members have the opportunity to pull together the information and insight gained, clarify the meaning of the group, and make plans for using the experience and learnings in their lives (Corey & Corey, 1992). Termination is a time for dealing with feelings of sadness and anxiety, giving and receiving feedback, and practicing new behaviors. Some groups may choose to combine the last session with a social activity such as a potluck meal. The focus of the group leader is on helping the members to separate from the group in a way that encourages them to function independently. It is important for the group leader to administer some type of group evaluation both the group process and individual changes. The group rating scales and scales for individual goals and target behaviors that were given during pretreatment or performing stages could be readministered. These instruments also assist the members to evaluate their progress and identify their future plans.

Beyers (1987/1988) emphasizes that group development stages are not discrete; overlap is common and recurs repeatedly throughout the life of the group. The group leader needs to be sensitive to where the members are in their development as group members. It is important to balance the freedom of group members to progress at their own pace, with the needs of the group as a whole to grow developmentally. Therefore, the leader should record anecdotal notes about the progress of the group and individuals in order to promote the group's development. The group leader can record these notes in the client/member record or chart.

Measurement of Outcomes

While theoretically and methodologically sound studies regarding the effectiveness of the group intervention do exist, anecdotal reports are more widespread and empirical evidence is scant and not developed systematically. Kahn and Kahn (1992) identified several problem areas with respect to group outcomes research, including lack of comparison groups, biased assignment to treatments, lack of standardized treatment techniques, and limitations of the outcome measurement indicators. Wilson (1992) suggests that for outcomes of group interventions to have meaning, groups must meet several standards: (a) the membership of the group must be well defined, (b) the group intervention must be clearly described so that it can be duplicated by others, (c) measurable outcome(s) of the group intervention must be identified, and (d) there must be meaningful comparison groups.

Nurses are beginning to systematically measure outcomes of group interventions. Nehls (1992) compared various therapist interventions which were related to successful group therapy. Abraham et al. (1992) compared the effects of three types of group interventions on cognition, depression, hopelessness, and life dissatisfaction among depressed nursing home residents. Heiney, Wells, and Gunn (1993) studied the effects of a support group on positive emotional changes of families grieving the death of a child with cancer. If groups, as an intervention, are to be used successfully across client populations and clinical settings, further clinical research is needed to validate the group's process and outcomes.

USES

Conditions/Populations

Nurses have incorporated many types of groups into their practice. For example, Burnside used reminiscence and life review groups with elderly residents of nursing homes (Burnside, 1986; Haight & Burnside, 1992). Kurek-Ovshinsky (1991) described the use of group therapy with patients on an acute inpatient psychiatric unit to repair self-esteem. Christman and Bingham (1989) discussed how nurse practitioners can influence their clients to stop smoking by developing group therapy programs for smoking cessation. Lovrin (1995) described a support group at a public school for 8-year-old girls who had lost a parent or sibling to AIDS.

As group interventions are refined, researchers and practitioners are working together to develop group treatment manuals for professionals that define specific approaches which are most likely to help clients improve their well-being. For example, Dr. Verona Gordon, a nurse, developed a structured manual for group therapy for women who are depressed (Gordon, Sumner, & McMichael, 1995). The University of California at Los Angeles (UCLA) social skills modules reliably teach social skills to schizophrenic patients in a reproducible method (Wallace, Liberman, MacKain, Blackwell, & Eckman, 1992). Table 26.2 presents a description of various types of groups and examples of specific populations/conditions for which nurses have used groups. Nurses will continue to use groups as an intervention, but in the future we will be required to standardize our group intervention and provide evidence of the effectiveness of this type of treatment.

Precautions

Although groups have been widely used, they should not be used with everyone. Loomis (1979) and Adrian (1980) stressed the importance of conducting an adequate assessment of the person before recommending that the person become a member of a group. Some persons need extensive one-to-one interaction before they can benefit from group interaction. Not only initial assessment, but also ongoing assessment is necessary to determine if the person is benefiting from participation in the group.

Loomis (1979) identified a number of disadvantages of groups. A group may be too large to achieve its stated purpose, causing members to become dissatisfied because they are unable to meet their goals for joining. Leading a group requires specific knowledge and skills. Too often groups are begun without the leader(s) having the requisite basic skills, particularly in resolving problems that may arise. Planning the environment and the number, length, and content of sessions is critical to the success of the group (Heiney & Wells, 1989).

FURTHER RESEARCH

Clinical research is needed to examine, specify, and expand the use of groups in nursing. Often such interventions as imagery, music, and dance are used within the context of a group; the interactive effects have not typically been examined. There are a number of areas in

TABLE 26.2 Types and Uses of Groups

Type of Group	Basic Goal	Uses	Examples
Group therapy	Improve psychological functioning and adjustment of individual members	Psychodynamic and cognitive-behavioral groups, interactional group therapy, behavior therapy	• Stroke (Adsit & Lee, 1986) • Siblings of oncology patients (Heiney, Goon-Johnson, Ettinger, R.S., & Ettinger, S., 1990) • Elderly nursing home patients (Williams-Barnard & Lindell, 1992) • Bipolar patients (Pollack, 1993) • Male incest offenders (Scheela & Stern, 1994)
Psychoeducational group	Help members gain self-understanding and im-prove their interpersonal skills	Skills-training seminars and workshops; medication groups	• Mothers of incest victims (DelPo & Koontz, 1991) • Head trauma (Dikengil, King & Monde, 1992) • Borderline personality (Nehls, 1992) • Women with AIDS/HIV (Haynes, 1993) • Anger management (Anderson-Mallico, 1994)
Self-help/Support group	Help members cope with or overcome specific problems or life crises	Alcoholics Anonymous, Weight Watchers, support groups for parents of terminally ill children	• Families of cancer patients (Whitman & Gustafson, 1989) • Depressed adolescents (Fine, Forth, Gilbert & Haley, 1991) • 8–year old girls (Lovrin, 1995)

Adapted from *Group Dynamics* (2nd ed., p. 462), by D. R. Forsyth, 1990, Pacific Grove, CA: Brooks/Cole.

which nursing research is needed to improve the use of groups as a practice intervention. The following projects are suggestions for research:

1. Define specific inclusion and exclusion criteria using standardized rating scales to select group members and monitor their progress.
2. Standardize the group intervention as treatment that can be used with various client populations.
3. Develop specific outcomes (e.g., patient, family, cost) for various types of groups and the instruments that measure those outcome.
4. Determine the cost/benefit ratio of groups as an intervention to reduce hospitalization and/or return to higher levels of nursing care.
5. Compare group treatment to other nursing interventions (e.g., supportive therapy, medication, home visits) in reducing morbidity and improving quality of life for our clients.

REFERENCES

Abraham, I. L., Neundorfer, M. M., & Currie, L. J. (1992). Effects of group interventions on cognition and depression in nursing home residents. *Nursing Research, 41,* 196–202.

Achmon, J., Granek, M., Golomb, M., & Hart, J. (1989). Behavioral treatment of essential hypertension: A comparison between cognitive therapy and biofeedback of heart rate. *Psychosomatic Medicine, 51*(2), 152–164.

Adrian, S. (1980). A systematic approach to selecting group participants. *Journal of Psychosocial Nursing, 18*(2), 37–41.

Adsit, P. A., & Lee, J. (1986). The use of art in stroke group therapy. *Rehabilitation Nursing, 11*(6), 18–19.

Anderson-Mallico, R. (1994). Anger management using cognitive group therapy. *Perspectives in Psychiatric Care, 30*(3), 17–20.

Beyers, B. (1987/1988). Dealing with divorce: A group therapy intervention for women. *Perspectives in Psychiatric Care, 3/4,* 91–100.

Buccheri, R., Trygstad, L., Kanas, N., Waldron, B., & Dowling, G. (1996). Auditory hallucinations in schizophrenia: Group experience in examining symptom management and behavioral strategies. *Journal of Psychosocial Nursing & Mental Health, 34*(2), 12–26, 44–45.

Burnside, I. (1986). *Working with the elderly: Group process and techniques* (2nd ed.). Boston: Jones and Bartlett.

Christman, C., & Bingham, M. (1989). The nurse practitioners' role in smoking cessation. *Journal of American Academy of Nurse Practitioners, 1*(2), 49–54.

Clark, C. C. (1989). *Nurse as group leader* (3rd ed.). New York: Springer.

Corey, M. S., & Corey, G. (1992). *Groups: Process and practice* (4th ed.). Pacific Grove, CA: Brooks/Cole.

Corey, G. (1995). *Theory and practice of group counseling* (4th ed.). Pacific Grove, CA: Brooks/Cole.

DelPo, E. G., & Koontz, M. A. (1991). Group therapy with mothers of incest victims: Structure, leader attributes, and countertransference. Part I. *Archives of Psychiatric Nursing, 5*(2), 64–69.

Dies, R. R., & Dies, K. R. (1993). The role of evaluation in clinical practice: Overview and group treatment illustration. *International Journal of Group Psychotherapy, 43*(1), 77–105.

Dikengil, A., King, C., & Monda, D. (1992). Communication functional skills group: An integrated group therapy approach to head injury rehabilitation. *Journal of Cognitive Rehabilitation, 10*(4), 28–31.

Evans, R. L., & Connis, R. T. (1995). Comparison of brief group therapies of depressed cancer patients receiving radiation treatment. *Public Health Reports, 110*(3), 306–311.

Fine, S., Forth, A., Gilbert, M., & Haley, G. (1991). Group therapy for adolescent depressive disorder: A comparison of social skills and therapeutic support. *Journal of the American Academy of Child & Adolescent Psychiatry, 30*(1), 79–85.

Forsyth, D. R. (1990). *Group dynamics* (2nd ed.). Pacific Grove, CA: Brooks/Cole.

Garfield, S. L. (1986). Research on client variables in psychotherapy. In S. L. Garfield & A. E. Bergin (Eds.), *Handbook of psychology and behavior change* (3rd ed., pp. 213–256). New York: Wiley.

Gordon, V., Sumner, J., & McMichael, C. (1995, February). Intervention for depression: Behavioral restructuring model that works. *Employee Assistance*, pp. 6–9, 30.

Haight, B. K., & Burnside, I. (1992). Reminiscence and life review: Conducting the process. *Journal of Gerontological Nursing, 18*(2), 39–42.

Haynes, Y. L. (1993). A women's issue: HIV/AIDS. *Perspectives in Psychiatric Care, 29*(1), 23–25.

Heiney, S. P., Goon-Johnson, K., Ettinger, R. S., & Ettinger, S. (1990). The effects of group therapy on siblings of pediatric oncology patients. *Journal of Pediatric Oncology Nursing, 7*(3), 95–100.

Heiney, S. P., & Wells, L. M. (1989). Strategies for organizing and maintaining support groups. *Oncology Nursing Forum, 16,* 803–809.

Heiney, S. P., Wells, L.M., & Gunn, J. (1993). The effects of group therapy on bereaved extended family of children with cancer. *Journal of Pediatric Oncology Nursing, 10*(3), 99–104.

Janosik, E. (1982). Aspects of group development. In E. Janosik & L. Phipps (Eds.), *Life cycle group work in nursing.* Monterey, CA: Wadsworth.

Kahn, E. M., & Kahn, E. W. (1992). Group treatment assignment for outpatients with schizophrenia: Integrating recent clinical and research findings. *Community Mental Health Journal, 28,* 539–550.

Kurek-Ovshinsky, C. (1991). Group psychotherapy in an acute inpatient setting: Techniques that nourish the self esteem. *Issues in Mental Health Nursing, 12*(1), 81–88.

Loomis, M. (1979). *Group process for nurses.* St. Louis: Mosby.

Lovrin, M. (1995). Interpersonal support among 8-year-old girls who have lost their parents or siblings to AIDS. *Archives in Psychiatric Nursing, 1*(2), 92–98.

Nehls, N. (1992). Group therapy for people with borderline personality disorder: Interventions associated with positive outcomes. *Issues in Mental Health Nursing, 13,* 255–269.

Pollack, L. E. (1993). Do inpatients with bipolar disorder evaluate diagnostically homogeneous groups? *Journal of Psychosocial Nursing, 31*(10), 26–31.

Sampson, E., & Marthas, M. (1990). *Group process for the health professions* (3rd ed.). Albany, NY: Delmar.

Scheela, R. A. & Stern, P. N. (1994). Falling apart: A process integral to the remodeling of male incest offenders. *Archives of Psychiatric Nursing, 8*(2), 91–100.

Tuckman, B. W. (1965). Developmental sequence in small groups. *Psychological Bulletin, 63,* 384–399.

Wallace, C. J., Liberman, R. P., MacKain, S. J., Blackwell, G., & Eckman, T. A. (1992). Effectiveness and replicability of modules for teaching social and instrumental skills to the severely mentally ill. *American Journal of Psychiatry, 149,* 654–658.

Weiner, M. F. (1992). Group therapy reduces medical and psychiatric hospitalization. *International Journal of Group Psychotherapy, 42*(2), 267–275.

Whitman, H. H., & Gustafson, J. P. (1989). Group therapy for families facing a cancer crisis. *Oncology Nursing Forum, 16,* 539–543.

Williams-Barnard, C. L., & Lindell, A. R. (1992). Therapeutic use of "prizing" and its effect on self-concept of elderly clients in nursing homes and group homes. *Issues in Mental Health Nursing, 13,* 1–17.

Wilson, W. H. (1992). Response to Kahn and Kahn: Group treatment assignment for outpatients with schizophrenia. *Community Mental Health Journal, 28,* 551–560.

Yalom, I. (1995). *The theory and practice of group psychotherapy* (4th ed.). New York: Basic Books.

Yesavage, J., Brink, T., Rose, T., & Lum, O. (1983). Development and validation of a geriatric depression rating scale: A preliminary report. *Journal of Psychiatric Research, 17,* 37–49.

27

Family Support

Michaelene P. Mirr

Inclusion of families in nursing care has occurred since the beginning of the nursing profession. However, this focus has had varying priorities within the profession over the centuries. During the past two decades, nursing has experienced a resurgence of the family as a priority in nursing care. Many professional organizations have developed standards of care that include the care of families. Previously, the emphasis on family nursing has been primarily within community health nursing, midwifery, and psychiatric nursing. The focus of care in acute care settings has traditionally been on individuals. Nurses are often self-conscious and feel uncomfortable in the presence of family members (Hopkins, 1994).

It is now time for all areas of nursing to recognize the importance of families in the care of the patient. What affects the patient affects the family; what affects the family has an impact on the patient (Bahnson, 1987; Engli & Kirsivali-Farmer, 1993; Leavitt, 1989). The patient does not live in isolation but exists in a system in which there are constant interactions of the patient, family, and environment (Wright & Leahey, 1994). Support of the family as a nursing intervention is one mechanism that can bridge the gap between nursing care of the patient and the family. This chapter will define family support within the context of nursing and demonstrate how family support can be incorporated into daily nursing care resulting in positive outcomes for patient, family, and nurse.

DEFINITION

A single definition of family support is not universally accepted. A fairly new concept within nursing, family support has been defined as assistance provided by nurses to patients and families. Family support is a family intervention that assists the family in realistically assessing the impact of the event on the patient and family (Rosenthal & Young, 1988). Family support, as a nurisng intervention, focuses on family members in relation to their effect on the patient. Although family support can mean support within the family unit, the emphasis of this nursing intervention focuses on how nurses can support families rather than how to use families to support patients. Family support includes the intervention of presence as an underlying component. Family support includes the family as a unit of care, but it is more episodic and informal in structure.

The term *family* also has a variety of definitions. Family is usually defined as the individual's closest biological relations or spouse. However, broader interpretations include whomever the individual is closest to or defines as his or her family (Buchanan & Brock, 1986). The extended family is also affected by situational or health crises and need to be considered in the plan of family support.

Family support should not be confused with family therapy. Family therapy is a formal therapeutic approach involving treatment of the entire family unit for problems that are disruptive to family functioning. Family therapy is an ongoing process with a qualified and licensed therapist. Family therapists require special skills such as interviewing families in conflict, assisting in resolving the conflict, supporting one family member against another, and facilitating change when resistance is strong (Gillis, Roberts, Highley, & Martinson, 1989).

Family support also differs from family protectiveness. Although Tapp (1993) defines family protectiveness as a defensive response on the part of the family as a safeguard against injury and loss, nurses can also "protect" a family rather than support the family. Family protectiveness implies that the family receives preferential treatment and the nurse or other individuals take over family responsibilities or decisions.

SCIENTIFIC BASIS

A review of nursing literature indicates an increasing number of manuscripts describing concerns and needs of families during periods of stress, crisis, developmental changes, chronic illness and hospitalizations (Campbell & Linc, 1996; Everitt, 1995; Frazier, Davis-Ali, & Dahl, 1995; Laizner, Yost, Barg, & McCorkle, 1993; Lopez-Fagin, 1995;

Mangini, Confessore, Girard, & Spadola, 1995; Mausner, 1995, Petr, Murdock, & Chapin, 1995; Watkins et al., 1996). The recognition of concern and care for families is more apparent, although research demonstrating the effect of nursing interventions, such as family support, remains minimal. The majority of research on family support is at an exploratory or descriptive level.

A large number of studies have been conducted examining various aspects of family coping and needs in an effort to identify nursing interventions that would benefit families during their time of need (Engli & Kirsivali-Farmer, 1993; Foss & Tenltolder, 1993; Gaws-Ens, 1994; Henneman & Cardin, 1992; Hickey & Rykerson, 1992; Jacono, Hicks, Antonioni, O'Brien, & Rasi, 1990; Kleiber et al., 1994; Koller, 1991; Leske, 1991, 1992; Lewandowski, 1992; Lynn-McHale & Bellinger, 1988, Miracle & Hovekamp, 1994; Simpson, 1989; Titler & Walsh, 1992). These studies have indicated that families need to have hope, close proximity to the patient, frequent and consistent information, assurance, and comfort. The ability to support the patient is increased by meeting family needs, thus improving patient outcomes (Boykoff, 1986; Brooten & Naylor, 1995; Gurley, 1995; Lynn-McHale & Bellinger, 1988; Mirr, 1991a, 1991b; Moser, 1994; Reider, 1994; Simpson, 1991; Stanik, 1990; Wright & Leahey, 1994).

One of the themes identified in the needs assessment studies is the necessity for family support during periods of stress, such as hospitalization or critical injury (Richmond & Craig, 1986). Because families are dealing with the stress of injury or illness, family support is often the only form of assistance people use during a time of high stress or crisis (Halm, 1990). The development of flexible visiting hours and family-centered critical care units are some examples of adapting the environment to provide family support.

Assessment of the need for family support during acute hospitalization or following a situational crisis is simple, because families are visibly distressed. However, one must keep in mind that family support is also needed during chronic illness, such as chronic mental illness or during developmental changes (Woods, Yates, & Primono 1989). Often, acute situational crises extend to become long-term situations; examples are recovery from traumatic brain injury or acute myocardial infarction. Transition between hospital and home or between hospital units may increase stress on family members (Bull & Maruyama, 1995).

Family support is more instrumental in chronic illness because families deal with stressors that are continuously present. The trend to discharge patients early leads to larger care responsibilities for family members. The nature of support needed is correlated with the demands of the illness or situation (Woods, Yates, & Primono, 1989). In this respect, family support by professional nurses can take on various dimensions, particularly if nurses care for families over a period of time. For example, during a period of high stress or crisis, emotional support may be needed by family members. As time progresses, emotional support may be replaced by cognitive support in the form of information or resource sharing. Depending on the situation, cognitive support may periodically change to material support as the nurse assists the family in finding appropriate resources. In time, organized family support groups may meet some of the needs previously provided by professional nurses.

INTERVENTION

In caring for patients in a holistic manner, family support becomes inherent in the care of the patient. Each patient is entitled to support being provided to his/her family because every patient originates from some type of family unit. Various techniqes or methods can be used in providing family support. Careful assessment of the family is needed to determine which technique best fits the particular family and situation. Consideration of cultural and ethnic influences are inherent in assessing family support (Meyers, 1992; Young, 1995). The techniques listed in Table 27.1 can be used in providing family support. The techniques listed are not meant to be exhaustive. Each of these techniques can be adapted for individual families. For example, in providing information to families (techniques 3, 4, 5), one nurse should be identified as the primary information provider to a particular family. Information needs to be offered frequently and presented in clear, understandable terms. Technical terms, such as the names of surgical or diagnostic procedures, need to be defined clearly and written down for families to refer to later. Nurses may struggle to determine what information family members need. Asking families if they have any questions is not adequate because families are often unaware of what information is needed. Offering information such as what the patient did during the day or night provides the background for families to begin asking questions. Families of patients in long-term care or home care also need to be contacted regularly even if the patient's status does not change significantly.

Families frequently use a literal interpretation of information. They

TABLE 27.1 Techniques for Family Support

1. Initiate contact with the family and introduce self. Inquire as to how the family members wish to be addressed and document this. Subsequent contacts should be frequent and build upon previous interactions.
2. Assess family functioning using established assessment tools.
3. Listen for and acknowledge fears or concerns that family members may have. Encourage family members to participate in resolving these concerns.
4. Provide unsolicited information on the patient's condition; do this in understandable terms. Repeat information as often as needed.
5. Verify to see if family members understand the information.
6. Offer information regarding patient's response during each family visit or contact.
7. Provide a comfortable environment for families of hospitalized patients when they are not in the patient's room. If the patient is critically ill, comfortable furniture in a quiet environment can provide periods of rest while still allowing the family to be close to the the ill family member.
8. Modify hospital or agency routines to provide normal routines for families as much as possible, e.g. visiting hours, sleeping facilities, or telephone hotline.
9. Initiate referrals for crisis intervention, family therapy, or other specialized family treatment when needed.
10. Work closely with the case manager or discharge personnel to provide for smooth transition to home or alternative placement.
11. Provide suggestions to family friends regarding ways to assist the family (e.g., provide a complete meal, mow lawn, care for siblings, etc.).
12. Facilitate family contact with families who have been in similar circumstances; this may give additional support.
13. Provide information on appropriate family support groups if they are available.
14. Provide information on computer networks that are available for electronic discussions or information.
15. Assess need for and provide relief/respite care for caregivers.

may define time in terms of hours and minutes, whereas health professionals use the term *time* more loosely. For example, one day may mean approximately 24 hours to a nurse whereas the family may understand it as exactly 24 hours. Families often set hopes based on literal interpretation of information. Therefore, in providing information nurses need to use caution in their choice of terms. A useful strategy for nurses may be to have a nurse listen to what another nurse is saying to a family and then give feedback about how remarks could be interpreted. Validation of the family's comprehension of information should be frequent, because families try to incorporate medical terminology in their discussions, yet often use these terms incorrectly.

Measurement of Effectiveness

A review of nursing literature does not reveal any research on outcome data or criteria that quantitatively measure the effectiveness of family support. Assessments of effectiveness can be validated with families via self-report and documentation (Sabo et al., 1989). Documentation of outcomes is extremely important in evaluating the effectiveness of the nursing intervention. Ongoing family assessment and validation will verify if information is comprehended. Several questions can assess the effectiveness of family support. For example, do family members seek out the nurses or address them by name? Do family members express their fears and concerns? Are family interactions with patients appropriate and nonstrained? Do families seek out nurses for support? Do verbal and nonverbal messages indicate successful intervention? These examples provide a basis for evaluating family support. Other questions can also be used to assess the effect of family support on the family. Until a valid and reliable tool is available to measure family support, the nurse must assume the responsibility for assessing and documenting outcomes.

Family support can also be measured in terms of the patient's physiological response to their presence and actions. Family support may decrease anxiety and help families be more relaxed in interactions. Several studies have shown positive physiological responses to family visitation and interactions (Giuliano & Giuliano, 1992; Hendrickson, 1987; Johnson, Omery, & Nikas, 1989; Kleman et al., 1993; Prins, 1989; Simpson, 1991; Simpson & Shaver, 1990).

USES

Family support can be used in a variety of settings and in a variety of ways. To provide family support, nurses need to shift from a patient-centered focus to a collaborative model that places families as central in the care of the patient (Ahmann, 1994). Family support can be instrumental in situational crises such as acute or critical illness, developmental life changes, chronic illness, long-term care, bereavement, and times of stress (Stewart, 1995). Although stress can never be totally eliminated, it is hypothesized that family support can be instrumental in reducing the amount of stress experienced by families. Families are traditionally shy in approaching care providers. Initiation of family support can open the door to meaningul family/nurse relationships. Use of family support in situational crises, developmental life changes, chronic illness and stressful periods will be discussed separately.

Populations/Conditions

Situational Crisis. Family support is an important intervention, particularly during situational crises. During times of acute or critical illness, families often feel alone in an unfamiliar environment. Feelings of warmth and of families may make an unpleasant experience less traumatic. Family emotions often resemble a rollercoaster and can benefit from external support. A personal routine that closely resembles the family's daily schedule can disrupt family life less than insistence on conforming to hospital or agency routines. Frequent informational sessions also decrease anxiety regarding the patient's condition, even if there is no significant change. This is particularly true regarding a patient undergoing surgery. Stanik (1990) found that interoperative reports are appreciated by families and decrease the intensity of feelings during the waiting period.

Developmental Life Changes. Developmental life changes provide an opportunity for family support. The birth of a child or adjustment to retirement can have an impact on families. Assistance in coping and adjusting to these changes as a family can lessen any traumatic transition that may occur. Educational opportunities as well as continued offerings of assistance can be supportive to families. Postdischarge contact or follow-up have also been found to be helpful.

Chronic Illness. Managing illnesses, particularly chronic or terminal illnesses, at home in preference to in hospitals is becoming more common. Caregiver stress associated with high acuity illness or chronic illness in the home is natural. The presence of long-term stress associated with care for persons with chronic illness is an opportunity for the intervention of family support. Family relations and interactions can become strained in the daily care and routine of caring for a chronically ill family member. The type and level of family support will change over time, necessitating frequent assessment of family needs. Some families have unique needs and require ongoing assessemnt and revision of intervention strategies. Community or church programs, such as relief or respite care, have been helpful for reducing the burden of caregiving (Mausner, 1995).

Stressful Periods.   Family support can be beneficial in times of stress. Stress can occur with the hospitalization of a family member, at the diagnosis of a chronic or terminal illness, or during periods of personal adjustment. Fear of death, uncertain outcomes, financial concerns, role changes and unfamiliar surroundings all increase family members' stress level (Leske, 1991; Titler et al., 1991). Recognition of a family's need for support by professional nurses can be instrumental in relieving or resolving family stress before it reaches a crisis level. Meeting family members' basic needs—comfort, sleep, hope, and food—are important support at this time.

Precautions

Nurses must be conscious of the fine line that may exist between family support and family therapy. Families who need long-term therapy or crisis intervention should be referred to appropriate sources. Good family assessment skills are useful in differentiating between the two needs.

Awareness of dependency needs is also necessary. The professional nurse must recognize the point in time when family support is no longer needed and when the family's own support systems and resources can take over. Periodic assessement of family functioning is desirable in order to determine if continued family support by the nurse is needed. Respect for the wishes of families who do not want family support must be acknowledged.

RESEARCH QUESTIONS

Family support, as an independent nursing intervention, is a comparitively new phenomenon within nursing. Efforts to resolve the following questions will provide a solid research base for use of family support as a nursing intervention:

1. What methods of family support are most effective? Which techniques are most helpful for families with specific problems or concerns?

2. When is family support most beneficial to families? How does the timing of support facilitate the achievement of positive outcomes?
3. What method or tool is most effective for evaluating family support? Evaluation tools are not currently available to effectively evaluate family support as an intervention. Development of a specific instrument to measure support to families remains a priority.
4. What models for family support are most effective? The method or framework in which the family support is provided may influence the effectiveness of the intervention.

REFERENCES

Ahmann, E. (1994). Family-centered care: Shifting orientation. *Pediatric Nursing, 20*(2), 113–117, 132–133.

Bahnson, C. (1987). The impact of life-threatening illness on the family and the impact of family on the illness: An overview. In M. Leahey and L. Wright (Eds.), *Families and life-threatening illness* (pp. 26–44). Springhouse, PA: Springhouse.

Boykoff, S. L. (1986). Visiting needs reported by patients with cardiac disease and their families. *Heart and Lung, 15,* 573–576.

Brooten, D., & Naylor, M. (1995). Nurses' effect on changing patient outcomes. *Image: Journal of Nursing Scholarship, 27*(2), 95–99.

Buchanan, A., & Brock, D. W. (1986). Deciding for others. *The Milbank Quarterly, 64*(Suppl. 2), 17–94.

Bull, M. J., Maruyama, G., & Luo, D. (1995). Testing a model for posthospital transition of family caregivers for elderly persons. *Nursing Research, 44*(3), 132–138.

Campbell, J. M., & Linc, L. G. (1996). Support groups for visitors of residents in nursing homes. *Journal of Gerontological Nursing, 22*(2), 30–35.

Engli, M., & Kirsivali-Farmer, K. (1993). Needs of family members of critically ill patients with and without acute brain injury. *Journal of Neuroscience Nurisng, 25*(2), 78–85.

Everitt, J. (1995). Schizophrenia and family support: Interventions to reduce relapse rate. *Mental Health Nursing, 15*(5), 12–15.

Foss, K., & Tenltolder, M. (1993). Expectations and needs of persons with family members in an intensive care unit as opposed to a general wards. *Southern Medical Journal, 86,* 380–384.

Frazier, P. A., Davis-Ali, S. H., & Dahl, K. E. (1995). Stressors, social support and adjustment in kidney transplant patients and their spouses. *Social Work in Health Care, 21*(2), 93–108.

Gaw-Ens, B. (1994). Informational support for families immediately after CABG surgery. *Critical Care Nurse, 14*(1), 41–42, 47–50.

Gillis, C. L., Roberts, B. M., Highley, B. L., & Martinson, I. M. (1989). What is family nusing. In C. L. Gillis, B. L. Highley, B. M. Roberts, & I. M. Martinson (Eds.), *Toward a science of family nursing* (pp. 64–73). Menlo Park, CA: Addison-Wesley.

Giuliano, K., & Giuliano, M. (1992). Cardiovascular responses to family visitation and nurse-physician rounds. *Heart & Lung, 21,* 290.

Gurley, M. (1995). Determining ICU visiting hours. *MEDSURG Nursing, 4,* 40–43.

Halm, M. A. (1990). Effects of support groups on anxiety of family members during critical illness. *Heart and Lung, 19,* 62–71.

Hendrickson, S. L. (1987). Intracranial pressure changes and family needs. *Journal of Neuroscience Nursing, 19,* 14–17.

Hennemann, E., & Cardin, S. (1992). Need for information. *Critical Care Nursing Clinics of North America, 4,* 615–621.

Hickey, P., & Rykerson, S. (1992). Caring for parents of critically ill infants and children. *Critical Care Nursing Clinics of North America, 4,* 565–571.

Hopkins, A., (1994). The trauma nurse role with families in crisis. *Critical Care Nurse, 14,* 35–43.

Jacono, J., Hicks, G., Antonionio, C., O'Brien, K., & Rasi, M. (1990). Comparison of perceived needs of family members between registered nurses and family members of critically ill patients in intensive care and neonatal intensive care units. *Heart and Lung, 19,* 72–78.

Johnson, S., Omery, A., & Nikas, D. (1989). Effects of conversation on intracranial pressure in comatose patients. *Heart and Lung, 19,* 56–63.

Kleiber, C., Halm, M., Titler, M., Montgomery, L., Johnson, S., Nicholson, A., Craft, M., Buckwalter, K., & Megivern, K. (1994). Emotional responses of family members during a critical hospitalization. *American Journal of Critical Care, 3*(1), 70–76.

Kleman, M., Bickert, A., Karpinski, A., Wantz, D., Jacobsen, B., Lowery, B., & Menapace, F. (1993). Physiologic responses of coronary care patients to visiting. *Journal of Cardiovascular Nursing, 7*(3), 52–62.

Koller, P. (1991). Family needs and coping strategies during illness crisis. *American Association of Critical Care Nurses: Clinical Issues in Critical Care Nursing, 2*(2), 338–345.

Laizner, A.M., Yost, L.M.S., Barg, F.K., & McCorkle, R. (1993). Needs of family caregivers of persons with cancer: a review. *Seminars in Oncology Nursing, 9*(2), 114–120.

Leavitt, M. (1989). Transitions to illness: The family in the hospital. In C. Gillis, B. Highley, B. Roberts, & I. Martinsen (Eds.), *Toward a science of family nursing* (pp. 262–283). Menlo Park, CA: Addison-Wesley.

Leske, J. (1991). Overveiw of family needs after a critical illness: From assessment to intervention. *AACN: Clinical Issues in Critical Care Nursing, 2*(2), 220–226.

Leske, J. (1992). Comparison ratings of need importance after critical illness from family members with varied demographic characteristics. *Critical Care Nursing Clinics of North America, 4,* 607–613.

Lewandowski, L. (1992). Needs of children during the critical illness of a parent or sibling. *Critical Care Nurisng Clinics of North America, 4,* 573–585.

Lopez-Fagin, L. (1995). Critical care family needs inventory: a cognitive research utilization approach. *Critical Care Nurse, 15*(4), 21, 23–26.

Lynn-McHale, D., & Bellinger, A. (1988). Need satisfaction levels of family members of critical care patients and accuracy of nurses' perception. *Heart & Lung, 17,* 117–453.

Mangini, L., Confessore, M.T., Girard, P., & Spadola, T. (1995). Pediatric trauma support program: supporting children and families in emotional crises. *Critical Care Nursing Clinics of North America, 7,* 557–567.

Mausner, S. (1995). Families helping families: an innovative approach to the provision of respite care for families of children with complex medical needs. *Social Work in Health Care, 21*(1), 95–106.

Meyers, C. (1992). Hmong children and their families: consideration of cultural influences in assessment. *American Journal of Occupational Therapy, 46,* 737–744.

Miracle, V., & Hovekamp, G. (1994). Needs of families and patients undergoing invasive cardiac procedures. *American Journal of Critical Care, 3*(2), 155–157.

Mirr, M. P. (1991a). Decisions made by family members of patients with severe head injury. *AACN Clinical Issues in Critical Care Nursing, 2*(2), 242–251.

Mirr, M. P. (1991b). Factors affecting decisions made by family members of patients with severe head injury. *Heart & Lung, 20,* 228–235.

Moser, D. (1994). Social support and cardiac recovery. *Journal of Cardiovascular Nursing, 9*(1), 27–39.

Petr, C. G., Murdock, B., & Chapin, R. (1995). Home care for children dependent on medical technology: The family perspective. *Social Work in Health Care, 21*(1), 5–22.

Prins, M. (1989). The effect of family visits on intracranial pressure. *Western Journal of Nursing Research, 11,* 281–297.

Reider, J. A. (1994). Anxiety during critical illness of a family member. *Dimensions of Critical Care Nurisng, 13*(5), 272–279.

Richmond, T. S., & Craig, M. (!986). Family-centered care for the neurotrauma patient. *Nurisng Clinics of North America, 21,* 641–651.

Rosenthal, M., & Young, T. (1988). Effective family intervention after traumatic brain injury: Theory and practice. *Head Trauma Rehabilitation, 3*(4), 42–50.

Sabo, K. A., Draay, C., Rudy, E., Abraham, T., Bender, M., Lewandowski, W., Lombardo, B., Turk, M., & Dawson, D. (1989). ICU family support sessions: Family members perceived benefits. *Applied Nursing Research, 2*(2), 82–89.

Simpson, T. (1989). Needs and concerns of families of critically ill patients. *Focus on Critical Care, 16*, 388–397.

Simpson, T. (1991). The family as a source of support for the critically ill adult. *AACN: Clinical Issues in Critical Care Nursing, 2*(2), 229–235.

Simpson, T., & Shaver, J. (1990). Cardiovascular responses to family visits in coronary care unit patients. *Heart & Lung, 19*, 344–351.

Smith, L., Kupferschmid, B., Dawson, C., & Briones, T. (1991). A family-centered critical care unit. *AACN: Clinical Issues in Critical Care Nursing, 2*(2), 258–268.

Stanik, J. (1990). Caring for the family of the critically ill surgical patient. *Critical Care Nurse, 10*(1), 43–46.

Stewart, E. S. (1995). Family matters. Family-centered care for the bereaved. *Pediatric Nursing, 21*(2), 181–184.

Titler, M., Cohen, M., & Craft, M. (1991) Impact of adult critical care hospitalization: Perceptions of patients, spouses, and nurses. *Heart & Lung, 20*, 623–632.

Titler, M., & Walsh, S. (1992). Visiting critically ill adults. *Critical Care Nursing Clinics of North America, 4*, 623–632.

Tapp, D.M. (1993). Family protectiveness: A response to ischemic heart disease. *Canadian Journal of Cardiovascular Nursing, 4*(2), 4–8.

Watkins, P. N., Cook, E. L., May, S. R., Still, J. M, Luterman, A., & Purvis, R. J. (1996). Postburn psychologic adaptation of family members of patients with burns. *Journal of Burn Care and Rehabilitation, 17*(1), 78–92.

Woods, N. F., Yates, B. C., & Primono, J. (1989). Supporting families during chronic illness. *Image: Journal of Nursing Scholarship, 21*(1), 47–50.

Wright, L., & Leahey, M. (1994). *Nursing and families: A guide to family assessment and intervention.*. Philadelphia: Davis.

Young, J. B. (1995). Black families with a chronically disabled family member: A framework for study. *Association of Black Nursing Faculty Journal, 6*(3), 68–73.

28

Advocacy

Margot L. Nelson

The nurse's role as advocate for the recipient of nursing care and the incorporation of advocacy into practice are integral to professional nursing. Although definitions have changed with the evolving discipline of nursing and debate continues about the congruence of various models with current nursing theory and practice, there are key concepts which have emerged to define the essence of advocacy in nursing.

DEFINITIONS

A central characteristic of advocacy in nursing is that it is a "way of being in relationship with a patient/client in a way which respects and promotes the uniqueness of the individual as a total human being in the context of his/her health experience" (Nelson, 1992, p. 263). (The terms *client, patient,* and *consumer* are used interchangeably throughout this chapter to refer to an individual or group recipient of health care in general or nursing care in particular.) Advocacy is a relational characteristic of the nurse, not just what he or she does. Watson (1989) refers to advocacy as an outgrowth of caring, that foundational aspect of nursing in which an authentic and intimate connection occurs between nurse and patient, enabling the patient to find his or her "own voice during life's most vulnerable moments" (p. 53).

Advocacy is viewed by some nurse authors (Curtin, 1979; Gadow, 1990) as an essential component of the philosophical basis for nursing. Curtin describes advocacy as integral to the nurse-patient relationship, one with its roots in a shared humanity and shared human rights (freedom, respect, and integrity). In an advocacy role, the nurse assists individuals to find meaning in their living or dying; and Curtin (1979) emphasizes that it is the patient's experience, meaning and values—not the experience, meaning, and values of the nurse or anyone else. Gadow identifies this philosophy as existential advocacy, whereby patients are enabled to determine the unique personal meaning of their health experiences and exercise self-determination in that context. Authentically exercising freedom of self-determination, according to Gadow, means reaching decisions that are truly one's own and reflect what one values and believes important about oneself and the world.

Kavanagh (1994) suggests an additional dimension for advocacy, cultural congruence. If a nurse engages in culturally congruent advocacy, she or he enables the patient to maintain the integrity of his or her own perspectives and ways of being. This involves a conscious effort not to impose the values of the dominant culture on clients from other cultures.

EVOLUTION OF THE ADVOCACY ROLE IN NURSING

In order to understand more fully the concept of advocacy and evaluate its current relevance for nursing, one should grasp the pattern of its historical development. In keeping with the evolution of professional nursing, advocacy has progressed from interceding for a client to acting as guardian of client rights to promoting autonomy and free choice for all health consumers (Nelson, 1988). Advocacy will continue to evolve along with the shift in health care toward a paradigm of health rather than illness, increasingly community-based care models, and further development of advanced practice roles in nursing.

Acting For or on Behalf of Another

Florence Nightingale, although she did not use the term *advocacy*, clearly implied the notion of the nurse as an actor for or an intercessor on behalf of the patient. In 1859, she defined the role of nursing as manipulating environmental factors "to put the patient in the best condition for nature to act upon him" (Nightingale, 1859/1969).

Nightingale's actions to reform care of the sick during and following the Crimean War, as well as the actions of nurse leaders such as Lillian Wald and Lavinia Dock, clearly reflected advocacy for recipients of health care on a community scale.

As the value placed upon individualism increased, objections were raised to this notion of advocacy. It clearly implied, according to Leddy and Pepper (1984), an active position for the advocate and a passive role for the client.

Advocacy for the client continued to evolve, despite strong counterthemes of loyalty and obedience in nursing. Winslow (1984) describes nursing education in the early 20th century as embedded in a military analogy for medicine and health care. The mandate for students of nursing in this framework was unquestioning respect for authority, and nurses were clearly positioned at the lower end of the health care provider hierarchy. The expectation of unquestioning obedience is reflected in Perry's (1906) declaration that a nurse must be trained to absolute accuracy and skill and "obliteration of self" (p. 451).

As early as 1910, there were questions, however timid, of the loyalty and obedience injunctions: "Is a nurse required to be untruthful or practice deceit to uphold the reputation of the physician at her own expense or that of the patient?" ("Where Does Loyalty End?", 1910, p. 230). A further challenge to loyalty as the underpinning for professional nursing was apparent in the first version of the American Nurses' Association "Suggested Code of Ethics for Nurses" (1926, p. 601): "Loyalty to the motive inspiring nursing should make the nurse fearless to bring to light any serious violation of the ideals (by another nurse)." It reflected the assumption of a more foundational commitment to the community and the well-being of the patient than to an erring colleague.

In spite of these signs of progress, loyalty to physician and hospital was (and still is) a strong influence on nurses' decision making, as illustrated by Murphy's (1983) study of nurses' moral reasoning. Nurses participating in the study described making decisions more often in accordance with physician advocacy than patient advocacy. Similar findings were reported even more recently by Millette (1993). In her sample of 222 practicing nurses, Millette found that two thirds of the sample indicated a preference for client advocacy versus bureaucratic and physician advocacy. Surprisingly, however, only a small number selected the actions of a client advocate as the best responses to case presentations. The predominant choices reflected greater concern for the institution than for the client (bureaucratic advocacy), particularly by nurses in management positions and practicing in acute care rather than community settings.

Nurse as Mediator

Despite undercurrents of loyalty and obedience, the nurse advocate role gradually evolved into that of mediator. Mediation involved coordination of services, explanation to the client of the roles and responsibilities of various health care providers, and clarification of communication by others. Later, the mediator role also embraced interpreting clients' needs to other members of the health team and informing clients and families of their rights (e.g., to information, privacy, and refusal) in keeping with the Patient's Bill of Rights movement (Annas & Healey, 1975).

Nurse as Proponent of Self-Determination

The most recent version of advocacy emphasizes the client's rights and autonomy in decision making as the unconditional first priorities. This role was officially sanctioned, and even termed "advocacy" in the 1985 version of the American Nurses' Association *Code for Nurses with Interpretive Statements*:

> Since clients themselves are the primary decision makers in matters concerning their own health, treatment, and well-being, the goal of nursing actions is to support and enhance the client's responsibility and *self-determination* to the greatest extent possible . . .
> Truth telling and the process of reaching informed choice underlie the exercise of *self-determination* which is basic to respect for persons . . .
> The nurse's primary commitment is to the health, welfare, and safety of the client. As an *advocate* for the client, the nurse must be alert to and take appropriate action regarding any instances of incompetent, unethical or illegal practice by any member of the health care team or the health care system, or any action . . . that places the rights or best interests of the client in jeopardy [italics added] (American Nurses' Association, 1985).

In a discussion of whether advocacy fits the realm of contemporary nursing practice, Rafael (1995) proposes the concept of empowerment as a better alternative. Empowerment refers to a liberating pedagogy described by Freire (1973) as a process of enabling oppressed people to develop their own responses to dehumanizing social and

TABLE 28.1   Types of Advocacy

Type	Role of the Advocate	Underpinnings
Legal advocacy	Guardian of patient rights	Individual rights (e.g. to informed consent, to refuse, to competent care and privacy)
Moral-Ethical advocacy	Preserver of patient values	Awareness of values and congruent decision making
Substitutive advocacy	Conservator of patient best interests	Preservation of rights for persons who are unable to speak for themselves
Political advocacy	Champion of social justice	Equal access to nursing and health care for everyone
Spiritual advocacy		Spiritual comfort and counsel in the quest for meaning

Note. Contents of this typology informed by the following sources: Curtin, L. L. (1979). The nurse as advocate: A philosophical foundation for nursing. *Nursing Science, 1,* 1–10; Fowler, M. D. M. (1989). Social advocacy. *Heart & Lung, 18,* 97–99.

cultural circumstances. In empowerment, clients would be viewed as active and equal partners. Rafael concedes, however, that the ethical basis for advocacy determines whether it is congruent with empowerment and thus with contemporary nursing practice. Gadow's existential advocacy, Watson's (1988) transpersonal caring as advocacy, Newman's rhythmic connecting (1994), and the nurse-client relational "process of mutuality and creative unfolding" described by Newman, Sime and Corcoran-Perry (1991, p. 4) are deemed ethically compatible with empowerment.

INTERVENTION

Types of Advocacy

Curtin (1979) and Fowler (1989) have proposed frameworks which incorporate different types or forms of advocacy. A comparison and synthesis of these frameworks is represented in Table 28.1 and includes five categories of advocacy: legal, moral-ethical, substitutive, political, and spiritual advocacy. The common goal of all forms of advocacy is to facilitate the client's self-determination related to health and to promote decision making congruent with who the person is, what he or she values, and the level of self-determination possible at a given point in time.

Legal Advocacy. Clients' legal rights form the basis for legal advocacy, including rights to be informed, to accept or refuse treatment, and to be protected from incompetent, illegal, or unethical practices. Actions empowering patients in their interaction with the health care system fit within this form of advocacy.

Segesten (1993) reported that the most common need for advocacy, based on the narrative accounts of expert nurses, involves patients' rights to decide for themselves. The criteria for informed consent apply in these situations: adequate information to make rational decisions, mental competence on the part of the decision maker, and uncoerced, freely given consent (Grodin, Kaminov, & Sassower, 1986).

Other legal rights which the nurse is obliged to protect are right of privacy, the right to refuse procedures or providers, and the freedom to leave an institution which is providing care. Privacy is protected by sharing personal information about clients only in the context of facilitating care provision and expecting other health care providers to treat such information with the same respect. Patients and families, perceiving the power differential between themselves and health care providers, are often unaware of the right to refuse medication, tests, procedures, treatments, or care providers. This makes it even more important for the nurse advocate to make these rights known.

The bottom line in legal advocacy is that rights belong to the patient, which means that he or she also has the right *not* to exercise those rights. It also means that patient choices must be accepted and support of the patient continued, even when the nurse disagrees with the choice.

Advocacy may take the form of ascertaining a client's competence to understand, being the primary purveyor of information, updating or clarifying information provided by another professional, and ascertaining understanding. Foss (Nelson, 1993a), a clinical nurse specialist, has described situations in which she found that patients and families were not getting the answers that they needed because they didn't don't know how to ask questions adequately of their care providers. Foss describes her role in helping people articulate these questions and serving as interpreter when other providers talked in complex medical terms to a family that needed to have things explained more simply.

Moral-Ethical Advocacy. Moral-ethical advocacy is based upon honoring patients' values and facilitating decision making which is congruent with those values. It requires that the patient desire self-determination and have the ability to participate in values exploration and decision making. In this type of advocacy, every encounter is viewed in the context of respect for the person and the situation in time. The intent of the nurse is to preserve or clarify patient values and assure autonomy in decision making while at the same time providing the professional assistance needed to make decisions. Nurses in this role often serve as the communication bridge among members of the health team, the patient, and the family (Copp, 1986). They act as what Jezewski (1993) has called a "culture broker," bridging the gaps in cultural meaning or understanding between two cultures: the culture of the client and that of the health care system.

A prerequisite for this type of advocacy is an existential relationship between nurse and client, wherein both parties are attuned to each other, expressing their wholeness and uniqueness in a clarification and sharing of values (Gadow, 1980). Objections have been raised to this authentic sharing of the nurse's personal views or even to pursuing clarification of patient values on the grounds that this may undermine the patient's decisional autonomy (Kohnke, 1982). The nurse advocate walks a fine line between "clarification" and "subtle manipulation" (p. 29). It is critical, therefore, to assure that the emphasis is upon the *client's values and desires*.

Miller (Nelson, 1993b), a geriatric clinical specialist, described her role as supporting clients as they clarify their values and desired outcomes, "letting them know it's okay for *them* to decide or to disagree with their doctor." Another useful intervention for clients of any age or condition is to invite and encourage their discussion of values related to life, health, and death and how these values inform their preferences for treatment in potentially life-threatening circumstances. It is important to consider these questions prior to situations of crisis or threat to life (Omery & Caswell, 1989). Such discussions might include the option of an advanced directive (living will or durable power of attorney for health care), specifying the kinds of medical intervention and the type of health care experience one would desire or wish to refuse under certain circumstances. Such dialogue provides a means for clients to exercise control over their destinies "before-the-fact" (Grady, 1989).

Substitutive Advocacy. Substitutive advocacy is relevant when the patient is unable to express his or her own wishes and an identified proxy decisionmaker is unavailable to speak on his or her behalf. The underlying principle is that the ultimate right to speak for oneself belongs to everyone, so advocacy as a substitute for the patient's own voice is not something to be embarked upon lightly.

In instances where mental incapacity or lack of responsiveness clearly precludes self-expression, it is important that someone verbalize the patient's preferences, if they are known. This is obviously much easier when discussions with that person have previously occurred. Benner (1981) and Wolff (1992) promote nurses as authentic voices for clients because of their privileged relationship with them and awareness of their abilities, concerns, values, and wishes.

Foss (Nelson, 1993a) describes "translating [clients'] issues and points of view to other players [on the health care team]." This may even be appropriate for mentally competent patients in some circumstances (e.g., helping family members and other care providers understand how shortness of breath and anxiety affect the life experience of a person with chronic lung disease). With the growth in numbers of people with chronic health conditions and increased care provision in the community (Hicks, Stallmeyer, & Coleman, 1992), this form of advocacy has even broader application through teaching self- and family care and linking families to resources across health care settings.

Changes in traditional patterns of care provision may also be viewed as a kind of substitutive advocacy. For example, some of the acute care practices which were routine early in the AIDS era have been modified to become less restrictive. In many settings where there was a policy of "family only" visiting, the client is now asked to identify those who constitute family and should have visiting privileges.

Substitutive advocacy, although not a desirable first option, is sometimes necessary because of circumstances prohibiting patients from acting on their own behalf. Nurses may be in prime positions to serve as a proxy voice.

Political Advocacy. Also referred to as the "champion of social justice" role, political advocacy is based on the ethic of justice (universal access to adequate nursing and health care). It calls for nurses to actively strive for change on behalf of individuals, groups, and communities so that inequities and inconsistencies are identified and corrected. This form of advocacy frequently requires action at a policy and legislative level. Nursing history is rich with nurse role models in this arena, including Florence Nightingale; Lavinia Dock, who addressed the problem of venereal disease through her writings and public health actions; and Margaret Sanger, who provided leadership in meeting the health needs of women and educating the public about birth control options.

Today political advocacy is more expedient through professional organizations than individual efforts, in order to influence change in such areas as health care quality and access. As an example, the American Nurses' Association (ANA) is attempting to improve health care accessibility and financing as well as availability of long-term care facilities, homes and apartment for persons with AIDS and other chronic illnesses. And Sohier (1992) calls nurses to respond to even broader Issues such as hunger, poverty, homelessness, and illiteracy. Nurses have a responsibility to respond to the fact that close to 45 million Americans receive little or no health care. Collectively, nurses are a large voting block and a potentially powerful lobby.

In order to take advantage of the opportunity for political advocacy, nurses must be willing to become politically sophisticated and to participate in organizations that utilize collective power. Membership in professional organizations and willingness to serve on health policy-making boards and councils constitute action on this level.

Spiritual Advocacy. This type of advocacy is based upon individual rights to spiritual comfort and access to the clergy of choice. Since the search for meaning is both an ethical and a spiritual task, spiritual advocacy could be considered a subcategory of moral-ethical advocacy. Gadow (1980) references this kind of advocacy when she discusses the nurse's interaction with the patient to determine the unique personal meaning a health experience has for that individual. Through advocacy, nurses communicate sensitivity to personal hopes and values and create an atmosphere of caring and a sense of the possible.

In addition to collaborating with and referring clients to clergy and counselors, nurses implement spiritual advocacy by being fully present and open to participate with and enter the "lifeworld" (Johnson, 1993) of patients in their search for meaning.

Advocacy for the Community's Health. Although the term *client* has been used to refer to individuals, groups, or communities, the health of the community is lifted up specifically because it is becoming a more central concern for nurses in the evolving health care system. All nurses must become more attuned to providing care in multiple settings and in the transitions between settings. Current nursing practice involves the identification of high-risk individuals, families, and groups (or aggregates) in the community and evaluation of the appropriateness of health policies, accessibility of health services, and environmental factors in the community. According to Zotti, Brown, and Stotts (1996), community-based nursing practice is evolving as an expectation for nurses in any setting. Community health nursing emphasizes another level in which the client is not the individual or groups within the community but the community itself.

Barriers to Advocacy

Although the needs of health care recipients for advocacy are well documented and its implementation is congruent with a nursing paradigm, there are barriers to its implementation. One barrier is the typical view of the physician or managed care organization as the authority and prime decision maker in health care. Physicians have tended to treat patients as their exclusive domain, a stance which effectively blocks advocacy by other providers as well as self-determination for the client. In such a scheme, the would-be nurse advocate may be viewed as a troublemaker rather than a meaningful contributor to patients' welfare (Nelson, 1988).

There are some additional theoretical counterarguments to the appropriateness of the advocacy role for nurses. Porter (1992), for example, sees nursing's professionalism as a contradiction to genuine advocacy. While professionalism stresses expert knowledge and might increase the knowledge and power differential between nurse and client, advocacy assumes partnership and sharing of knowledge and power. A related concern has been raised concerning the position of most nurses as a part of the system against which consumers may need protection (Allmark & Klarzynski, 1992; Segesten, 1993). Further, when a nurse cannot advocate for all, how should the choice be made (e.g., mother vs. fetus, adult vs. child on a transplant list)?

There is no doubt that in some circumstances the nurse is cast as a "double agent," attempting to represent both patient and physician, more than one patient, or patient and health care institution (Nelson, 1988). Nevertheless, nursing's paradigm entails a basic ethical commitment to the rights and well-being of patients (ANA, 1985) and to understanding human health experiences through the eyes of those who live them (Newman, Sime, & Corcoran-Perry, 1991). These professional underpinnings make advocacy for the client a first priority, even in situations where fulfilling this priority may need to be delegated to another person in order for the client's cause to be most fairly represented.

Measurement of Effectiveness

Since advocacy includes a significant ethical dimension, one approach to its evaluation is through the use of ethical principles as standards. For example, if one uses nonmaleficence (the principle of causing no harm) as a guide, one of the most basic expected outcomes of advocacy is that the client not be hurt by advocacy interventions. If beneficence serves as a standard, advocacy should in some way promote the well-being of the client. If autonomy is a guiding principle, the client's self-determination must be included as a measure of effectiveness. If justice is a priority, a measure of fairness or equity in distributing health resources is in order. Fidelity suggests that one should evaluate fulfillment of obligations, such as commitments to provide care until a satisfactory alternative is found and the degree to which privacy and confidentiality are honored.

The typology of advocacy discussed earlier supplies a more precise framework for posing evaluative questions about whether advocacy behaviors have been effective (see Table 28.1). Each form of advocacy provides somewhat different guidelines and questions.

For legal advocacy, the client's legal rights must be upheld and he or she must be able to verbalize understanding of those rights and resources available to assist with their protection. Specific rights and related questions are:

1. *Informed consent.* Has the client been provided the desired information about treatment or other health-related alternatives? Is he or she competent to give consent or been provided the opportunity to identify a proxy decisionmaker? Barring this, have earnest attempts been made to determine the substance of previously written or verbalized advanced directives? Does the client feel free to choose or decide without penalty or pressure from health care providers?
2. *Acceptance or refusal of treatment.* Can the client verbalize understanding of his or her right to refuse? Are the client's expressions of doubt or ambivalence given opportunity for expression and exploration?
3. *Protection from incompetent or unethical practices.* Are quality assurance measures in place to assure client safety and the compe-

tence of health care providers? Are procedures in place (and utilized) to intervene when there are threats to client safety or rights? Does the client know whom to contact with concerns about the quality of care?

For moral-ethical advocacy, the nurse-client relationship and the client's opportunity to be authentic with himself and a caring other (the nurse) are the focus of evaluation. Has the client been given the opportunity to explore personal values that are relevant to the present health situation? Have opportunities been provided for considering advanced directives regarding future life, health, and death decisions? Does the client feel he or she has as much control over health planning as desired?

For substitutive advocacy, the major concern is that the best interests of the client are protected when he or she is unable to participate actively in the planning process. Have attempts been made to determine what wishes the client would express? Have the safety and dignity of the client been maintained? Have significant others been allowed and assisted to participate in care and decision making?

For political advocacy, nurses need to participate individually and collectively in actions to promote such goals as a healthy environment and accessible and affordable health care for all. Are nurses visible in community, state, regional, and national organizations and agencies that promote societal awareness of threats to health, seek health-related policy and legislative changes, and strive for resolution of economic and health care inequities?

For spiritual advocacy, clients must be supported as they search for meaning in their health experiences, living, and dying. Is the nurse open and present with the client in such a way that meaningful interchange about spiritual concerns can occur? Is there an attitude of caring and hope on the part of the nurse? Are clients' unique personal meanings sought and respected? Are opportunities provided for client contact with the clergy of choice? Has communication been maintained despite the client's level of response?

Some of these questions can be answered through information in the client's health record, others subjectively by the client, the family, and/or the nurse. Others, such as those pertaining to spiritual advocacy, can only be intuited by an observer or perhaps only by the participants in a nurse-client relationship.

USES

A Case Study

Edwin Dawes was 43 when he was diagnosed with pancreatic cancer. By the time it was discovered, his disease was in an advanced stage. He elected to have surgery to resect his pancreas and a portion of his liver and create a jejunostomy through which he would be able to take nourishment. He also elected to have aggressive chemotherapy from which he experienced multiple side effects: nausea, vomiting, diarrhea, leukopenia, anemia, and severe stomatitis. Mr. Dawes lived at home with his wife, Gwen, and children (Ben, age 8; Martha, age 10; and Arthur. age 15). He also had the intermittent care and support of a visiting nurse service for a few months after his diagnosis. After several rounds of chemotherapy and increasing weakness and weight loss, Ed and Gwen agreed that he should stop the treatments. Marion, the visiting nurse who had worked with Ed and Gwen for several months, allowed them to think through their options and encouraged them to talk about how and where they would like Ed to die and what were the most important aspects of the life he had remaining. She was authentically present for them, providing information only to clarify alternatives and explain how the health care team could help them deal with the issues of greatest concern to Ed and Gwen: pain management, Gwen's need for support, and pressure from Ed's mother and siblings to continue treatment. Ed's physician had also encouraged them to consider another form of chemotherapy. They were able to make the decision to stop treatment but were insecure about whether Ed should remain at home. Marion brought in a nurse to discuss home hospice care with them, but Ed was unwilling to die at home in the presence of his children. After lengthy discussion, Ed and Gwen opted for institutional hospice care. It was not the choice Marion had hoped they would make, but she allowed them to choose in a way that was congruent with their meanings and values, not hers.

FURTHER RESEARCH

There has been little research related to advocacy in nursing, with the exception of some early attempts to identify role priorities for physicians and nurses in specific settings and Murphy's (1983) and Millette's (1993) study of nurses' decision making according to advocacy preferences. Research is needed to refine the concept further, ascertain nurses' commitment to advocacy roles, explicate the ways in which advocacy can be operationalized, and document client outcomes. A few of the relevant questions which might be asked are these:

1. To what extent do nurses perceive themselves as advocates and for whom (clients, families, communities, institutions, or physicians)?
2. What are the needs for advocacy in specific population groups?
3. To what extent do clients expect and desire nurses to serve as their advocates? How are specific advocacy interventions received?
4. How do advocacy behaviors on the part of the nurse affect the congruence between clients' values and their health-related decisions? other potential outcomes?
5. What is the experience of the nurse as advocate? How is this experienced by the client?

Advocacy fits well with the evolution of the nursing discipline, and needs for advocacy are apparent in the uncertain but rapidly changing health care system. The way of being which constitutes advocacy in nursing is congruent with some of the major nursing theories. Advocacy is present in what Watson (1988) describes as a transpersonal caring relationship, encompassing "high regard for the whole person and their being-in-the-world" (p. 63) and basic concern for human dignity. It is also reflected in Parse's (1992) description of the process of becoming as on in which individuals freely choose personal meaning and in the emphasis on quality of life from the individual's own perspective. Advocacy as honoring persons' meanings as they are revealed in the unfolding patterns of identity is reflected in Newman's theory of health as expanding consciousness (1994). These theories, and perhaps others, could therefore be used as the foundation for research related to advocacy in nursing and as a basis for nursing practice which encompasses advocacy.

REFERENCES

Allmark, P., & Klarzynski, R. (1992). The case against nurse advocacy. *British Journal of Nursing, 2,* 33–36.
American Nurses' Association. (1985). *Code for nurses with interpretive statements* [Brochure]. Kansas City, MO: Author.

American Nurses' Association, Ethical Standards Committee. (1926). A suggested code. *American Journal of Nursing, 26,* 599–601.

Annas, G. J., & Healey, J. (1975). The patient rights advocate. In *Fundamental Issues in Nursing* (pp. 78–84). Wakefield, MA: Contemporary.

Benner, P. (1981). Commentary. *American Journal of Nursing, 81,* 82.

Copp, L. A. (1986). The nurse as advocate for vulnerable persons. *Journal of Advanced Nursing, 11,* 255–263.

Curtin, L. L. (1979). The nurse as advocate: A philosophical foundation for nursing. *Advances in Nursing Science, 1,* 1–10.

Fowler, M. D. M. (1989). Social advocacy. *Heart & Lung, 18,* 97–99.

Freire, P. (1973). *Pedagogy of the oppressed.* New York: Continuum.

Gadow, S. (1990). Existential advocacy: Philosophical foundations of nursing. In T. Pence & J. Cantrell (Eds.), *Ethics in nursing: An anthology* (pp. 41–52). New York: National League for Nursing.

Gadow, S. (1980). Existential advocacy: Philosophical foundation of nursing. In S. F. Spicker & S. Gadow (Eds.), *Nursing, images and ideals: Opening dialogue with the humanities* (pp. 79–89). New York: Springer.

Grady, C. (1989). Ethical issues in providing nursing care to human immunodeficiency virus-infected populations. *Journal of Advanced Nursing, 14,* 513–514.

Grodin, M., Kaminov, P., & Sassower, R. (1986). Ethical issues in AIDS research. *Quarterly Review Bulletin, 10,* 347–352.

Hicks, L., Stallmeyer, J. M., & Coleman, J. R. (1992). Nursing challenges in managed care. *Nursing Economics, 10,* 265–276.

Jezewski, M. A. (1993). Culture brokering as a model for advocacy. *Nursing & Health Care, 14,* 78–85.

Johnson, R. (1993). Nurse practitioner-patient discourse: Uncovering the voice of nursing in primary care practice. *Scholarly Inquiry for Nursing Practice, 7,* 143–157.

Kavanagh, K. H. (1994). Transcultural nursing: Facing the challenges of advocacy and diversity/universality. *Journal of Transcultural Nursing, 5,* 4–13.

Kohnke, M. F. (1982). *Advocacy: Risk and reality.* St. Louis: Mosby.

Leddy, S., & Pepper, J. M. (1984). *Conceptual bases of professional nursing.* Philadelphia: Lippincott.

Millette, B. E. (1993). Client advocacy and the moral orientation of nurses. *Western Journal of Nursing Research, 15,* 607–618.

Murphy, C. P. (1983). Models of the nurse-patient relationship. In C. P. Murphy & H. Hunter (Eds.), *Ethical problems in the nurse-patient relationship* (pp. 8–24). New York: Allyn & Bacon.

Nelson, M. L. (1988). Advocacy in nursing. *Nursing Outlook, 36,* 136–141.

Nelson, M. L. (1992). Advocacy. In M. Snyder (Ed.), *Independent nursing interventions* (2nd ed., pp. 262–275. Albany: Delmar.

Nelson, M. L. (1995). Client advocacy. In M. Snyder & M. P. Mirr (Eds.), *Advanced practice nursing: A guide to professional development* (pp. 103–116). New York: Springer.

Nelson, M. L. (1993a). [Interview with Nancy Foss, pulmonary clinical nurse specialist]. Unpublished raw data.

Nelson, M. L. (1993b). [Interview with Doreen S. Miller, geriatric clinical specialist]. Unpublished raw data.

Newman, M. A. (1994). *Health as expanding consciousness* (2nd ed.). New York: National League for Nursing.

Newman, M. A., Sime, A. M., & Corcoran-Perry, S. A. (1991). The focus of the discipline of nursing. *Advances in Nursing Science, 14,* 1–6.

Nightingale, F. (1969). *Notes on nursing: What it is and what it is not.* Dover, NY: Lippincott. (Original published 1859)

Omery, A., & Caswell, D. (1989). Ethical perspectives. *Critical Care Nursing Clinics of North America, 1,* 165–173.

Parse, R. R. (1992). Human becoming: Parse's theory of nursing. *Nursing Science Quarterly, 5,* 35–42.

Perry, C. M. (1906). Nursing ethics and etiquette. *American Journal of Nursing, 6,* 448–452.

Porter, S. (1992). The poverty of professionalization: A critical analysis of strategies for the occupational advancement of nursing. *Journal of Advanced Nursing, 17,* 720–726.

Rafael, A. R. F. (1995). Advocacy and empowerment: Dichotomous or synchronous concepts? *Advances in Nursing Science, 18,* 25–32.

Segesten, K. (1993). Patient advocacy: An important part of the daily work of the expert nurse. *Scholarly Inquiry for Nursing, 7,* 129–135.

Sohier, R. (1992). Feminism and nursing knowledge: The power of the weak. *Nursing Outlook, 40,* 62–66, 93.

Watson, J. (1988). *Nursing: Human science and human care, a theory of nursing.* New York: National League for Nursing.

Watson, J. (1989). Transformative thinking and a caring curriculum. In E. O. Bevis & J. Watson (Eds.), *Toward a caring curriculum: A new pedagogy for nursing.* New York: National League for Nursing.

Winslow, G. R. (1984). From loyalty to advocacy: A new metaphor for nursing. *Hastings Center Report, 14,* 32–40.

Where does loyalty end? [editorial]. (1910). *American Journal of Nursing, 10,* 230–231.

Wolff, T. L. (1992). The community health nurse as advocate. *Home Healthcare Nurse, 10,* 14–17, 78–79.

Zotti, M. E., Brown, P., & Stotts, R. C. (1996). Community-based nursing versus community health nursing: What does it all mean? *Nursing Outlook, 44,* 211–217.

Index

Vasodilation from heat therapy, 90
Ventilation, positioning affecting, 183
Vibration strokes in massage, 64, 67
Vipassana meditation, 128

Walking programs, 27–28
Wandering, validation therapy in, 238
Warm-up exercises, 26–27
Weight reduction, contracting in, 302–303
Well-being
    journal writing affecting, 207, 208

prayer affecting, 264
Working touch, 150
Wound healing, therapeutic touch affecting, 53, 58, 59
Writing of journals, 203–209. *See also* Journal writing

Yin-yang principles of Tai chi/movement therapy chi, 38, 40
Yoga, breathing techniques in, 15, 17

Zazen, 123

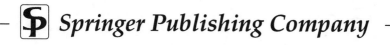
Springer Publishing Company

Wellness Practitioner
Concepts, Theory, Research, Strategies, and Programs, 2nd Edition

Carolyn Chambers Clark, EdD, ARNP

Now in a second edition, this is a comprehensive resource on health maintenance, disease prevention, and alternative health practices. The author explores conceptual bases and practical techniques for a wide range of programs, activities, and therapies that promote wellness. Topics include relaxation and stress management, nutrition, exercise, herbal remedies, massage, imagery, affirmations, reflexology, aromatherapy, natural healing, and self care measures for conditions ranging from hay fever to multiple sclerosis.

Environmental influences and community wellness are each addressed in a separate chapter. Learning exercises are included with each chapter to facilitate integration of the material. A useful resource for nurses, physicians, and other health professionals — both traditional and alternative.

Partial Contents
- Introduction to Wellness Theory
- Beginning to Move Toward Wellness
- Positive Relationship Building
- Stress Management
- Nutritional Wellness
- Exercise and Movement
- Self-Care, Touch, and Wellness

1996   354pp   0-8261-5151-5   hardcover

536 Broadway, New York, NY 10012-3955 • (212) 431-4370 • Fax (212) 941-7842

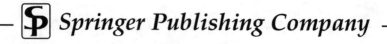
$\boxed{\text{S}}$ Springer Publishing Company

Alternative Therapies
Expanding Options in Health Care

Rena J. Gordon, PhD, **Barbara Cable Nienstedt,** DPA,
Wilbert M. Gesler, PhD, Editors

"By focusing on medical, political, social, cultural, and economic factors, [the] editors have enabled readers to better understand the movement's growing popularity....I would recommend this work for health professionals, students, and consumers of the alternative therapy movement." —Rosalie F. Young, PhD
Associate Professor and Director, Health and Aging Program
Wayne State University School of Medicine

In this volume, an interdisciplinary team of scholars and social scientists address the ramifications of the increasing utilization of alternative and complementary medicine. The book provides a scholarly and theoretical discussion of salient issues within this new field. Topics discussed include: the changing medical market place, political and legal aspects of practice, influential cultural factors, and clinical and educational issues.

The many case examples that appear throughout the text illustrate how alternative health care relates to everyday life. The book serves as a primer for an array of health professionals and students, and provides new insights to those familiar with alternative health practices.

Contents:
- **Part I.** Introduction
- **Part II.** Politics and the Law
- **Part III.** The Changing Medical Marketplace
- **Part IV.** The Culture Complex
- **Part V.** Toward Complementary Medicine

1998   296pp   0-8261-1164-5   hardcover

536 Broadway, New York, NY 10012-3955 • (212) 431-4370 • Fax (212) 941-7842